PROGRESS IN PERITONEAL DIALYSIS

Edited by **Raymond Krediet**

Progress in Peritoneal Dialysis
Edited by Raymond Krediet

Published by InTech

Janeza Trdine 9, 51000 Rijeka, Croatia

Publishing Process Manager Niksa Mandic

Technical Editor Teodora Smiljanic

Cover Designer InTech Design Team

Additional hard copies can be obtained from orders@intechopen.com

Progress in Peritoneal Dialysis, Edited by Raymond Krediet
p. cm.
ISBN 978-953-307-390-3

For EU product safety concerns:
IN TECH d.o.o., Prolaz Marije Krucifikse Kozulić 3, 51000 Rijeka, Croatia,
info@intechopen.com or visit our website at intechopen.com.

Meet the editor

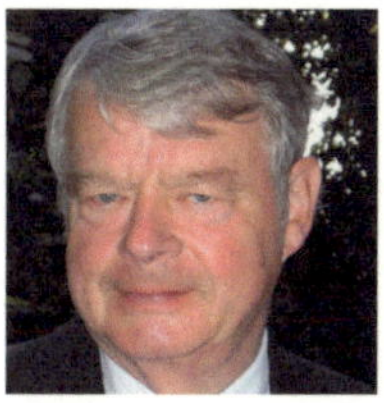

Dr. Raymond (Ray) Krediet graduated in 1973 at the University of Amsterdam. In 1978 he completed his training as an internist-nephrologist and became Head of Nephrology at the Binnengasthuis in 1979 where he introduced treatment with continuous ambulatory dialysis (CAPD). In 1986 he was promoted on a PhD thesis, entitled "Peritoneal permeability in continuous ambulatory peritoneal dialysis patients". In 1999 he became Professor and Head of the Department of Nephrology at the Academic Medical Centre, University of Amsterdam. Professor Krediet supervised the research of 26 PhD students and is author of 470 publications in scientific journals. His h-index is 51. Among others, he is former chairman of the Dialysis Group Netherlands, the International Society for Peritoneal Dialysis and the Nephrology Section of the European Union for Medical Specialists. He retired in October 2010, but is still involved in research and a number of academic and organisational activities.

Contents

Preface

Continuous peritoneal dialysis was first introduced by Popovich and Moncrief in 1976. It gained popularity as a form of home dialysis in the eighties in Canada, USA, Western Europe and Hong-Kong. Since the nineties Eastern Europe followed and from 2000 onward the main growth was in the so-called third-world countries. As a consequence, the level at which peritoneal is practiced differs very much amongst countries. This translates into research that is focused either on in-vitro studies, some studies in animals, mathematics and, most-importantly, clinical studies in patients. This makes the scope of interest in peritoneal dialysis related studies very wide.

The aim of the present publication was not to create a comprehensive reference book on all aspects of peritoneal dialysis with invited authors, recognized as authorities in part of the field. Rather, the objective was to make a collection of various actual subjects, highlighted by authors from all over the world, who had shown their interest in a specific item by submitting an abstract. These abstracts were reviewed and chosen based on the quality of their contents. The chapters which emerged reflect the world-wide progress in peritoneal dialysis during the last years.

Five of the twelve chapters comprise clinical issues, two are on kinetic modelling, and the others show the results of the mainly in-vitro studies of the authors and their collaborators. Consequently the interested reader is likely to find state-of the art essays on the subject of his/her interest. I hope this book on Progression in peritoneal dialysis will contribute to spreading the knowledge in this interesting, but underused modality of renal replacement therapy.

Raymond T Krediet, MD, PhD
Emeritus Professor of Nephrology
Academic Medical Center,
University of Amsterdam,
The Netherlands

1

Representations of Peritoneal Tissue – Mathematical Models in Peritoneal Dialysis

Magda Galach[1], Andrzej Werynski[1],
Bengt Lindholm[2] and Jacek Waniewski[1]
[1]*Institute of Biocybernetics and Biomedical Engineering, Polish Academy of Sciences, Warsaw*
[2]*Divisions of Baxter Novum and Renal Medicine, Department of Clinical Science, Intervention and Technology, Karolinska Institutet, Stockholm*
[1]*Poland*
[2]*Sweden*

1. Introduction

During peritoneal dialysis solutes and water are transported across the peritoneum, a thin "membrane" lining the abdominal and pelvic cavities. Dialysis fluid containing an "osmotic agent", usually glucose, is infused into the peritoneal space, and solutes and water pass from the blood into the dialysate (and vice versa). The complex physiological mechanisms of fluid and solute transport between blood and peritoneal dialysate are of crucial importance for the efficiency of this treatment (Flessner, 1991; Lysaght &Farrell, 1989).

The major transport barrier is the capillary endothelium, which contains various types of pores. Capillaries are distributed in the tissue. Across the capillary walls, mainly diffusive transport of small solutes between blood and dialysate occurs. As the osmotic agent creates a high osmotic pressure in the dialysis fluid - exceeding substantially the osmotic pressure of blood - water is transported by osmosis from blood to dialysate and removed from the patient with spent dialysis fluid. At the same time the difference in hydrostatic pressures between dialysate (high hydrostatic pressure) and peritoneal tissue interstitium (lower hydrostatic pressure) causes water to be transported from dialysate to blood. In addition, there is a continuous lymphatic transport from dialysate and peritoneal tissue interstitium to blood.

In this chapter a brief characteristic of the two most popular simple models describing transport of fluid and solutes between dialysate and blood during peritoneal dialysis is presented with the focus on their application and techniques for estimation of parameters which may be used to analyze clinically available data on peritoneal transport.

2. Membrane representation of transport barrier

This rather complicated transport system of water and solutes can be described with sufficient accuracy for practical purposes with a simple, membrane model based on thermodynamic principles of fluid and solutes transport across an "apparent" semipermeable membrane that represents various transport barriers in the tissue (Kedem &Katchalsky, 1958; Lysaght &Farrell, 1989; Waniewski et al., 1992; Waniewski, 1999). In this model no specific structure of the membrane is assumed (the "black box" approach). The membrane model allows an accurate description of diffusive and convective transport of solutes and osmotic transport of water between blood and dialysate, but it must be supplemented by fluid and solute absorption from dialysate to blood.

2.1 Estimation of fluid absorption rate from dialysate to peritoneal tissue and determination of dialysate volume during dialysis

Transport of fluid from blood to dialysate (ultrafiltration) and from dialysate to peritoneal tissue (absorption) occurs at the same time. Estimation of fluid absorption can be done using a so-called "volume marker" - a substance added to the dialysate in low concentration (so that this addition does not influence the transport of other solutes) which might be distinguished from the solutes produced by the body (and transported to dialysis fluid), to calculate its disappearance from dialysis fluid (Waniewski et al., 1994).

Two processes: convection and diffusion take part in the transport of the volume marker from dialysate. The convective transport consists of lymphatic transport and fluid absorption from peritoneal cavity caused by dialysate hydrostatic pressure which is higher than that of interstitium. Because of a high molecular weight of the volume marker, its diffusion is negligible and the determination of its elimination rate, K_E, can serve as an estimation of fluid absorption rate from dialysate to peritoneal tissue, Q_A. However, it should be remembered that even small diffusion of a marker creates an error in determination of K_E (and Q_A). Therefore substantial decrease of marker's diffusive transport is of great importance and can be achieved by selection of macromolecular solutes, as the diffusive transport decreases with increasing molecular weight. For this reason only high molecular weight protein (albumin and hemoglobin) and dextrans of molecular weight from 70000 to 2 millions have been applied as a volume markers (De Paepe et al., 1988; Krediet et al., 1991; Waniewski et al., 1994).

K_E (and consequently Q_A) can be calculated using a simple, one compartment mathematical model representing dialysate of variable volume V_D caused by fluid transport from and to the peritoneal cavity. The applied model is based on the assumption that the rate of decrease of volume marker mass in the peritoneal cavity is proportional to the volume marker concentration in the intraperitoneal dialysis fluid. Applying the mass balance equation one gets (Waniewski et al., 1994):

$$\frac{dM_z}{dt} = -K_E C_z, \tag{1}$$

where M_z is mass and C_z concentration of the volume marker. After integration, Eqn (1) can be presented in the following form:

$$M_z(t_0) - M_z(t_{end}) = -K_E \int_{t_0}^{t_{end}} C_z(t)dt = K_E(t_{end} - t_0)\overline{C}_z(t_{end}), \tag{2}$$

where t_0 and t_{end} denoted the time of the beginning and the end of a peritoneal dialysis dwell, respectively (therefore $t_{end} - t_0$ is the time of dialysis) and $\overline{C}_z(t_{end})$ is an average concentration of volume marker in dialysate during the session, which can be calculated using frequent measurements of volume marker concentration in dialysate. Measurements should be done more frequently at the beginning of dialysis when concentration changes of the volume marker are more rapid. Mass of volume marker at the beginning of dialysis, $M_z(t_0)$, is equal to the mass in the fresh dialysis fluid in the peritoneal cavity, whereas mass at the end of dialysis, $M_z(t_{end})$, can be calculated knowing dialysate volume and marker concentration at the end of dialysis. It must be also remembered that dialysate volume at the end of dialysis is a sum of the volume removed and the residual volume remaining in the peritoneal cavity, which may be calculated using a short (5 min) rinse dwell just after the end of the dialysis session:

$$V_{res}C_z^{before} = (V_{res} + V_{rinse})C_z^{after}, \tag{3}$$

where V_{res} is the sought residual volume, V_{rins} is the rinse volume, C_z^{before} is the concentration of the marker before the rinse and C_z^{after} is the marker concentration after the rinse. Therefore:

$$V_{res} = V_{rinse}C_z^{after} \big/ \left(C_z^{before} - C_z^{after}\right), \tag{4}$$

Thus, as the other terms in this equation are known, K_E can be calculated from Eqn (2) as follows:

$$K_E = \left(C_z(t_0)V_D(t_0) - C_z(t_{end})\left(V_D(t_{end}) + V_{res}\right)\right) \big/ \left((t_{end} - t_0)\overline{C}_z(t_{end})\right). \tag{5}$$

Thereafter, knowing K_E and having data concerning marker concentration changes during the session (measured as a radioactivity), using Eqn (2) written not for duration of dialysis, t_{end}, but for a selected time during dialysis, t, dialysate volume during dialysis can be calculated. Expressing the mass of volume marker, $M_z(t)$, as the product of dialysate volume, $V_D(t)$, and marker concentration $C_z(t)$ one gets (Figure 1):

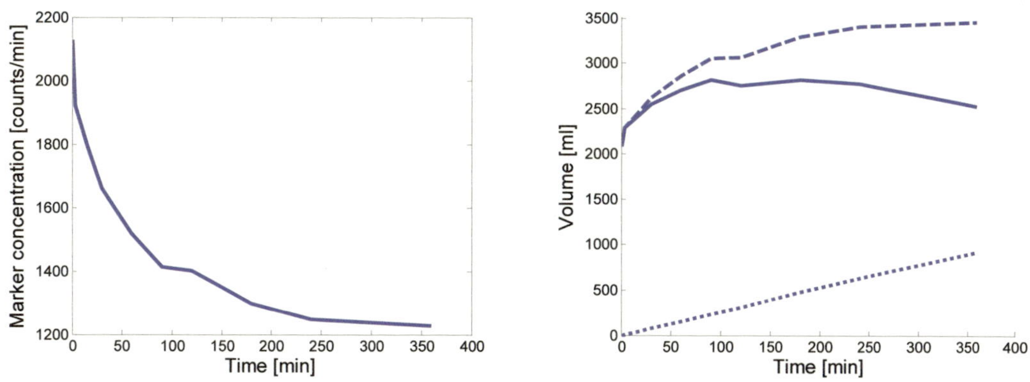

Fig. 1. Marker dialysate concentration during peritoneal dialysis dwell (left panel) and comparison of volumes calculated from marker concentration using Eqn (6) (right panel): dialysate volume (solid line), apparent volume calculated without the correction for the absorption of marker (dashed line) and absorbed volume (K_E = 2.29, dotted line).

$$V_D(t) = \underbrace{\frac{M_z(t_0)}{C_z(t)}}_{\text{APPARENT VOLUME}} \underbrace{-K_E t \frac{\overline{C}_z(t_{end})}{C_z(t)}}_{\text{ABSORPTION}}. \tag{6}$$

It is worth noting that the first part of the right hand side of Eqn (6) is the formula for calculation of dialysate volume using dilution of the volume marker without marker absorption taken into account. The second part is the correction for marker absorption (Figure 2).

2.2 Description of fluid transport in peritoneal dialysis

For low molecular weight osmotic agents, as glucose or amino acids, the value of osmotically induced ultrafiltration flow, Q_U, is proportional to the difference of osmotic pressure between dialysate and blood, $\Pi_D - \Pi_B$ (Waniewski et al., 1996b). The coefficient of proportionality, a_{os}, is called osmotic conductance. The mass balance equation for fluid is then as follows (Chen et al., 1991):

$$\frac{dV_D}{dt} = Q_V = Q_U - Q_A = a_{os}(\Pi_D - \Pi_B) - Q_A. \tag{7}$$

where: Q_V is the net rate of peritoneal dialysate volume change, Q_U is the rate of ultrafiltration flow ($Q_U = a_{os}(\Pi_D - \Pi_B)$) and Q_A is the fluid absorption rate.

Since V_D and Q_A (with the assumption that $Q_A = K_E$) can be estimated from Eqns (2) and (6), whereas Π_D and Π_B can be measured, thus Eqn (7) can be used for determination of osmotic conductance (Figure 2, left panel). Note however, that $Q_A = K_E$ is only a simplified assumption. Thus if both parameters (a_{os} as well as Q_A) are fitted, then the fitted Q_A value may not have a value comparable to K_E (Figure 2, right panel). All clinical data shown in this chapter are from Karolinska Institutet, Stockholm, Sweden.

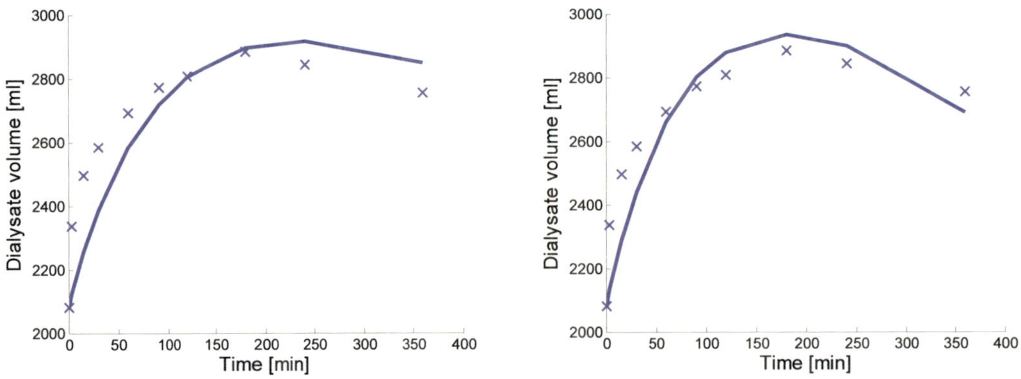

Fig. 2. Dialysate volume (x) calculated from marker concentration using Eqn (6) and osmotic model (solid line) with one fitted parameter and assumption $Q_A = K_E$ (left panel, a_{os} = 0.105, K_E = 1.93), and with two fitted parameters (right panel, a_{os} = 0.134, Q_A = 3.48).

As shown in Figure 2, the osmotic model underestimates dialysate volume during the first phase of dialysis dwell. This is the result of the assumption that osmotic conductance is constant that generally is only a simplification (Stachowska-Pietka et al., 2010; Waniewski et al., 1996a).

The fluid transport may be also described by a simple phenomenological formula proposed by Pyle et al. (Figure 3 shows example of patient with ultrafiltration failure defined as net ultrafiltration volume at 4 hour of the dwell less than 400 ml), and applied also by other investigators (Stelin &Rippe, 1990):

$$Q_V(t) = a_p e^{-k_p(t-t_0)} - b_p, \tag{8}$$

where t_0 is the start time of the dialysis, and a_p, b_p and k_p are the constants.

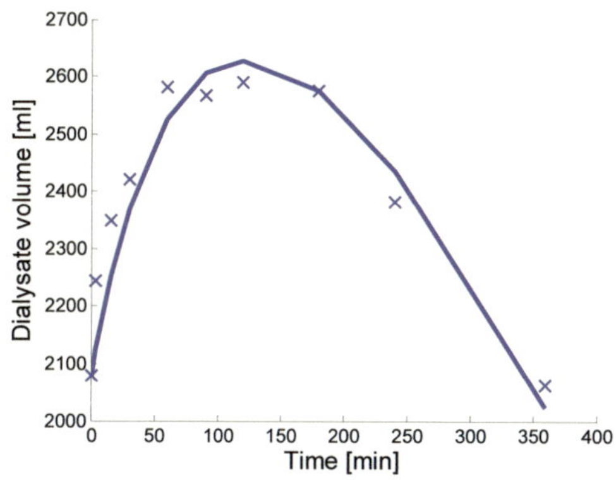

Fig. 3. Dialysate volume: clinical data (x) and Pyle model (solid line, a_p = 19.6, k_p = 0.022, b_p = 2.5).

2.3 Transport of low molecular solutes in peritoneal dialysis

Analysis of transport of low molecular weight solutes, such as urea, creatinine or glucose, from blood to dialysate (or in opposite direction) is of special importance in the evaluation of the quality of dialysis (Lysaght &Farrell, 1989; Waniewski et al., 1995). One of the methods used for assessment of the transport barrier between blood and dialysate is application of the so-called thermodynamic transport parameters. For the estimation of these parameters there is a need for frequent measurement of dialysate volume (i.e. volume marker concentration) during dialysis as well as concentrations of other solutes in the dialysate and blood, and then calculation of the rate of solutes mass change caused by their transport from blood to dialysate (or in opposite direction).

Solute transport occurs in three ways: a) diffusion of solute caused by the differences in solute's concentration in dialysate and blood; b) convective transport with fluid flow from blood to dialysate (ultrafiltration); c) convective transport with fluid absorbed from dialysate to the subperitoneal tissue and lymphatic vessels (absorption). In the description of these processes it is assumed that generation of solutes in the subperitoneal tissue and peritoneal cavity as well as the interaction between solutes are negligibly small.

All of these transport components are governed by specific forces (often described as thermodynamic forces) the effects of which, measured as a rate of solute flow, depends not only on the value of the force, but also on transport parameters characterizing the environment in which the solute transport occurs. Thus, the rate of diffusive solute transport is proportional to the difference of solute's concentration between blood and dialysate, $C_B - C_D$, with the rate coefficient K_{BD}, called diffusive mass transport coefficient.

The other two transport components are convective. The fluid flux, caused by the difference of osmotic pressures and the difference of hydrostatic pressures, carries solutes across the membrane characterized by its sieving coefficient. Sieving coefficient, S, determines the selectivity of this process: a sieving coefficient of 1 indicates an unrestricted solute transport while for S equal 0 there is no transport. Note also, that for a given membrane each solute has its specific sieving coefficient. Therefore, for the second transport component, the rate of convective flow is proportional to the rate of water flow (ultrafiltration), Q_U, to the average solute concentration in blood and dialysate C_R, and to sieving coefficient S. For the membrane model of peritoneal tissue C_R is expressed as follows:

$$C_R = (1-F)C_B + FC_D, \tag{9}$$

where C_B and C_D are concentrations in blood plasma and dialysate, respectively, and F is:

$$F = \frac{1}{Pe} - \frac{1}{e^{Pe} - 1}, \tag{10}$$

where Pe is Peclet number which is the ratio of terms characterizing the convective and diffusive transport:

$$Pe = \frac{SQ_U}{K_{BD}}. \tag{11}$$

In clinical investigations it has been demonstrated that for low molecular weight solutes it can be assumed that $F \approx 0.5$ and for proteins $F = 1$. The illustration of this estimation of F can be done using clinical data concerning the dwell study with 1.36% glucose solution published in (Olszowska et al., 2007). In this paper the values of K_{BD} for small solutes were found to be between 8 ml/min (glucose) and 25 ml/min (urea) and S of 0.68. Using these data it is possible to calculate F, yielding the values between 0.46 (for K_{BD} = 8 ml/min) and 0.65 (for K_{BD} = 25 ml/min).

For the third component, the rate of solutes absorption is proportional to the rate of fluid absorption rate, Q_A, and the solute concentration in dialysate. In this case the sieving coefficient is taken as equal to one. It is justified by experimental investigations in which no sieving effect (even for proteins) was demonstrated.

The total solute flow between blood and dialysate is the sum of all the described components. Thus, using the thermodynamic description, the following mass balance equation can be written (Waniewski et al., 1995):

$$\frac{dV_D C_D}{dt} = -K_{BD}(C_B - C_D) + SQ_U C_R - Q_A C_D. \tag{12}$$

In this equation there are two transport coefficients: diffusive mass transport coefficient, K_{BD}, and sieving coefficient, S, which characterize membrane properties of peritoneal tissue. All other variables in Eqn (12) can be measured or calculated from the measured values. In principle Eqn (12) can be used for estimation of S and K_{BD}. For practical reasons (decrease of the impact of measurement errors on parameters estimation) it is better to use Eqn (12) in its integral form (Waniewski et al., 1995):

$$V_D(t)C_D(t) = V_D(t_0)C_D(t_0) + K_{BD}(\bar{C}_B - \bar{C}_D)\Delta t + S\overline{Q_U C_R}\Delta t - Q_A \bar{C}_D \Delta t, \tag{13}$$

where the bar above symbols denotes averaged values for the time period from t_0 to t and $\Delta t = t - t_0$. The parameters K_{BD} and S can be estimated from Eqn (13) using two dimensional linear regression. The theoretical curves for solute concentrations that can be obtained by this procedure are compared to the measured concentrations in dialysis fluid in Figure 4.

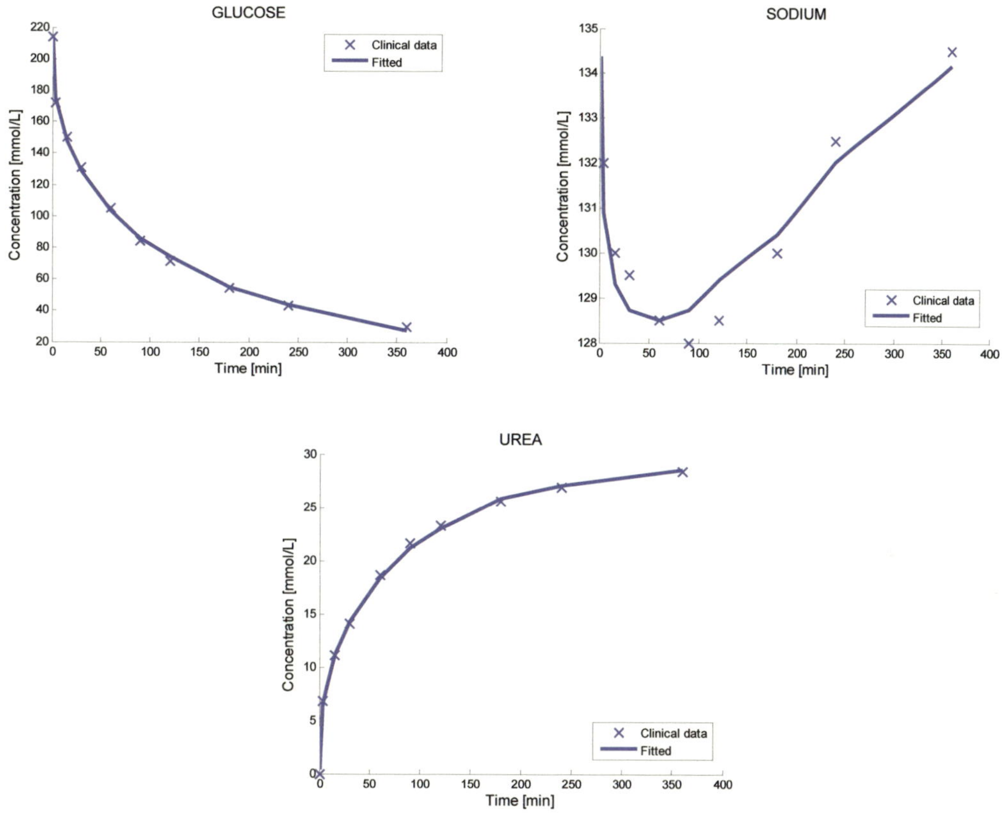

Fig. 4. Solute concentrations during peritoneal dialysis: clinical data vs. fitting curve (Eqn (13)) for: glucose (K_{BD} = 10.2 , S = -0.62), sodium (K_{BD} = 11.6, S = 0.73) and urea (K_{BD} = 14.0, S = 1.82)

It must be remembered that there are following limitations for the values of estimated parameters:

$$0 \le K_{BD} \text{ and } 0 \le S \le 1 . \tag{14}$$

The estimated values of K_{BD} are typically positive, but the limitations for S are often violated in experimental investigations (Waniewski et al., 1996d), as for the case depicted in Figure 4.

The reason for the problem with estimation of S is the assumption used in the estimation procedure that the transport parameters (K_{BD} and S) are constant during the whole dwell time (Imholz et al., 1994; Krediet et al., 2000; Waniewski et al., 1996c). Additionally, in normal condition of peritoneal dialysis the convective transport is much smaller than the diffusive one. In experimental conditions this problem can be overcome by choosing the concentration of the investigated solute in dialysate close to that in blood. In this way the diffusive transport component is substantially decreased and is similar to the convective component. In these conditions application of two-dimensional linear regression results in estimation of K_{BD} and S which are within the theoretical limits. The other advantages of this approach is the possibility of simplification of expression for convective transport in which the average value of substance concentration C_R can be substituted with solute blood plasma concentration and in this way, the problem of estimation of F can be eliminated.

2.4 Parameter estimation: An example

In the paper by Olszowska et al (Olszowska et al., 2007), data from a clinical study on dwells lasting 4 hours with glucose based (1.36%) and amino acids based (1.1%) solutions in 20 clinically stable patients on peritoneal dialysis are presented. With frequent sampling of dialysate, three samples of blood and with dialysate volume and fluid absorption rate obtained using macromolecular volume marker (RISA, radioiodinated serum albumin) it was possible to apply Eqn (13) and two-dimensional linear regression for estimation of diffusive mass transport coefficient, K_{BD}, and sieving coefficient, S, for glucose, potassium, creatinine, urea and total protein. The results demonstrate slightly higher values of K_{BD} obtained for dwells with amino acid solution as compared with glucose based solution (e.g. for glucose K_{BD} = 8.3 ml/min, S = 0.62 vs. K_{BD} 8.1 ml/min, S = 0.21 and for urea K_{BD} = 28.2 ml/min, S = 0.48 vs. K_{BD} 25.3 ml/min, S = 0.39). It seems that the amino acid based solution exerts a specific impact on peritoneal tissue which causes slight increases of diffusive and convective transport. It is worth to note that, for substances specified above, values of K_{BD} and S, estimated using two-dimensional linear regression, were in acceptable range ($K_{BD}>0$, $0 \le S \le 1$). However, for amino acids themselves estimation of S failed and the estimation of K_{BD} was performed with assumption that for these solutes S was 0.55 and therefore one-dimensional linear regression was applied. In this condition the estimated averaged values of K_{BD} for essential amino acids was 10.32±0.51 ml/min and for nonessential amino acids was 10.6±1.33 ml/min. Similar results was also described in (Douma et al., 1996).

In contrast to this assumption, the estimation of parameters performed for shorter periods of time demonstrated that estimated parameters have higher values at the beginning of the dwells than at the end (Waniewski, 2004), and it was proposed that the parameters values estimated for dwell time change with time as described by the function $f(t) = 1 + 0.6875e^{-t/50}$ (t is time in minutes). A more detailed evaluation of this variability (vasoactive effect) can be found in (Imholz et al., 1994; Waniewski, 2004; Douma et al., 1996).

3. Pore representation of peritoneal transport barrier

In the membrane model of the peritoneal barrier, no structure of this barrier is considered. It is simply assumed that blood and dialysate are separated by a semipermeable membrane and that the transport phenomena can be described using the thermodynamic theory of the transport processes. The pore model is more complex and derived from the field of capillary physiology. The basic idea of this model is the assumption that the capillary wall in the subperitoneal tissue is heteroporous and that the transport through the pores may be evaluated using the hydrodynamic theory of transport along a cylindrical pipe (Deen, 1987) which describes how much the solute and fluid transport is affected due to presence of the pores comparing to a uniform, semipermeable membrane.

In 1987, Rippe et al proposed the so-called two-pore model to describe solute and fluid transport during peritoneal dialysis (Rippe &Haraldsson, 1987; Rippe &Stelin, 1989; Rippe et al., 1991b; Rippe &Haraldsson, 1994). According to this model, the membrane is heteroporous with two size of pores: large pores (radius 250 Å), and small pores (radius 43 Å). A large number of small pores makes the membrane permeable to most small solutes, whereas a very small number of large pores allows for the transport of macromolecules (proteins) from blood to peritoneal cavity. However, this model could not describe the phenomenon of sieving of small solutes, such as sodium, for which one observes a marked decline of dialysate concentration, reflecting a water-only (free of solutes) pathway. After discovery of the existence of aquaporins, the model was extended with a third type of pore, the ultrasmall pore, allowing an accurate description of the low sieving coefficients of small solutes (Figure 5). As it has been shown by Ni et al. (Ni et al., 2006) the ultrasmall pores are an analog of aquaporin-1 in endothelial cells of peritoneal capillaries and venules.

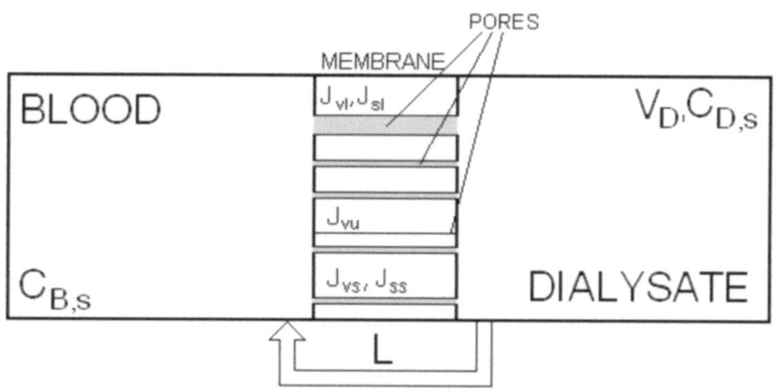

Fig. 5. Scheme of the three-pore model: J – flow of the fluid (subscript 'v') or solute (subscript 's') through the pore (subscript '*s*' – small pore, '*l*' – large pore or '*u*' – ultrasmall pore), L – lymphatic absorption from the peritoneal cavity, C_B – blood concentration. C_D – dialysate concentration, V_D – dialysate volume.

3.1 Three-pore model

According to the three-pore model (Figure 5), the change of the peritoneal volume (V_D) depends on the sum of the fluid flows through the three types of pores (J_{Vpore}, *pore*: *u* - ultrasmall, *s* - small, *l* - large) and the peritoneal lymph flow, *L*, (Rippe &Levin, 2000). Thus (Rippe &Stelin, 1989; Rippe et al., 1991a; Rippe et al., 1991b; Rippe &Levin, 2000):

$$\frac{dV_D}{dt} = J_{V_U} + J_{V_S} + J_{V_L} - L, \tag{15}$$

and J_{Vpore} is governed by the hydrostatic and osmotic pressures as follows (Rippe &Levin, 2000):

$$J_{V_{pore}} = a_{pore} L_p S \left[\Delta P(V_D) - \sum_{solute} \sigma_{solute,pore} \Delta\pi_{solute}(t) \right], \tag{16}$$

where: L_pS is the membrane ultrafiltration coefficient, α_{pore} is the part of L_pS accounted for the specific type of pore, ΔP is the hydrostatic pressure difference between the blood capillaries and the peritoneal cavity (which depends on the fluid volume in the peritoneal cavity: $\Delta P(V_D) = \Delta P(V_0) - {}^{V_D(t)-V_0}\!/_{490}$, V_0 is the initial dialysate volume, 490 is an empirical coefficient, (Twardowski et al., 1983)), $\sigma_{solute,pore}$ is the *solute* osmotic reflection coefficient describing osmotic efficiency of the *solute* in the *pore*, and $\Delta\pi_{solute}$ is the *solute* crystalloid osmotic pressure gradient ($\Delta\pi_{solute}(t) = RT[C_{solute,B} - C_{solute,D}]$, R - gas constant, T - absolute temperature, $C_{solute,B}$ and $C_{solute,D}$ - *solute* concentration in blood and dialysate, respectively).
Solutes are transported only through the large and small pores and by the lymphatic flow, and therefore the solute mass change in the peritoneal cavity ($M_{solute,D}$) is described by the following mass balance equation (Rippe &Levin, 2000):

$$\frac{dM_{solute,D}}{dt} = J_{S_{solute,S}} + J_{S_{solute,L}} - LC_{solute,D}. \tag{17}$$

where $J_{S_{solute,pore}}$ - *solute* flow through the *pore*

The solute flow, $J_{S_{solute,pore}}$, is by diffusion and convection, and is defined as:

$$J_{S_{solute,pore}} = \underbrace{-PS_{solute,pore}(C_{solute,D} - C_{solute,B})}_{\text{diffusion}} + \underbrace{J_{v_{pore}}(1 - \sigma_{solute,pore})\bar{C}_{solute}}_{\text{convection}}, \tag{18}$$

where: $PS_{solute,pore}$ is a *solute* permeability surface area for the specific type of pore, $\bar{C}_{solute}$ is the mean membrane solute concentration, $\bar{C}_{solute} = (1 - F_{solute})C_{solute,B} + FC_{solute,D}$, and $F_{solute} = 1/Pe_{solute,pore} - 1/(e^{Pe_{solute,pore}} - 1)$ is a function of the ratio of convective to diffusive transport given by the Peclet number $Pe_{pore,solute}$ (Rippe &Levin, 2000):

$$Pe_{solute,pore} = J_{V_{pore}} \frac{1 - \sigma_{solute,pore}}{PS_{solute,pore}}, \tag{19}$$

compare to Eqns (9)-(12). Note that $1 - \sigma_{solute,pore}$ is sieving coefficient for these particular *pore* and *solute*.
In the previous approach based on the membrane model, there were two transport coefficients: diffusive mass transport coefficient (K_{BD}) and sieving coefficient (S) which both characterize membrane properties of peritoneal tissue and can be estimated from clinical or experimental data. The analogues of these parameters in the three-pore model are, respectively, the permeability surface area coefficient ($PS_{solute,pore}$) and the solute's osmotic reflection coefficient ($\sigma_{solute,pore}$) which may be calculated using the following formulas (Rippe &Levin, 2000):

$$PS_{solute,pore} = D_{solute} \left(\frac{A_0}{\Delta x} \right)_{pore} \left(\frac{A}{A_0} \right)_{solute,pore}, \tag{20}$$

$$\sigma_{solute,pore} = 1 - \frac{(1-\lambda)^2[2-(1-\lambda)^2](1-\lambda/3)}{1-\lambda/3+2/3\lambda^2}, \tag{21}$$

where: D_{solute} represents the free solute diffusion coefficient, $A_0/\Delta x$ is the unrestricted (nominal) pore area over unit diffusion distance, A/A_0 is the restriction factor for diffusion defined as the ratio of the effective surface pore area over unrestricted (nominal) pore area, and λ = solute radius/pore radius.

3.2 Parameter estimation: Problems and pitfalls

The three-pore model is more complicated than the membrane model and it is not possible to find analytical or integrated solutions and to estimate parameter values using linear regression. Therefore the model has to be solved numerically using a computer software with ODE (ordinary differential equation) solver (e.g. Matlab®, Berkeley-Madonna or JSim) and with some parameter estimation techniques (Freida et al., 2007; Galach et al., 2009; Galach et al., 2010). For example, in Matlab the estimation of parameters may be done using function *fminsearch* (Nelder-Mead type simplex search method) with the aim to minimize the difference between numerical predictions and clinical data (usually, absolute difference or the squared difference). Therefore, the aim is to find the global minimum of the error function, and, thus, the values of parameters that describe the predicted curves as close to the clinical data as possible (Freida et al., 2007; Galach et al., 2009; Galach et al., 2010).
It should however be noted that, with the increasing number of estimated parameters or decreasing number of data points, the chance that not global but local minimum is attained is growing (Juillet et al., 2009). The results are often strongly dependent on starting values of the fitted parameters (in particular on their difference from those that describe the global minimum (Juillet et al., 2009)), see an example in Section 3.3. To deal with these problems, one can lower the number of fitted parameters using the sensitivity analysis to find parameters with the highest influence on numerical results, and use not one but many initial sets of parameter values to check parameter space extensively, avoid local minima and hit the global minimum. Additionally, to avoid calculation problems when fitted parameters have different order of magnitude (i.e. in chosen set of parameters there are very small as well as large values), it is to be preferred to fit not the parameter itself but its multiplier:

$$Par_{fitted} = x \cdot Par_{initial}, \tag{22}$$

where Par_{fitted} is the sought value of the parameter, $Par_{initial}$ is a basal value of the parameter and x is the fitted coefficient. Then all fitted coefficients (x) have a similar order of magnitude.
Another important issue is an appropriate selection of parameters set, because it is often possible to obtain similar predictions with much different sets of fitted parameters (see an example in Section 3.3). Therefore, any final conclusions should be drawn with the utmost caution.

3.3 Parameter estimation: An example

Clinical data of patients on six hour peritoneal dialysis dwell with glucose 3.86% solution (Karolinska Institutet, Stockholm, Sweden) were used to estimate the parameters of the three-pore model. More detailed description of the clinical data can be found in (Galach et al., 2010). The model was solved using *ode45* solver of Matlab® v. R2010b software

(MathWorks Inc., USA) based on an explicit 4th and 5th order Runge-Kutta formula. The data of each patient separately were used as target values for estimation of the model parameters done using Matlab® function *fminsearch* (Nelder-Mead type simplex search method) with the aim to minimize the function f_{min} that described the sum of fractional absolute differences between theoretical predictions and clinical data scaled to the experimental values:

$$f_{\min}=\sum_i\frac{|V_D^{\exp}(T_i)-V_D^{sim}(T_i)|}{V_D^{\exp}(T_i)}+\sum_i\frac{|C_{U,D}^{\exp}(T_i)-C_{U,D}^{sim}(T_i)|}{C_{U,D}^{\exp}(T_i)}+\sum_i\frac{|C_{Na,D}^{\exp}(T_i)-C_{Na,D}^{sim}(T_i)|}{C_{Na,D}^{\exp}(T_i)}+\ldots$$
$$\ldots+\sum_i\frac{|C_{G,D}^{\exp}(T_i)-C_{G,D}^{sim}(T_i)|}{C_{G,D}^{\exp}(T_i)}, \quad (23)$$

where $V_D(T_i)$ is dialysate volume at time T_i, $C_{s,D}(T_i)$ is dialysate solute concentration at time T_i ('s': 'G' - glucose, 'Na' - sodium), *'exp'* stands for clinical data, and *'sim'* stands for simulation results. The chosen f_{min} function depends, of course, on dialysate volume and on glucose, urea and sodium as a representative of small solutes: glucose is an osmotic agent, urea is a marker of uremia, and sodium is a solute for which the so-called "sodium dip" (indicating sodium sieving as water passes the ultra-small pores) is observed during the peritoneal dwell. The influence of the other substances is taken into account only through their impact on dialysate volume.

Six parameters were estimated by fitting the three-pore model to clinical data: *LpS* (membrane UF-coefficient), *L* (peritoneal lymph flow), *PS* (permeability surface area coefficient) for glucose, sodium and urea and, alternatively, r_{small} (small pore radius, Set 1), or α_{small} (the part of L_pS accounted for the small pores, Eqn (16), Set 2), see Table 1. Other parameters were calculated from the estimated ones or their values were assumed based on previous investigations (Rippe &Levin, 2000), Table 1. The choice between two different sets

Three-pore model parameters	
Set 1	Set 2
Fitted parameters	
LpS, L, $PS_{small,G}$, $PS_{small,Na}$, $PS_{small,U}$, r_{small}	LpS, L, $PS_{small,G}$, $PS_{small,Na}$, $PS_{small,U}$, α_{small}
Assumed parameters (Rippe &Levin, 2000)	
$\alpha_{ultrasmall}$ α_{small} α_{large}, r_{large}, r_{solute}	α_{large}, r_{small}, r_{large}, r_{solute}, $\sigma_{solute, small}$
Parameters calculated from the fitted values	
$PS_{large,solute}$, in proportion to the fitted values for small pores, $\sigma_{solute, small}$ (dependent on r_{small})	$PS_{large,solute}$ in proportion to the fitted values for small pores, $\alpha_{ultrasmall}$ to achieve $\sum_{pore}\alpha_{pore}=1$

Table 1. Division of the three-pore model parameters according to the source of their values.

of parameters that describe the three pore structure of the transport barrier used in estimation procedure is the choice between two different hypotheses about the variation of this structure among patients. The first hypothesis (Set 1) is based on the assumption that the radius of the small pore may vary from patient to patient but the fractional contribution of these pores to the hydraulic permeability, α_{small}, is the same in all patients. The other alternative with α_{small} varying between patients but the size of small pores being the same is investigated when Set 2 is selected. In general, both parameters may be expected to vary among patients, and, moreover, a similar variability may be considered for the remaining types of pores (large and ultrasmall). However, one cannot estimate all the parameters from the limited data and therefore, based on the previous experience with the model, the values of some of them need to be selected before the estimation procedure starts. The impact of the assumptions on the large pores on the simulations is less than those on the small pores. Thus, it was assumed that the radii of large and ultrasmall pores as well as the percentage input of large pores to the hydraulic permeability were constant. Note that the fraction of ultrasmall pores was related to the fraction of small and large pores by the condition that the sum of all coefficients α should be one.

It may happen that each single run of the fitting procedure (*fminsearch* function) for different starting parameter values yields different final sets of parameters and also different predictions for the simulated curves (Figure 6), which not necessarily are good approximations of the clinical data (Figure 6, right middle panel). It is also worth to mention that, usually, the fitting procedure is not sensitive to single data errors and may yield a smooth curve based on the other points (Figure 6, left panels).

As in the previous studies (Galach et al., 2009; Waniewski et al., 2008), the results of the simulations and estimations show that the three-pore model with fitted parameters is capable of reproducing clinical data concerning peritoneal dialysis with glucose solution rather well (Figures 6-9), but the parameter values are substantially different for different patients (Tables 2-3).

Parameters	Initial 2 hour	Dwell 6 hour	
	Set 1	Set 1	Set 2
LpS	0.0610	0.0870	0.0890
L	0.1624	2.9127	3.7367
PS_G	12.53	10.45	9.76
PS_{Na}	9.77	15.21	12.78
PS_U	23.05	31.83	31.37
r_{small}	43.8	48.5	43.0 (not estimated)
α_{small}	0.90 (not estimated)	0.90 (not estimated)	0.9799

Table 2. Values of estimated parameter for patient No 1; Estimation procedure: data concerning initial 2 hours of the dwell and Set 1 of the estimated parameters (Table 1), data concerning the whole dwell and Set 1 of the estimated parameters, data concerning the whole dwell and Set 2 of the estimated parameters

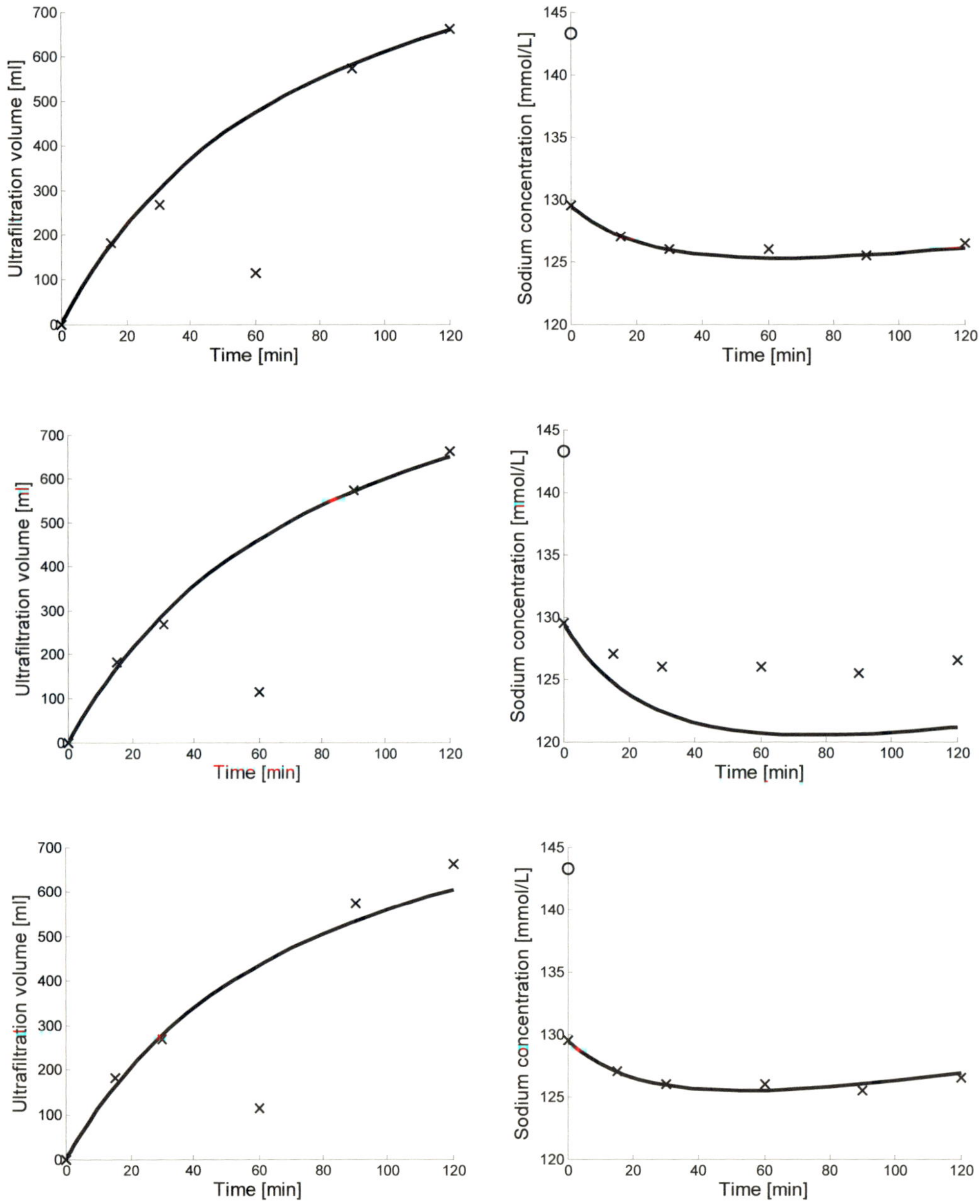

Fig. 6. Ultrafiltration volume and sodium concentration during initial 2 hours of the session for the patient No 1 and following starting points (x values) in the fitting procedure (*fminsearch*): [0.95,0.74,1.10,1.14,1.35,1.52] (top), [1.24,2.48,0.59,2.27,2.33,2.09] (middle) and [0.71,1.03,1.18,1.86,0.78,1.95] (bottom).

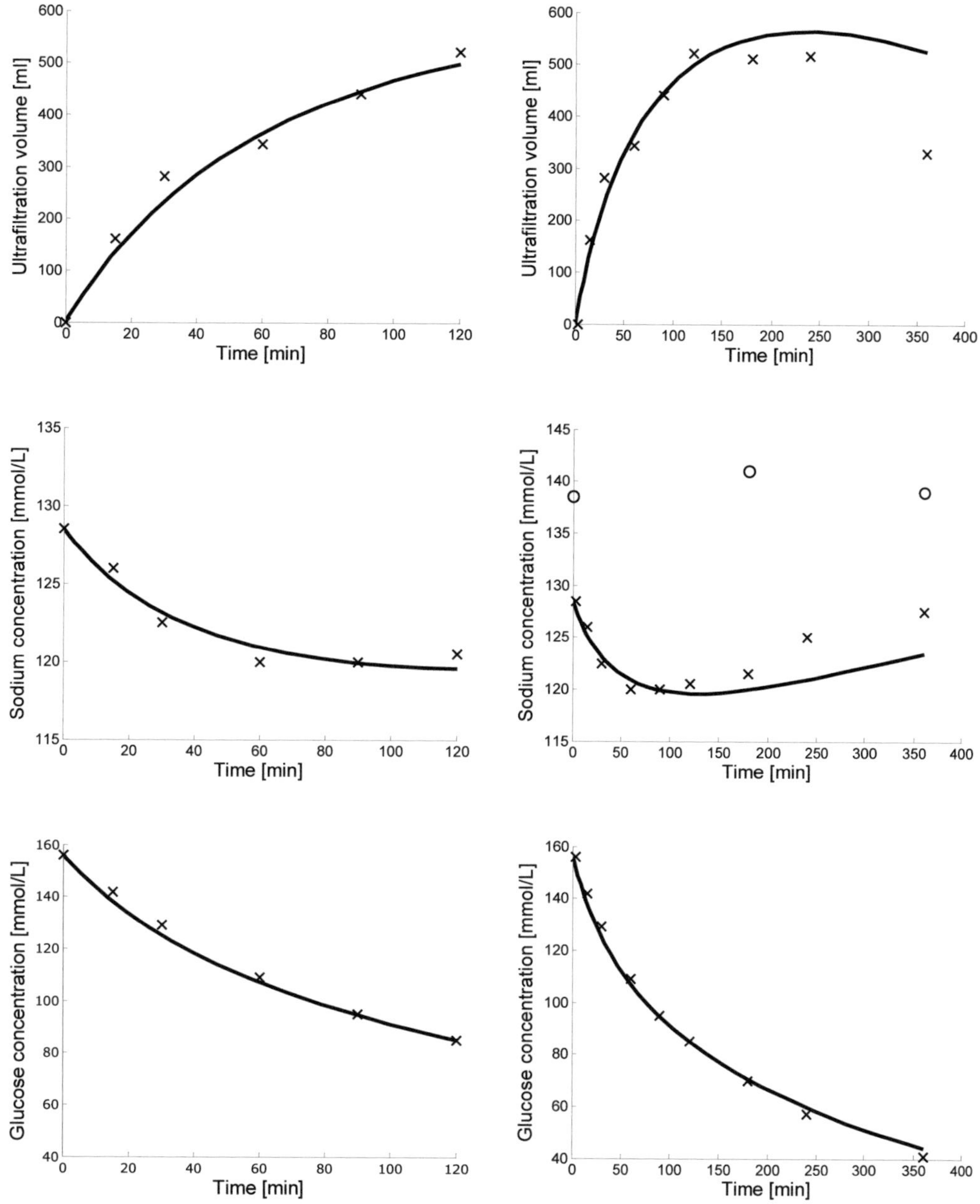

Fig. 7. Ultrafiltration volume, sodium concentration and glucose dialysate concentration during initial 2 hours of the session (left panel) and during the whole dwell (right panel) for the patient No 2 and for the same parameter values estimated from the initial 2 hours of the dwell; —- simulation result, x - dialysate data, o - blood data.

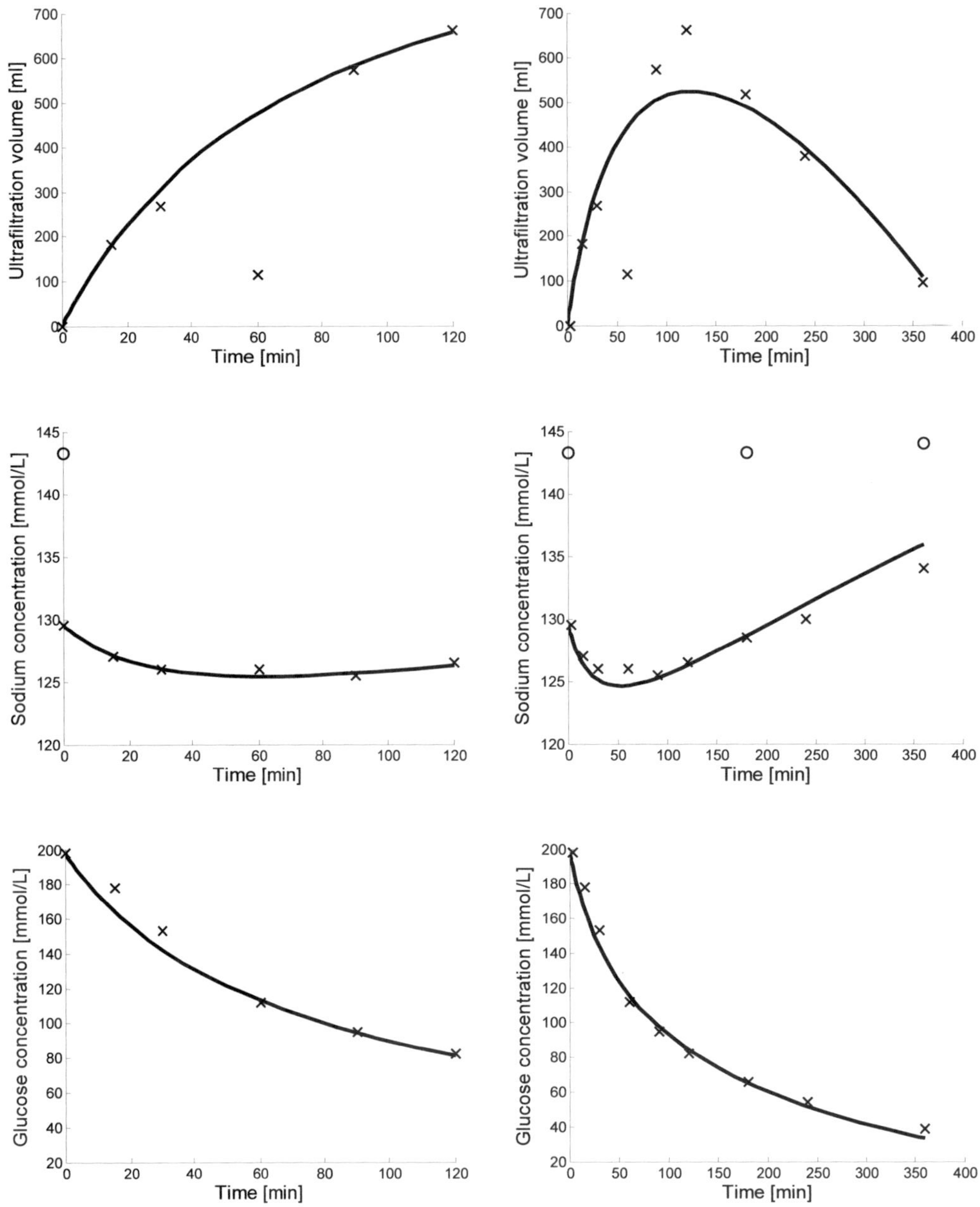

Fig. 8. Ultrafiltration volume, sodium concentration and glucose dialysate concentration during initial 2 hours of the session (left panel) and during the whole peritoneal dialysis dwell (right panel) for the patient No 1 and Set 1 of the estimated parameters (parameters from Table 2, column 1 and 2); — - simulation result, x - dialysate data, o - blood data

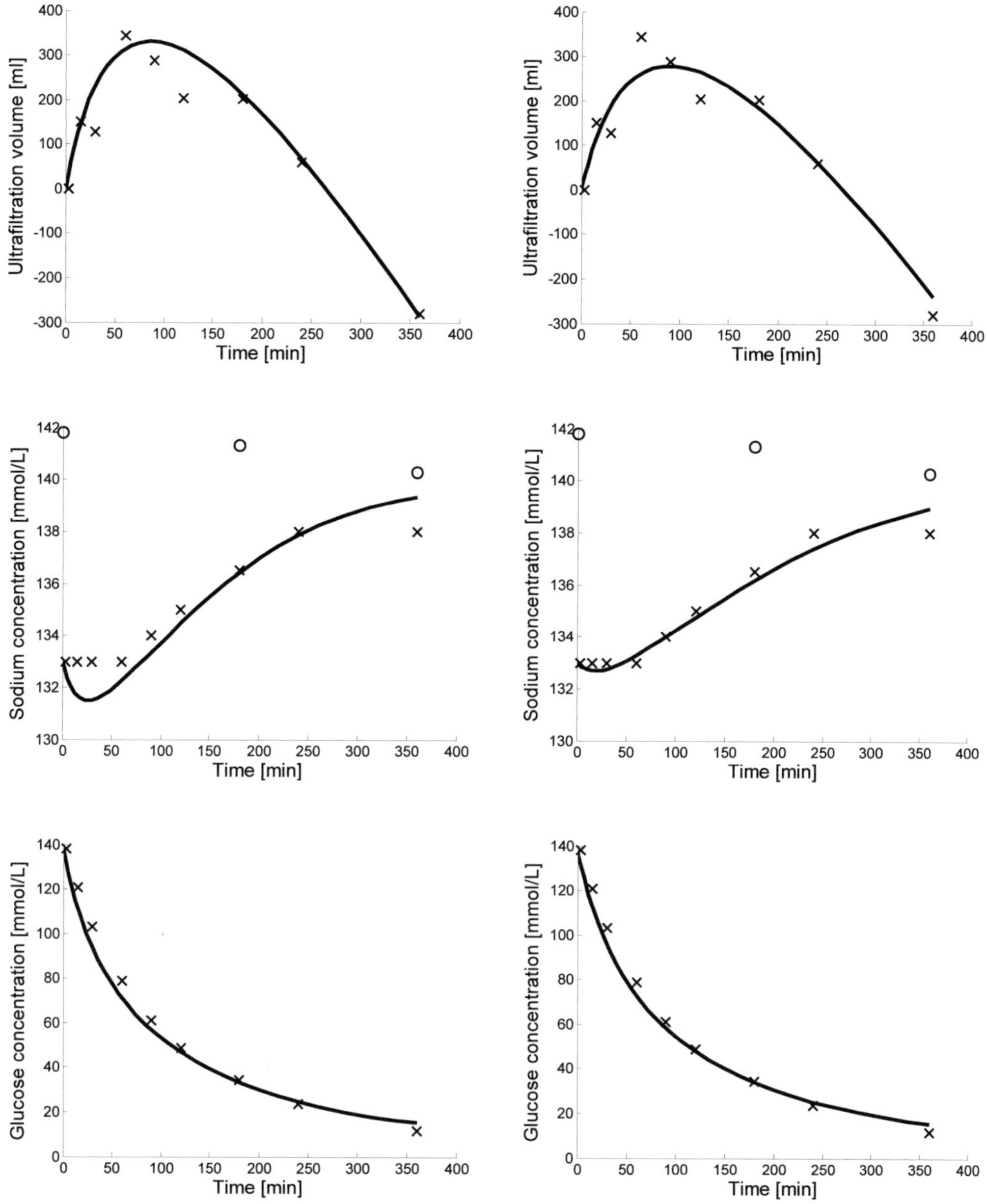

Fig. 9. Ultrafiltration volume, sodium and glucose concentration during 6 hour peritoneal dialysis dwell for the patient No 3 and Set 1 (left panel) or Set 2 (right panel) in fitting procedure; — - simulation result, x - dialysate data, o - blood data.

The assumption that the parameter values are constant during the whole dwell is only a simplification (Imholz et al., 1994; Krediet et al., 2000; Stachowska-Pietka et al., 2010; Waniewski et al., 1996a, 1996d). The transport processes occurring during the first part of dialysis dwell are much more rapid than in the later part, and therefore the parameters estimated using data from the first part of the dwell only may not be correct for the whole dwell (Figure 6); thus, the values of parameters estimated from the partial data and the whole set of data may differ (Figures 7-8, Table 2).
It is also worth noting that the selection of the assumptions, and consequently selection of the proper set of parameters for estimation procedure, is of high importance and has influence on all fitted parameters values and simulation results (Figure 9, Tables 2 and 3). The results of the simulations for different sets of estimated parameters may all give a good approximation of clinical data (Figure 9, results of the simulations for Set 1 and 2), however the fitted parameter values in these sets are different (Tables 3). But it may vary according to the patient. For example: for the patient No 1 the differences between fitted values of the parameters for Set 1 and 2 do not exceed 30% (Figure 8, Table 2), whereas for the patient No 3 the differences for 2 parameters were greater than 60% and for one parameter even than 100% (Figure 9, Table 3). Thus it is always very important to compare parameters fitted with the same assumptions or to discuss the differences in assumed hypotheses.

Parameters	Dwell 6 hour	
	Set 1	Set 2
LpS	0.0371	0.0862
L	2.5976	2.5026
PS_G	16.8806	17.05821
PS_{Na}	16.6024	27.5764
PS_U	30.2129	24.1114
r_{small}	26.7370	43 (not estimated)
α_{small}	0.9 (not estimated)	0.9799

Table 3. Values of estimated parameter for patient No 3 using data for whole dwell with two sets of the estimated parameters (Table 1).

4. Conclusions

Peritoneal dialysis is an interesting and important area for mathematical modeling. In fact peritoneal dialysis treatment as we know it today is the result of kinetic modeling leading to the concept of continuous ambulatory peritoneal dialysis. The first mathematical models describing peritoneal dialysis were based on a simple idea of a semipermeable peritoneal barrier between blood and dialysate allowing solute and fluid transport characterized by the so-called transport parameters (Imholz et al., 1994; Krediet et al., 2000; Waniewski et al., 1995; Waniewski, 1999). Such models were - and still are - useful in evaluation of peritoneal dwell studies and their various versions have been widely applied especially for analysis of solute transport (Heimburger et al., 1992; Pannekeet et al., 1995; Smit et al., 2005; Waniewski et al., 1991, 1992). Despite the fact that they were used to demonstrate and interpret new transport phenomena, many questions concerning the mechanisms for the transport process could not be answered using this simple mathematical modeling because, although such models can be well fitted to the data and used to estimate transport parameters separately for fluid and each solute, however they cannot reliably predict the results of dialysis session and indicate the relationship between the parameters for different solutes and fluid. Therefore, another type of model, with additional and more physiological assumptions about the structure of the peritoneal membrane, was proposed (Rippe &Haraldsson, 1987; Rippe et al., 1991a; Rippe &Haraldsson, 1994). The pore model derived the description and relationships between the transport parameters from the solute size and the structure of the transport barrier (size of pores, number of pores etc.). The mentioned models of peritoneal transport were included into practical methods and computer programs for the evaluation of the efficacy and adequacy of peritoneal dialysis (Haraldsson, 2001; Van Biesen et al., 2003; Van Biesen et al., 2006; Vonesh et al., 1991; Vonesh &Keshaviah, 1997; Vonesh et al., 1999).

In this chapter these two most popular models describing peritoneal transport of fluid and solutes were presented and compared as regards their basic ideas and aims as well as their applicability. The membrane model provides a simple relationship between the rates of fluid and solute flows and their respective driving forces, whereas the three-pore model gives a quantitative relationship between the transport coefficients for various solutes and between fluid and solute transport coefficients. Additionally, the parameters estimation techniques and the possible problems with parameter estimation were discussed.

5. References

Chen, T.W., Khanna, R., Moore, H., Twardowski, Z.J. &Nolph, K.D. (1991). Sieving and reflection coefficients for sodium salts and glucose during peritoneal dialysis in rats. *Journal of the American Society of Nephrology*, Vol. 2, No. 6, pp. (1092-1100)

De Paepe, M., Belpaire, F., Schelstraete, K. &Lameire, N. (1988). Comparison of different volume markers in peritoneal dialysis. *J Lab Clin Med*, Vol. 111, No. 4, pp. (421-429)

Deen, W.M. (1987). Hindered transport of large molecules in liquid-filled pores. *AIChE Journal*, Vol. 33, No. 9, pp. (1409)

Douma, C.E., de Waart, D.R., Struijk, D.G. &Krediet, R.T. (1996). Effect of amino acid based dialysate on peritoneal blood flow and permeability in stable CAPD patients: a potential role for nitric oxide? *Clin Nephrol*, Vol. 45, No. 5, pp. (295-302)

Flessner, M.F. (1991). Peritoneal transport physiology: insights from basic research. *J Am Soc Nephrol*, Vol. 2, No. 2, pp. (122-135)

Freida, P., Galach, M., Divino Filho, J.C., Werynski, A. &Lindholm, B. (2007). Combination of crystalloid (glucose) and colloid (icodextrin) osmotic agents markedly enhances peritoneal fluid and solute transport during the long PD dwell. *Perit Dial Int*, Vol. 27, No. 3, pp. (267-276)

Galach, M., Werynski, A., Waniewski, J., Freida, P. &Lindholm, B. (2009). Kinetic analysis of peritoneal fluid and solute transport with combination of glucose and icodextrin as osmotic agents. *Perit Dial Int*, Vol. 29, No. 1, pp. (72-80)

Galach, M., Waniewski, J., Axelsson, J., Heimburger, O., Werynski, A. &Lindholm, B. (2010). Mathematical modeling of the glucose-insulin system during peritoneal dialysis with glucose-based fluids. *Asaio J*, Vol. 57, No. 1, pp. (41-47)

Haraldsson, B. (2001). Optimization of peritoneal dialysis prescription using computer models of peritoneal transport. *Perit Dial Int*, Vol. 21 Suppl 3, pp. (S148-151)

Heimburger, O., Waniewski, J., Werynski, A. &Lindholm, B. (1992). A quantitative description of solute and fluid transport during peritoneal dialysis. *Kidney Int*, Vol. 41, No. 5, pp. (1320-1332)

Imholz, A.L., Koomen, G.C., Struijk, D.G., Arisz, L. &Krediet, R.T. (1994). Fluid and solute transport in CAPD patients using ultralow sodium dialysate. *Kidney Int*, Vol. 46, No. 2, pp. (333-340)

Juillet, B., Bos, C., Gaudichon, C., Tome, D. &Fouillet, H. (2009). Parameter estimation for linear compartmental models--a sensitivity analysis approach. *Ann Biomed Eng*, Vol. 37, No. 5, pp. (1028-1042)

Kedem, O. &Katchalsky, A. (1958). Thermodynamic analysis of the permeability of biological membranes to non-electrolytes. *Biochim Biophys Acta*, Vol. 27, No. 2, pp. (229-246)

Krediet, R.T., Struijk, D.G., Koomen, G.C. &Arisz, L. (1991). Peritoneal fluid kinetics during CAPD measured with intraperitoneal dextran 70. *ASAIO Trans*, Vol. 37, No. 4, pp. (662-667)

Krediet, R.T., Lindholm, B. &Rippe, B. (2000). Pathophysiology of peritoneal membrane failure. *Perit Dial Int*, Vol. 20 Suppl 4, pp. (S22-42)

Lysaght, M.J. &Farrell, P.C. (1989). Membrane phenomena and mass transfer kinetics in peritoneal dialysis. *Journal of Membrane Science*, Vol. 44, No. 1, pp. (5)

Ni, J., Verbavatz, J.M., Rippe, A., Boisde, I., Moulin, P., Rippe, B., Verkman, A.S. &Devuyst, O. (2006). Aquaporin-1 plays an essential role in water permeability and ultrafiltration during peritoneal dialysis. *Kidney Int*, Vol. 69, No. 9, pp. (1518-1525)

Olszowska, A., Waniewski, J., Werynski, A., Anderstam, B., Lindholm, B. &Wankowicz, Z. (2007). Peritoneal transport in peritoneal dialysis patients using glucose-based and amino acid-based solutions. *Perit Dial Int*, Vol. 27, No. 5, pp. (544-553)

Pannekeet, M.M., Imholz, A.L., Struijk, D.G., Koomen, G.C., Langedijk, M.J., Schouten, N., de Waart, R., Hiralall, J. &Krediet, R.T. (1995). The standard peritoneal permeability analysis: a tool for the assessment of peritoneal permeability characteristics in CAPD patients. *Kidney Int*, Vol. 48, No. 3, pp. (866-875)

Rippe, B. &Haraldsson, B. (1987). Fluid and protein fluxes across small and large pores in the microvasculature. Application of two-pore equations. *Acta Physiol Scand*, Vol. 131, No. 3, pp. (411-428)

Rippe, B. &Stelin, G. (1989). Simulations of peritoneal solute transport during CAPD. Application of two-pore formalism. *Kidney Int*, Vol. 35, No. 5, pp. (1234-1244)

Rippe, B., Simonsen, O. &Stelin, G. (1991a). Clinical implications of a three-pore model of peritoneal transport. *Adv Perit Dial*, Vol. 7, pp. (3-9)

Rippe, B., Stelin, G. &Haraldsson, B. (1991b). Computer simulations of peritoneal fluid transport in CAPD. *Kidney Int*, Vol. 40, No. 2, pp. (315-325)

Rippe, B. &Haraldsson, B. (1994). Transport of macromolecules across microvascular walls: the two-pore theory. *Physiol Rev*, Vol. 74, No. 1, pp. (163-219)

Rippe, B. &Levin, L. (2000). Computer simulations of ultrafiltration profiles for an icodextrin-based peritoneal fluid in CAPD. *Kidney Int*, Vol. 57, No. 6, pp. (2546-2556)

Smit, W., Parikova, A., Struijk, D.G. &Krediet, R.T. (2005). The difference in causes of early and late ultrafiltration failure in peritoneal dialysis. *Perit Dial Int*, Vol. 25 Suppl 3, pp. (S41-45)

Stachowska-Pietka, J., Waniewski, J., Vonesh, E. &Lindholm, B. (2010). Changes in free water fraction and aquaporin function with dwell time during continuous ambulatory peritoneal dialysis. *Artif Organs*, Vol. 34, No. 12, pp. (1138-1143)

Stelin, G. &Rippe, B. (1990). A phenomenological interpretation of the variation in dialysate volume with dwell time in CAPD. *Kidney Int*, Vol. 38, No. 3, pp. (465-472)

Twardowski, Z.J., Prowant, B.F., Nolph, K.D., Martinez, A.J. &Lampton, L.M. (1983). High volume, low frequency continuous ambulatory peritoneal dialysis. *Kidney Int*, Vol. 23, No. 1, pp. (64)

Van Biesen, W., Carlsson, O., Bergia, R., Brauner, M., Christensson, A., Genestier, S., Haag-Weber, M., Heaf, J., Joffe, P., Johansson, A.C., Morel, B., Prischl, F., Verbeelen, D. &Vychytil, A. (2003). Personal dialysis capacity (PDC(TM)) test: a multicentre clinical study. *Nephrol Dial Transplant*, Vol. 18, No. 4, pp. (788-796)

Van Biesen, W., Van Der Tol, A., Veys, N., Lameire, N. &Vanholder, R. (2006). Evaluation of the peritoneal membrane function by three letter word acronyms: PET, PDC, SPA, PD-Adequest, POL: what to do? *Contrib Nephrol*, Vol. 150, pp. (37-41)

Vonesh, E.F., Lysaght, M.J., Moran, J. &Farrell, P. (1991). Kinetic modeling as a prescription aid in peritoneal dialysis. *Blood Purif*, Vol. 9, No. 5-6, pp. (246-270)

Vonesh, E.F. &Keshaviah, P.R. (1997). Applications in kinetic modeling using PD ADEQUEST. *Perit Dial Int*, Vol. 17 Suppl 2, pp. (S119-125)

Vonesh, E.F., Story, K.O. &O'Neill, W.T. (1999). A multinational clinical validation study of PD ADEQUEST 2.0. PD ADEQUEST International Study Group. *Perit Dial Int*, Vol. 19, No. 6, pp. (556-571)

Waniewski, J., Werynski, A., Heimburger, O. &Lindholm, B. (1991). Simple models for description of small-solute transport in peritoneal dialysis. *Blood Purif*, Vol. 9, No. 3, pp. (129-141)

Waniewski, J., Werynski, A., Heimburger, O. &Lindholm, B. (1992). Simple membrane models for peritoneal dialysis. Evaluation of diffusive and convective solute transport. *Asaio J*, Vol. 38, No. 4, pp. (788-796)

Waniewski, J., Heimburger, O., Park, M.S., Werynski, A. &Lindholm, B. (1994). Methods for estimation of peritoneal dialysate volume and reabsorption rate using macromolecular markers. *Perit Dial Int*, Vol. 14, No. 1, pp. (8-16)

Waniewski, J., Heimburger, O., Werynski, A., Park, M.S. &Lindholm, B. (1995). Diffusive and convective solute transport in peritoneal dialysis with glucose as an osmotic agent. *Artif Organs*, Vol. 19, No. 4, pp. (295-306)

Waniewski, J., Heimburger, O., Werynski, A. &Lindholm, B. (1996a). Osmotic conductance of the peritoneum in CAPD patients with permanent loss of ultrafiltration capacity. *Peritoneal Dialysis International*, Vol. 16, No. 5, pp. (488-496)

Waniewski, J., Heimburger, O., Werynski, A. &Lindholm, B. (1996b). Simple models for fluid transport during peritoneal dialysis. *Int J Artif Organs*, Vol. 19, No. 8, pp. (455-466)

Waniewski, J., Heimburger, O., Werynski, A. &Lindholm, B. (1996c). Diffusive mass transport coefficients are not constant during a single exchange in continuous ambulatory peritoneal dialysis. *Asaio J*, Vol. 42, No. 5, pp. (M518-523)

Waniewski, J., Heimburger, O., Werynski, A. &Lindholm, B. (1996d). Paradoxes in peritoneal transport of small solutes. *Perit Dial Int*, Vol. 16 Suppl 1, pp. (S63-69)

Waniewski, J. (1999). Mathematical models for peritoneal transport characteristics. *Perit Dial Int*, Vol. 19 Suppl 2, pp. (S193-201)

Waniewski, J. (2004). A Mathematical Model of Local Stimulation of Perfusion by Vasoactive Agent Diffusing from Tissue Surface. *Cardiovascular Engineering*, Vol. 4, No. 1, pp. (115)

Waniewski, J., Debowska, M. &Lindholm, B. (2008). How accurate is the description of transport kinetics in peritoneal dialysis according to different versions of the three-pore model? *Perit Dial Int*, Vol. 28, No. 1, pp. (53-60)

2

Distributed Models of Peritoneal Transport

Joanna Stachowska-Pietka and Jacek Waniewski
Institute of Biocybernetics and Biomedical Engineering
Polish Academy of Sciences, Warsaw
Poland

1. Introduction

There are several methods to model the process of water and solute transport during peritoneal dialysis (PD). The characteristics of the phenomena and the purpose of modelling influence the choice of methodology. Among others, the phenomenological models are commonly used in clinical and laboratory research. In peritoneal dialysis, the compartmental approach is widely used (membrane model, three-pore model). These kinds of models are based on phenomenological parameters, sometimes called "lumped parameters", because one parameter is used to describe the net result of several different processes that occur during dialysis. The main advantage of the compartmental approach is that it decreases substantially the number of parameters that have to be estimated, and therefore its application in clinical research is easier. However, in the compartmental approach, it is usually very difficult to connect the estimated parameters with the physiology and the local anatomy of the involved tissues. Therefore, these models have limited applications in the explanation of the changes that occur in the physiology of the peritoneal transport. For example, the membrane models describe exchange of fluid and solute between peritoneal cavity and plasma through the "peritoneal membrane". However, this approach does not take into account the anatomy and physiology of the peritoneal transport system and cannot be used for the explanation of the processes that occur in the tissue during the treatment.

Basic concepts and previous applications of distributed models are summarized in Section 2. A mathematical formulation of the distributed model for fluid and solute peritoneal transport is also presented in Section 2. The effective parameters, which characterize transport through the peritoneal transport system, PTS (i.e. the fluid and solute exchange between the peritoneal cavity and blood), can be estimated from the local physiological parameters of the distributed models. The comparisons between transport parameters applied in phenomenological description and those derived using a distributed approach, are presented in Sections 3 and 4 for fluid and solute transport, respectively. Typical distributed profiles of tissue hydration and solutes concentration in the tissue are presented in Section 5.

2. Distributed modelling of peritoneal transport

The first applications of the distributed model are dated to the early 1960s and were limited to the diffusive transport. Pipper et al. studied the exchange of gases between blood and artificial gas pockets within the body (Piiper, Canfield, and Rahn 1962). The transport of gases between subcutaneous pockets and blood was studies in rats and piglets (Van Liew 1968; Collins 1981). The theory of heat and solute exchange between blood and tissue was investigated using distributed approach by Perl (Perl 1963, 1962). The first application of the distributed model for the description of the diffusive transport of small solutes was proposed by Patlak and Fenstermacher, in order to describe the transport from cerebrospinal fluid to the brain (Patlak and Fenstermacher 1975). The diffusive delivery of drugs to the human bladder during intravesical chemotherapy, as well as drug delivery from the skin surface to the dermis, has been also studied in normal and cancer tissue using distributed approach (Gupta, Wientjes, and Au 1995; Wientjes et al. 1993; Wientjes et al. 1991). The distributed model was also applied for the theoretical description of fluid and solute transport in solid tumors (Baxter and Jain 1989, 1990, 1991).

The need of the model that could relate the anatomy and local physiological processes with the observed outcome of the peritoneal transport was mentioned by Nolph, Miller, and Popovich (Nolph et al. 1980). One of the attempts in this direction was proposed by Dedrick, Flessner and colleagues. They considered a distributed approach, in which the spatial structure of the tissue with blood capillaries and lymphatics distributed at different distance from the peritoneal cavity, was taken into account (Dedrick et al. 1982; Flessner 2005; Flessner, Dedrick, and Schultz 1985). Another approach, based on the three-pore model, assumes existence of serial layers of two kinds: tissue and "peritoneal membrane" (Venturoli and Rippe 2001).

The application of distributed models in intraperitoneal therapies was initiated in the early eighties of the 20th century. Initially, the diffusive transport of gases between intraperitoneal pockets and blood was studied by Collins in 1981 (Collins 1981). In the peritoneal dialysis field the distributed approach was introduced by Dedrick, Flessner and colleagues (Dedrick et al. 1982; Flessner, Dedrick, and Schultz 1984). The distributed modelling of diffusive solute transport during peritoneal dialysis was also studied by Waniewski (Waniewski 2002). Further applications of the model in the peritoneal dialysis field were related to the transport of small, middle and macro -molecules in animal studies as well as in CAPD patients (Dedrick et al. 1982; Flessner 2001; Flessner, Dedrick, and Schultz 1985; Flessner et al. 1985; Flessner, Lofthouse, and Zakaria el 1997). The initial models of peritoneal solute transport considered interstitium as a rigid, porous medium with constant fluid void volume and intraperitoneal and interstitial hydrostatic pressures (Flessner, Dedrick, and Schultz 1984). This theoretical description was validated with experimental data from rats (Flessner, Dedrick, and Schultz 1985). In the later model of IgG peritoneal transport, the changes in interstitial and intraperitoneal pressure were taken into account according to experimental studies (Flessner 2001). The process of intraperitoneal drug delivery, especially for anticancer therapies, was also described using the distributed approach (Flessner 2001; Collins et al. 1982; Flessner 2009). The so far mentioned models were applied for diffusive and convective solute transport. Seames, Moncrief and Popovich were the first who investigated osmotically driven fluid and solute transport during peritoneal dwell (Seames, Moncrief, and Popovich 1990). However, their attempt was later disproved by animal experiments (Flessner et al. 2003; Flessner 1994). Further investigations by Leypoldt and Henderson were focused on solute transport driven by diffusion and ultrafiltration from blood and interactions of the solute with the tissue (Leypoldt 1993; Leypoldt and Henderson 1992). A new attempt to apply a distributed approach to model impact of chronic peritoneal inflammation from sterile solutions and structural changes within the tissue on the solute and water transport was undertaken recently by Flessner et al. (Flessner et al. 2006).

The distributed model of fluid absorption was proposed by Stachowska-Pietka et al. and applied for the analysis changes in the tissue caused by infusion of isotonic solution into the peritoneal cavity (Stachowska-Pietka et al. 2005; Stachowska-Pietka et al. 2006). This model can be applied to describe situation at the end of a dwell with hypertonic solution, when the osmotic pressure decreases and the intraperitoneal hydrostatic pressure is the main transport force. The osmotically driven glucose transport was modelled by Cherniha, Waniewski and co-authors (Cherniha and Waniewski 2005; Waniewski et al. 2007; Waniewski, Stachowska-Pietka, and Flessner 2009). These authors where able to predict high ultrafiltration from blood to the peritoneal cavity and positive interstitial pressure profiles assuming a high value of reflection coefficient for glucose in the capillary wall and a low value of reflection coefficient for glucose in the tissue. Further extensions of this model were suggested (Stachowska-Pietka, Waniewski, and Lindholm 2010; Stachowska-Pietka 2010; Stachowska-Pietka and Waniewski 2011). In this new approach, the variability of dialysis fluid volume, hydrostatic pressure and solute concentrations with dwell time were additionally taken into account and yielded a good agreement of the theoretical description and clinical data. A distributed model that takes into account also the two phase structure of the tissue and allows for the modelling of bidirectional fluid and macromolecular transport during PD was recently formulated (Stachowska-Pietka, Waniewski, and Lindholm 2010; Stachowska-Pietka 2010).

2.1 Basic concepts

The distributed approach takes into account the spatial distribution of the peritoneal transport system (PTS) components. Typically, this concept includes the microcirculatory exchange vessels that are assumed to be uniformly distributed within the tissue. However, this simplifying assumption can in general be omitted and the variability of the tissue space and structure can be taken into account. In order to describe the distributed structure of PTS, the methods of partial differential equation (instead of ordinary differential equations) should be applied. As a result, the changes in the spatial distribution of solutes and fluid in the tissue with time can be modelled.

Peritoneal fluid and solute exchange concerns all the organs that surround peritoneal cavity. It is assumed that tissue is perfused with blood by capillaries, which are placed at different distance from the peritoneal surface (Figure 1).

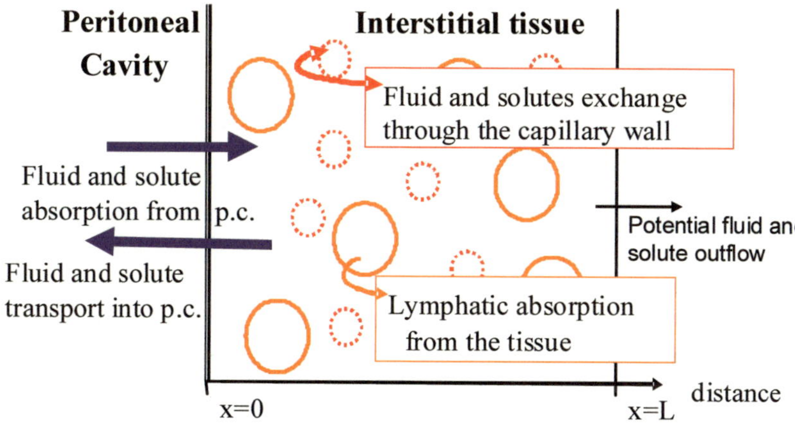

Fig. 1. Fluid and solute transport pathways during peritoneal dialysis: dashed, red circles - blood capillaries walls, solid, orange circles - lymphatic capillaries

Lymphatic absorption plays an important role in the process of regulation of fluid and solute transport within the tissue. The tissue properties, including the spatial distribution of blood and lymph capillaries, are idealized in the distributed modelling by the assumption that blood and lymph capillaries are uniformly distributed within the tissue and that the interstitium is a deformable, porous medium, see Figure 1 (Flessner 2001; Waniewski 2001). The difference in solute concentration between blood and dialysis fluid results in a quasi-continuous spatially variable concentration profile. Moreover, fluid infusion into the peritoneal cavity induces increase of interstitial hydrostatic pressure and results in fluid transport within the tissue. The tissue hydrostatic pressure equilibrates with the intraperitoneal hydrostatic pressure at the peritoneal surface, and decreases with the distance from the peritoneal cavity.

2.1.1 Structure of the peritoneal transport systems and its barriers

Once water and solutes leave the peritoneal cavity and enter the adjacent tissue they penetrate to its deeper parts, c.f. Figure 1. In the tissue, fluid and solute partly cross the heteroporous capillary wall and are washed out by the blood stream, whereas another part is absorbed from the tissue by local lymphatics. A part of the fluid and solute accumulates in the tissue. In some situations, fluid and solutes can leave the tissue on its other side, as in the case of the intestinal wall or in some experiments with the impermeable outer surface (skin) removed (Flessner 1994). Figure 1 summarizes the fluid and solute transport pathways.
Two main transport barriers for peritoneal fluid and solute transport are considered in the distributed approach. On the basis of experimental data it was found that: 1) the heteroporous structure of the capillary wall, and 2) interstitium, are significant barriers of the peritoneal transport system (Flessner 2005). The experimental studies showed that interstitium is the most important barrier for the transport of fluid and selected solutes across the tissue. In contrast, some authors considered also the mesothelium as a substantial transport barrier and modeled it as a semipermeable membrane with the properties analogous to the that of the endothelium (Seames, Moncrief, and Popovich 1990). They analyzed the transport of water, BUN, creatinine, glucose and inulin. They fitted the model to the data on intraperitoneal volume and solute concentrations in dialysate and blood and predicted negative values of interstitial hydrostatic pressure (Seames, Moncrief, and Popovich 1990). However, later studies disproved this assumption and found the positive interstitial pressure profiles in the tissue (Flessner et al. 2003).

2.1.2 Fluid and solute void volume

The fluid space within the interstitium can be described using the interstitial fluid void volume ratio, θ, that is defined as the fraction of the interstitial space that is available for interstitial fluid (non-dimensional, being the ratio of volume over volume). Typically, at physiological equilibrium, this value remains around 15% - 18%, and may be doubled during peritoneal dialysis (Zakaria, Lofthouse, and Flessner 2000, 1999). The fraction of solute interstitial void volume, θ_S, i.e., the fraction of tissue volume effectively available to the solute S, depends on the solute molecular size, and in the case of large macromolecules can be significantly smaller than that for fluid. Experimental studies showed that distribution of the solute macromolecules can be restricted to even 50% of θ (Wiig et al. 1992). Therefore, in general $\theta_S \leq \theta$.
The interstitial fluid void volume ratio as a function of interstitial hydrostatic pressure derived on the basis of experimental studies is presented in Figure 2, c.f. (Cherniha and Waniewski 2005; Stachowska-Pietka et al. 2005; Stachowska-Pietka et al. 2006).

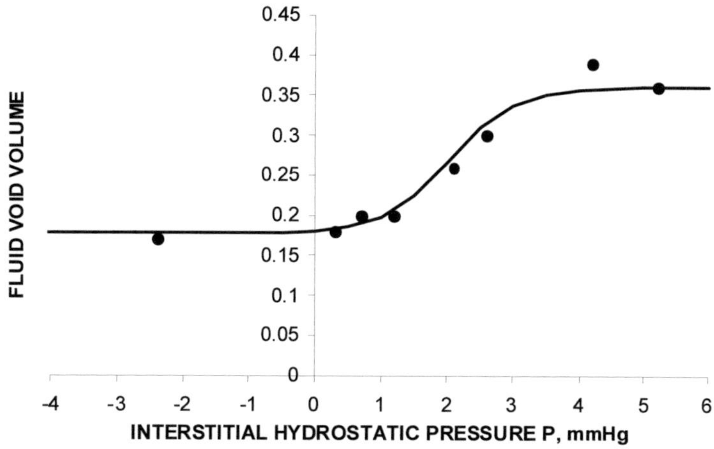

Fig. 2. The experimental data of interstitial fluid void volume ratio measured in the rat skeletal muscle and signed by solid circles (Zakaria, Lofthouse, and Flessner 1999) and the fitted interstitial fluid void volume ratio curve, θ, as a function of interstitial pressure, P.

This approach reflects the experimental findings showing that interstitial fluid void volume ratio may increase initially rapidly (for positive, low values of interstitial pressure), whereas there is no effect of further increasing of P if θ reaches its maximal value, θ_{MAX}. The interstitial fluid void volume, θ, can be mathematically described as (Stachowska-Pietka et al. 2006):

$$\theta = \theta_{MIN} + \frac{\theta_{MAX} - \theta_{MIN}}{1 + \left(\frac{\theta_{MAX} - \theta_{MIN}}{\theta_0 - \theta_{MIN}} - 1 \right) e^{-\beta(P - P_0)}} \tag{1}$$

where $\theta_{MIN} = 0.177$ and $\theta_{MAX} = 0.36$ are respectively minimal and maximal values of the fluid void volume, $\theta_0 = 0.18$ is the fluid void volume for $P = P_0 = 0$ mmHg, $\beta = 2.019$ mmHg^{-1}, and P_0 is the initial value of interstitial hydrostatic pressure measured in mmHg, see Figure 2. A particular case of this general formula was considered previously by An and Salathe (An and Salathe 1976). They were the first, who proposed the explicit formula for the fluid void volume as a function of interstitial pressure, assuming erroneously that $\theta_{MIN} = 0$ and $\theta_{MAX} = 1$.

2.2 Distributed model of fluid transport

The changes in the total tissue volume are considered to be small enough to assume the constant total tissue volume. Therefore, the whole tissue is considered as not expendable, whereas the interstitial compliance and changes in the tissue hydration are taken into account. Under this condition, the equation for the changes in the fraction of the interstitial fluid void volume ratio can be described using the volume balance of the interstitium as follows (Stachowska-Pietka et al. 2006; Stachowska-Pietka et al. 2005; Flessner 2001):

$$\frac{\partial \theta}{\partial t} = -\frac{\partial j_V}{\partial x} + q_V \tag{2}$$

where θ is the fraction of the interstitial fluid volume over the total tissue volume, further on called as the void volume, j_V is the volumetric fluid flux across the interstitium, q_V is the rate of the net fluid flow into the tissue from the internal sources (sinks) such as blood or lymphatic capillaries per unit tissue volume, t is the dwell time, and x is the distance measured from the peritoneal cavity. Note, that volumetric flux, j_V, is defined as volumetric flow (in ml/min) per unit surface (in cm^2) perpendicular to its direction, i.e., the unit of flux is cm/min. The unit of local volumetric flow density, q_V, is 1/min, i.e., as for volumetric flow (in ml/min) per unit volume (in mL). The orientations of specific fluid fluxes are presented in Figure 3.
Fluid flux across the interstitium depends on the local tissue hydraulic conductivity, K, and local interstitial hydrostatic pressure gradient, $\partial P / \partial x$. Moreover, the osmotic agent (crystalloid or colloid) may exert osmotic effect on the fluid. These effects can be taken into account by including the role of local tissue osmotic gradients into the model. In particular, the impact of the oncotic gradient exerted by proteins was previously included in the Darcy formula by Taylor et al. (Taylor, Bert, and Bowen 1990). Thus, the volumetric fluid flux across the interstitium may be calculated by the extended Darcy law as follows (Waniewski, Stachowska-Pietka, and Flessner 2009; Waniewski et al. 2007):

$$j_V = -K\left(\frac{\partial P}{\partial x} - \sum_{S=1,\dots,N} \sigma_S{}^T \cdot RT \cdot \frac{\partial C_S}{\partial x}\right) \quad (3)$$

where $\sigma_S{}^T$ is the reflection coefficient (positive for osmotically active solutes in the tissue), C_S is the concentration of solute in the tissue, and solutes are indexed by S from 1 to N.

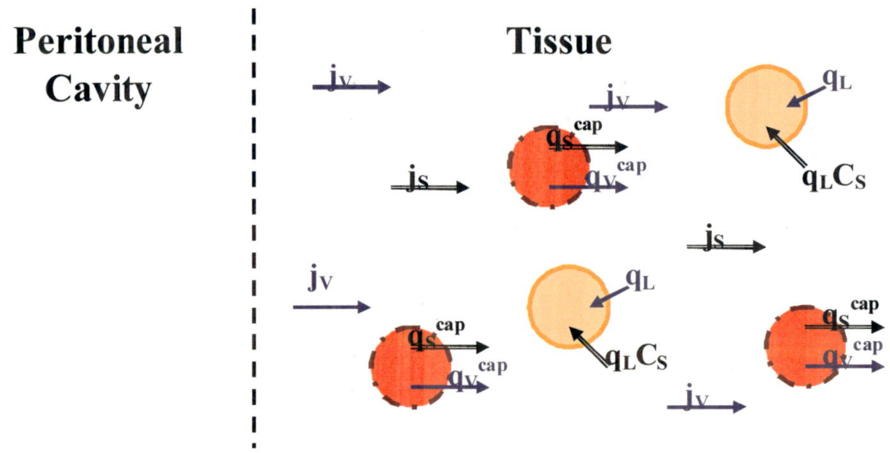

Fig. 3. Scheme of fluid and solute transport and positive orientations of each flux as modelled by the distributed approach: dashed circles - blood capillaries walls, solid circles - lymphatic capillaries.

Fluid flow between tissue and circulatory system, $q_V{}^{cap}$, can occur through the capillary wall in both directions: into and from the tissue. In addition, the final net inflow of fluid to the tissue is typically smaller due to the local tissue lymphatic absorption. Therefore, the net fluid inflow into the tissue is given as:

$$q_V = q_V^{cap} - q_L \tag{4}$$

where q_V^{cap} is the net fluid flow through the capillary wall into the tissue, and q_L is the rate of lymphatic absorption in the tissue. For the calculation of the fluid flow across capillary wall, the three-pore model or the membrane model can be applied. According to both approaches, the fluid flow across the capillary wall, q_V^{cap}, is driven by the hydrostatic (first term) and osmotic pressure (second term) differences that are exerted through the capillary wall. In particular, if the membrane model is applied for the microvascular exchange of fluid, net fluid flow across the capillary wall to the tissue can be calculated as (Stachowska-Pietka et al. 2006; Waniewski, Stachowska-Pietka, and Flessner 2009):

$$q_V^{cap} = L_P a(P_B - P) - L_P a \sum_{S=1,\dots,N} \sigma_S^{cap} \cdot RT \cdot (C_{B,S} - C_S) \tag{5}$$

where P_B and $C_{B,S}$ are the hydrostatic pressure and solute concentration in the blood, respectively, P and C_S are interstitial hydrostatic pressure and solute concentration in the tissue, respectively, $L_P a$ and σ_S^{cap} are the capillary wall hydraulic conductance and reflection coefficient of the capillary wall, respectively. If the three-pore model for the microvascular exchange across capillary wall is applied, the fluid transport through each type of pore should be calculated separately, and summed up.
Equation (1) specifies the interstitial fluid void volume, θ, as a function of interstitial pressure, P. Therefore, the rate of change of θ can be transformed as $\frac{\partial \theta}{\partial t} = \frac{d\theta}{dP} \cdot \frac{\partial P}{\partial t}$ and equation (2) for time evolution of variable θ can be converted to the following equation for the time evolution of variable P (Stachowska-Pietka et al. 2006):

$$\frac{d\theta}{dP} \cdot \frac{\partial P}{\partial t} = -\frac{\partial}{\partial x} j_V + q_V \tag{6}$$

In order to find theoretical solution, these equations must be combined with equations for the transport of solutes. In general, the transport parameters in equations (2) - (5), such as K, q_L, $L_P a$, σ_S^T, σ_S^{cap} can be assumed constant for some approximate considerations (Waniewski 2001; Flessner 2001). However, physiological data suggest that in more realistic modelling, the relationship between the parameters and the tissue properties should be taken into account. In particular, the dependence of tissue hydration, hydraulic conductivity, or lymphatic absorption on the interstitial hydrostatic pressure as well as the vasodilation induced by hyperosmotic dialysis fluid should be considered. Therefore, in numerical simulations of distributed models, some of the transport parameters (such as K, q_L, $L_P a$) are typically functions of model variables (solute concentration in the tissue, C_S, interstitial hydrostatic pressure, P, and also indirectly of interstitial fluid void volume ratio, θ) and dwell time, t. The specific forms of these functions can be found elsewhere (Stachowska-Pietka et al. 2006; Waniewski, Stachowska-Pietka, and Flessner 2009; Stachowska-Pietka 2010). Initial and boundary conditions for this problem are well define and were previously discussed in details (Stachowska-Pietka et al. 2006; Stachowska-Pietka 2010; Stachowska-Pietka et al. 2005).

2.3 Distributed model of solute transport

The solute concentration profiles within the tissue can be derived from the equation on the local solute mass balance using a partial differential equation for local solute balance as (Stachowska-Pietka et al. 2007; Waniewski 2002; Waniewski, Stachowska-Pietka, and Flessner 2009; Flessner 2001):

$$\frac{\partial(\theta_S \cdot C_S)}{\partial t} = -\frac{\partial j_S}{\partial x} + q_S \tag{7}$$

where θ_S is the fraction of interstitial fluid void volume ratio, θ, available for the distribution of solute S, C_S is the solute concentration in the interstitial fluid, j_S is the solute flux across the tissue, q_S is the rate of the net solute inflow to the tissue from the external sources/sinks, such as blood or lymph, x is the distance measured from the peritoneal surface, and t is time. The solute flux across the tissue, j_S, is defined as the solute flow (in mmol/min) per unit surface (in cm^2) perpendicular to its direction, i.e., the unit of flux is mmol/min/cm^2. The unit of local solute flow density, q_S, is mmol/min/mL, i.e., as for solute flow (in mmol/min) per unit volume (in mL). The orientations of solute fluxes are presented in Figure 3.

Solute flux across the tissue comprises two components. The diffusive transport of solute depends on the local concentration gradient, whereas fluid flux across the tissue induces its convective transport. Therefore, the solute flux across the tissue can be calculated as follows (Stachowska-Pietka et al. 2007; Waniewski 2002; Waniewski, Stachowska-Pietka, and Flessner 2009; Flessner 2001):

$$j_S = -D_S{}^T \frac{\partial C_S}{\partial x} + s_S{}^T \cdot j_V \cdot C_S \tag{8}$$

where $D_S{}^T$ is the diffusivity of solute S in the tissue, $s_S{}^T$ is sieving coefficient of solute in the tissue, and j_V is the volumetric fluid flux across the tissue. Note, that for homogenous structure $\sigma_S{}^T = 1 - s_S{}^T$ is the tissue reflection coefficient of solute S.

The net changes in the solute amount in the tissue are considered to be caused by the local microvascular exchange between blood and tissue through the capillary wall, decreased by the solute absorption from the tissue by local lymphatics:

$$q_S = q_S{}^{cap} - q_L \cdot C_S \tag{9}$$

where $q_S{}^{cap}$ in the net solute flux across the capillary wall into the tissue, and q_L is the rate of local lymphatic absorption. Depending on the purpose of the study, the solute transport between blood and tissue can be calculated according to the three-pore model or the membrane model. In general, solute flux across the capillary wall is driven by the solute concentration difference between blood and tissue, $C_{B,S} - C_S$, and by the convective fluid flow across the capillary wall, $q_V{}^{cap}$. In particular, if the membrane model is applied for the microvascular exchange, the solute net flux across the capillary wall to the tissue can be calculated as (Waniewski et al. 2007; Waniewski, Stachowska-Pietka, and Flessner 2009):

$$q_S{}^{cap} = p_S a\left(C_{B,S} - C_S\right) + s_S{}^{cap} \cdot q_V{}^{cap} \cdot \left[f C_{B,S} + (1-f) \cdot C_S\right] \tag{10}$$

where $p_S a$ is the diffusive permeability of solute S through the capillary wall, s_S^{cap} is sieving coefficient for solute in the capillary wall, and f is the weighting factor within the range from 0 to 1, which in general can be calculated from the fluid flow across the capillary wall according to the formula for Peclet number. Note, that $\sigma_S^{cap} = 1 - s_S^{cap}$ is the capillary wall reflection coefficient for solute S. In the case of a three-pore model for the microvascular exchange across the capillary wall it can be described as the sum of solute fluxes through each type of the pore.

Equation (7) together with equations (8) - (10) for j_S and q_S may be analyzed theoretically for constant values of θ_S, constant transport parameters such as D_S^T, s_S^T, $p_S a$, s_S^{cap}, and for given fluid transport characteristics j_V and q_V^{cap}. However, in the general case, equation (7) must be coupled with equation (6) for time evolution of P, in order to calculate θ and then θ_S. Furthermore, the dynamic changes in the transport parameters, caused by the changes in tissue hydration and vasodilation of the capillary bed, make D_S^T and $p_S a$ functions of P (or θ), C_S and dwell time, t. The specific forms of these functions can be found elsewhere (Stachowska-Pietka 2010; Stachowska-Pietka et al. 2006; Waniewski, Stachowska-Pietka, and Flessner 2009). The details concerning initial and boundary conditions for solute and fluid peritoneal transport can be found elsewhere (Stachowska-Pietka and Waniewski 2011; Stachowska-Pietka 2010; Waniewski, Stachowska-Pietka, and Flessner 2009, Waniewski 2001, 2002).

3. Modelling of fluid transport

The purpose of this section is to present relationships between the net fluid transport parameters for the transport between blood and dialysis fluid in the peritoneal cavity (as estimated using phenomenological models of peritoneal dialysis in clinical and experimental studies), and the separate characteristics of the capillary wall and interstitial transport barriers as well as the distributed geometry of peritoneal transport system (PTS). Two simplified versions of the distributed model for fluid peritoneal transport are analysed assuming steady state conditions. The effective permeability of the tissue is analysed for the simplified model in which fluid transport is driven by hydrostatic pressure difference, causing fluid absorption. In order to present osmotic properties of PTS, the distributed model of osmotic fluid flow is presented, in which water absorption from the peritoneal cavity is neglected.

In order to evaluate effective transport parameters from the distributed model, which can be compare with the experimental values, one should refer to the net fluid flow instead of fluid flux. In general, the net fluid flow can be calculated from the fluid flux by multiplying by the effective peritoneal surface area A in cm². Therefore $J_V = A \cdot j_V$ is the fluid flow described in mL/min, and $A \approx 6000$ cm². More details concerning results presented in this section can be found in (Waniewski, Stachowska-Pietka, and Flessner 2009).

3.1 Effective hydraulic conductivity

A simple version of the distributed model with fluid flow induced only by hydrostatic pressure may be applied for the derivation of the description of the flux across the tissue peritoneal surface, $j_V\left(t_{steady}, x = 0\right) = j_V^{perit}$, and the effective hydraulic conductivity for fluid at time t_{steady}, when the system reaches its steady-state. Therefore, equation (3) for fluid transport across tissue can be simplified to the from $j_V = -K\frac{\partial P}{\partial x}$, whereas fluid transport across capillary wall is given by $q_V^{cap} = L_P a(P_B - P)$. In this case, the fluid flow across the peritoneal surface (i.e. fluid flux multiplied by effective peritoneal surface area) depends on the hydrostatic pressure difference between peritoneal cavity and the tissue and can be described by the following formula (Waniewski, Stachowska-Pietka, and Flessner 2009):

$$J_V^{perit} = memL_P a\left(P_D - P^{eq}\right) \tag{11}$$

where P_D and P^{eq} are hydrostatic pressures in the peritoneal cavity and tissue, respectively, and $memL_P a$ is the effective hydraulic conductivity for transport between blood and dialysate that is calculated as:

$$memL_P a = A \cdot \tanh(\varphi)\sqrt{K \cdot L_P a} \tag{12}$$

with $\varphi = L / \Lambda_F$, L - tissue width, and $\Lambda_F = \sqrt{K / L_P a}$ - fluid penetration depth in the tissue, K - tissue hydraulic conductivity, $L_P a$ - hydraulic conductance of capillary wall, A - effective peritoneal surface area. Furthermore, assuming that tissue width is much higher than the fluid penetration depth, $\Lambda_F << L$, i.e. $\varphi >> 1$, one can get the following, simplified formula for the effective hydraulic conductivity for transport between blood and dialysate:

$$memL_P a = A\sqrt{K \cdot L_P a} \tag{13}$$

Some exemplary values of fluid penetration depth, effective hydraulic conductivity of PTS and the corresponding values of tissue and capillary wall transport are presented in Table 1.

Remark 1. Formula (13) can be transformed to $memL_P a = A \cdot L_P a \cdot \Lambda_F$, which means that the fluid transport may be considered, according to the distributed model, as proceeding directly between blood and dialysis fluid across the total capillary wall surface within the tissue layer of the width Λ_F with hydraulic conductance $L_p a$, as this capillary would be immersed directly in dialysis fluid (Waniewski, Stachowska-Pietka, and Flessner 2009).

Remark 2. Formula (13) can be alternatively transformed to $memL_P a = A \cdot K / \Lambda_F$ indicating that the same fluid transport may be considered also as proceeding between blood and dialysis fluid across the tissue layer with hydraulic conductivity K and width Λ_F (which is fluid penetration depth) without any interference from blood flow in the capillaries; however, Λ_F depends on $L_p a$ (Waniewski, Stachowska-Pietka, and Flessner 2009).

Remark 3. The maximal possible value of $memL_P a$ is $A \cdot L_P a \cdot L$, which would happen if the fluid penetrated fully the whole tissue layer, and in this case the effective hydraulic conductivity of distributed system would be equal to the total hydraulic conductance for the whole capillary bed in the tissue (Waniewski, Stachowska-Pietka, and Flessner 2009).

Parameter	Range of values
Assumed/adjusted:	
$K\,10^4$, cm²min⁻¹mmHg⁻¹	0.139
$L_p a\,10^4$, ml·min⁻¹mmHg⁻¹g⁻¹	1.48 - 3.66
Derived:	
Λ_F, cm	0.19 - 0.31
$memL_p a$, ml·min⁻¹mmHg⁻¹	0.27 - 0.43

Table 1. Theoretical values of transport parameters assumed in computer simulations and the corresponding values of effective transport parameters of PTS estimated for A = 6000 cm²: K – tissue hydraulic conductivity, $L_p a$ - capillary wall hydraulic conductance, A – effective peritoneal surface area, Λ_F - fluid penetration depth, $memL_p a$ - effective hydraulic conductivity of PTS (Waniewski, Stachowska-Pietka, and Flessner 2009).

3.2 Effective reflection coefficient and osmotic conductance

In this section a model with a single osmotic agent that induces osmotic fluid flow between blood and the peritoneal cavity is discussed. The hydrostatic pressure gradient in the tissue also contributes to the fluid flow, but the hydrostatic pressure difference across the capillary wall is neglected by assuming, for example, that it is approximately balanced by oncotic pressure difference. This approximation may be used only for the description of osmotic ultrafiltration induced by a high concentration of a crystalloid osmotic agent. Therefore, in the case of a single osmotic agent (as glucose), equation (3) for fluid flux across the tissue is $j_V = -K\left(\frac{\partial P}{\partial x} - \sigma^T \frac{\partial C}{\partial x}\right)$, and equation (5) is $q_V{}^{cap} = L_p a \cdot \sigma^{cap} RT(C_B - C)$. Note, that for the sake of simplicity, in the case of single solute, the bottom index S for solute can be omitted. If the solute (e.g., glucose) concentration profile in the tissue may be approximately described by the exponential function with the solute penetration depth Λ, i.e. as $C = C_B + (C_D - C_B)\exp(-x/\Lambda)$, the steady state fluid flow across the peritoneal surface can approximated by the following formula (Waniewski, Stachowska-Pietka, and Flessner 2009):

$$J_V{}^{perit} = -memL_p a \cdot \sigma^{eff} \cdot RT\left(C_D - C^{eq}\right) \tag{14}$$

where $memL_p a$ is the effective hydraulic conductivity of the peritoneal transport system, C_D and C^{eq} are solute concentrations in dialysate and tissue, respectively, and σ^{eff} is the effective reflection coefficient for solute transport between peritoneal cavity and blood given by (Waniewski, Stachowska-Pietka, and Flessner 2009):

$$\sigma^{eff} = \frac{\sigma^{cap}}{\alpha}\left(1 - e^{-L/\Lambda}\right) \tag{15}$$

where $\alpha = \Lambda_F / \Lambda$ is the ratio of fluid to solute penetration depth, σ^{cap} is the capillary wall reflection coefficient to solute S. Moreover, assuming that the tissue width is much higher than the solute penetration depth, i.e. $L >> \Lambda$, one can get the following simplified formula for the effective reflection coefficient of PTS (Waniewski, Stachowska-Pietka, and Flessner 2009):

$$\sigma^{eff} = \frac{\sigma^{cap}}{\alpha} \qquad (16)$$

Remark 1. The value of the effective reflection coefficient for particular solute transport between peritoneal cavity and blood, σ^{eff}, can not exceed the value of the capillary wall reflection coefficient for this solute, σ^{cap}, i.e. $\sigma^{eff} \le \sigma^{cap}$.
Remark 2. The effective reflection coefficient can be calculated from the capillary wall reflection coefficient, after dividing by the ratio of fluid to solute penetration depth. Moreover, if necessary, this value should be additionally decreased by the formula $\left(1-e^{-L/\Lambda}\right)$. As the result, the distributed geometry of the capillary bed yields a substantial decrease in the effective reflection coefficient for crystalloid osmotic agents compared with their reflection coefficient in the capillary wall. Numerical simulations suggest 7-20 times lower values of σ^{eff} if compared to σ^{cap} (see, Table 2 and (Waniewski, Stachowska-Pietka, and Flessner 2009)).
Remark 3. The effective reflection coefficient for the transport between peritoneal cavity and blood depends not only on the sieving properties of the capillary wall, but is also related to the tissue transport properties, since both fluid and solute penetration depths depends on the local tissue and capillary wall permeabilities.
Remark 4. The effective osmotic conductance for the transport between peritoneal cavity and blood depends on both tissue and capillary wall transport characteristics and can be calculated as the effective hydraulic conductivity described by equation (13), multiplied by the effective reflection coefficient, described by equation (15), c.f. equation (14) (Waniewski, Stachowska-Pietka, and Flessner 2009):

$$memOsmCond = \sigma^{eff} memL_p a \qquad (17)$$

In Table 2, some typical values of effective reflection coefficient and osmotic conductance of PTS are derived for glucose in the case of clinical dialysis.

Parameter	Range of values
Assumed/adjusted:	
σ^{cap}	0.16 - 0.46
Derived:	
Λ, cm	0.015 - 0.017
α	11.40 - 20.86
σ^{eff}	0.014 - 0.022
memOsmCond, (ml/min)/(mmol/l)	0.116

Table 2. Theoretical values of glucose transport parameters assumed in computer simulations and the corresponding values of effective transport parameters of PTS (Waniewski, Stachowska-Pietka, and Flessner 2009): σ^{cap} - capillary wall reflection coefficient, Λ - solute penetration depth, α - ratio of fluid to solute penetration depth, σ^{eff} - effective reflection coefficient of PTS, *memOsmCond* – effective osmotic conductance of PTS.

4. Modelling of solute transport

During peritoneal dialysis solutes, such as osmotic agents, buffer solutes, additives and drugs, are transported from dialysis fluid to the tissue, and inside the tissue are absorbed to blood and lymph. On the other hand, solutes, which are to be removed with peritoneal dialysis, are transported first from blood to the tissue and there they are partly absorbed with lymph and partly transported to dialysis fluid. The contribution of blood and lymph flows to the solute gradient, created within the tissue due to the presence of dialysis fluid at the tissue surface, results in characteristic solute concentration profiles within the tissue. For some solutes, diffusive transport prevails (as for small molecules), but the role of convective transport through the capillary wall and (convective) absorption with lymph increases with the increased molecular weight. In particular, in the case of macromolecules, both types of convective transport should be considered.

Therefore, for small molecules such as urea, creatinine, the simplified version of the distributed model with pure diffusive transport can be considered. In this case, simple relationships between net solute transport characteristics such as effective diffusivity across PTS, solute penetration depth and effective blood flow, and corresponding local distributed parameters are presented. The impact of combined diffusive and convective transport on derived effective characteristics is analysed in Section 4.2. In particular, the comparison between diffusive and convective penetration depth, as well as the analysis of effective sieving coefficient for macromolecules is analysed.

Note, that all results presented in this section were derived for the steady state conditions. Moreover, to compare the effective solute transport parameters with the experimental one, the solute flux from the peritoneal cavity is multiplied by the effective peritoneal surface area, A. This transforms the equation for solute flux, j_S, into the equation for solute flow, $J_S = A \cdot j_S$, expressed in mmol/min. More details concerning models and the derivation of the expressions for effective transport parameters can be found in (Waniewski 2002, 2001). The bottom index S, which denotes solute, was omitted in this section for the sake of simplicity.

4.1 Diffusive solute transport between blood and the peritoneal cavity

In this section the relationships between the net diffusive mass transport coefficients for the solute transport between blood and dialysis fluid and the local physiology based transport parameters of distributed models are analyzed. Moreover, the formulas for the solute diffusive penetration depth and effective peritoneal blood flow are derived. Therefore, a simplified model of pure diffusive transport across the tissue is analysed at the steady state with the solute flux across the tissue given by $j_S = -D^T \frac{\partial C}{\partial x}$ and solute transport across capillary wall described by equation (10). Note, that equation (10) can be grouped in the following way: $q_S{}^{cap} = k^{cap} C_B - k^T C$, where $k^{cap} = p_S a + s^{cap} q_V{}^{cap} f$ is a unidirectional clearance for transport between blood and tissue, and $k^T = p_S a + s^{cap} q_V{}^{cap}(1-f)$ is a unidirectional clearance for transport from tissue to blood (Waniewski 2002).

4.1.1 Effective diffusive mass transport parameter

At the steady state, the solute flow from the peritoneal cavity to the tissue can be presented in analogy to the membrane models in the following way (Waniewski 2002):

$$J_S{}^{perit} = memKBD_S (C_D - \kappa C_B) \tag{18}$$

where C_D and C_B are solute concentrations in dialysate and blood, respectively, $memKBD_S$ is the effective diffusive mass transport parameter for solute *S*, and κ describes the ratio of the equilibrium concentration of solute in the tissue over its concentration in blood and can be calculated as $\kappa = k^{cap} / \left(k^T + q_L\right)$. In this case, the effective diffusive mass transport parameter for solute *S* can be approximated from the formula (Waniewski 2002, 2001):

$$memKBD_S = A\sqrt{D^T\left(k^T + q_L\right)} \tag{19}$$

Theoretical values of effective diffusive mass transport parameter derived from the distributed model compared with the experimental values are presented in Figure 4 and in Tables 3 and 4.

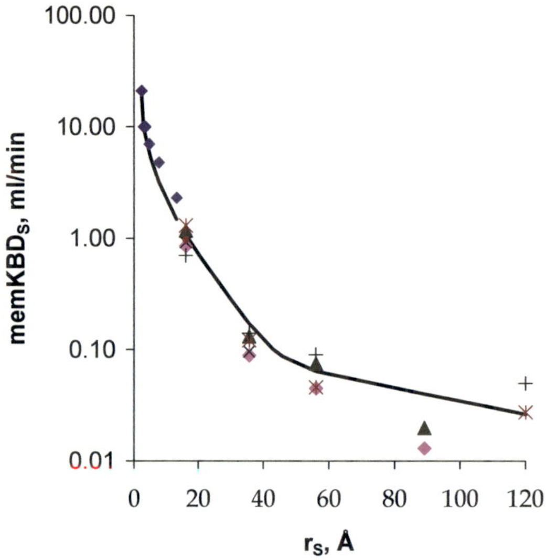

Fig. 4. Theoretical values of effective diffusive mass transport parameter derived from the distributed model (solid line, assuming A=1 m²) and the experimental values: * (Rippe and Stelin 1989), + (Kagan et al. 1990), ▲ (Imholz et al. 1993), ♦ (Pannekeet et al. 1995), after (Waniewski 2001).

Remark 1. If one neglects convective transport across the capillary wall and the tissue lymphatic absorption, the effective diffusive mass transport parameter for solute *S* can be calculated from a simplified formula (Dedrick et al. 1982):

$$memKBD_S = A\sqrt{D^T \cdot p_S a} \tag{20}$$

Remark 2. The important difference between equations (18) and the corresponding equation for diffusive solute transport according to the phenomenological membrane approach is the presence of coefficient κ in equation (18). Therefore, according to the distributed model (equation (18)), the equilibration level for a solute in dialysate is not its concentration in blood, C_B, as it is in the membrane model, but its equilibrium concentration in the tissue $C^{eq} = \kappa C_B$. In typical physiological conditions of the transport through the capillary wall, κ

is close to 1 for small and middle molecules, but substantially lower than 1 for macromolecules (Waniewski 2002, 2001). Therefore, the correction for κ is practically important only for macromolecules. In this case, the membrane model may underestimate the effective diffusive mass transport parameter. In fact, the equilibrium level for total protein five times lower than blood concentration was observed in experiments in dogs with prolonged accumulation of the lost protein in dialysate (Rubin et al. 1985). The typical values of κ for proteins are presented in Table 3.

Solute	MW	Λ_{Dif}, mm	κ	$memKBD_S$, ml/min
β_2-microglobulin	11 800	0.385	0.986	1.091
myoglobin	17 000	0.465	0.961	0.704
α-globulin	45 000	0.652	0.811	0.348
albumin	68 000	0.731	0.656	0.262
transferin	90 000	0.746	0.475	0.212
haptoglobin	100 000	0.732	0.430	0.202
IgG	150 000	0.667	0.351	0.182
α_2-macroglobin	820 000	0.529	0.277	0.144
IgM	900 000	0.456	0.212	0.124

Table 3. Solute diffusive penetration depth, Λ_{Dif}, the ratio of the equilibrium concentration of solute in the tissue over its concentration in blood, κ, and effective diffusive transport parameter, $memKBD_S$, estimated from the distributed model assuming A=1 m^2 (Waniewski 2002).

4.1.2 Diffusive solute penetration depth

The solute concentration distribution within the tissue (assuming only diffusive transport across the tissue) is described in the steady state by the following equation:

$$\frac{\partial^2 C}{\partial x^2} = \left(C^{eq} - \kappa C_B\right) / \Lambda_{Dif}^2 \tag{21}$$

where C^{eq} is the solute concentration in the tissue at equilibrium, and Λ_{Dif} is diffusive penetration depth given by (Waniewski 2001):

$$\Lambda_{Dif} = \sqrt{D^T / \left(k^T + q_L\right)} \tag{22}$$

where D^T is tissue diffusivity, k^T is unidirectional clearance for transport from tissue to blood, and q_L is tissue lymphatic absorption. The penetration depth for solutes with different molecular weight is presented in Tables 3 and 4.

Remark 1. In the case of purely diffusive transport across the capillary wall and the tissue, and neglected lymphatic absorption from the tissue, one can get a simplified formula $\Lambda_{Dif} = \sqrt{D^T / p_S a}$ (Dedrick et al. 1982), which shows that purely diffusive penetration depth for solutes depends on the square root of their diffusivity in the tissue divided by their diffusivity across capillary wall.

Remark 2. The diffusive solute penetration depth depends not only on the diffusive properties of both transport barriers. The additional correction for the lymphatic absorption from the tissue, q_L, fluid transport across the capillary wall, $q_V{}^{cap}$, and sieving properties of the capillary wall, s^{cap}, should be additionally taken into account resulting in further decrease of the solute penetration depth.

Remark 3. Formula (19) can be transformed to $memKBD_S = A\left(k^T + q_L\right)\cdot\Lambda_1$, which means that the effective diffusive mass transport parameter for solute transport may be considered, according to the distributed model, as proceeding directly between blood and dialysis fluid across the total capillary wall surface within the tissue layer of the width $\Lambda_1 = \Lambda_{Dif}\tanh\left(L/\Lambda_{Dif}\right)$ (where L is tissue width) with the transport parameter equal to $k^T + q_L$, and these capillaries can be considered as immersed directly in dialysis fluid (Waniewski 2002; Waniewski, Werynski, and Lindholm 1999). For small solutes, $k^T + q_L$ is approximately equal to $p_S a$ (Waniewski, Werynski, and Lindholm 1999).

Remark 4. Formula (19) can be alternatively transformed to $memKBD_S = A\cdot D^T/\Lambda_2$ indicating that the same solute transport may be considered also as proceeding between blood and dialysis fluid across the tissue layer with solute tissue diffusivity D^T and width $\Lambda_2 = \Lambda_{Dif}/\tanh\left(L/\Lambda_{Dif}\right)$ without any interference from blood flow in the capillaries (Waniewski 2002; Waniewski, Werynski, and Lindholm 1999).

Remark 5. Note, that for $L >> \Lambda_{Dif}$, $\Lambda_1 \approx \Lambda_2 \approx \Lambda_{Dif}$.

4.1.3 Effective peritoneal blood flow

In the context of peritoneal dialysis it is usually assumed that only a relatively thin layer of the tissue that is adjacent to the peritoneal surface participates effectively in the exchange of solutes between dialysate and blood. The rate of blood flow in this layer is called the effective peritoneal blood flow (EPBF). Some investigators attempted to evaluate EPBF using quickly diffusing gases, others considered the gas clearances as an overestimation of EPBF and pointed out the possibility of much lower values for EPBF as well as different EPBF values for solutes of different transport characteristics (Nolph and Twardowski 1989).

The effective peritoneal blood flow, EPBF, can be defined according to the distributed model as the blood flow in a tissue layer of the depth equal to the solute penetration depth, that is (Waniewski, Werynski, and Lindholm 1999):

$$EPBF = A\cdot q_B\cdot\Lambda_{Dif} \tag{23}$$

where A is effective peritoneal surface area, q_B is perfusion rate (in ml/min/g), and Λ_{Dif} is solute diffusive penetration depth. An alternative approach to the definition of EPBF can be found in (Waniewski, Werynski, and Lindholm 1999; Waniewski 2002).

4.2 Combined diffusive and convective solute transport

In this section the relationships between the net diffusive mass transport coefficients for the solute transport between blood and dialysis fluid and the local physiology based transport parameters of distributed models are analyzed for combine diffusive and convective solute

transport. Inclusion of convective solute transport across the tissue is especially important in the case of macromolecules. In this section, the impact of the convective flow on the solute penetration depth as well on the effective reflection coefficient of peritoneal transport system is analyzed.
Remark 1. The effective peritoneal blood flow is different for different solutes, see Table 4.

Solute	Λ_{Dif}, mm	$memKBD_S$, ml/min	$EPBF$, ml/min
H_2	0.68	269.6	269.6
CO_2	0.39	154.6	154.6
Urea	0.18	19.8	52.7
Creatinine	0.18	14.7	53.8
Glucose	0.19	11.6	55.1
Sucrose	0.19	7.9	57.7
Vitamin B_{12}	0.21	4.1	63.4
Inulin	0.24	1.9	71.2

Table 4. Theoretical values of solute penetration depth, diffusive mass transport coefficient, and perfusion rate calculated according to the distributed model assuming perfusion rate $q_B = 0.3$ ml/min/g (Waniewski, Werynski, and Lindholm 1999).

In the commonly applied phenomenological membrane models, the solute flow from dialysate to blood is typically evaluated using the following equation (Waniewski 2006, 2001):

$$J_S = KBD_S(C_D - C_B) + SJ_V[(1-F)C_D + FC_B], \tag{24}$$

where KBD_S is membrane diffusive mass transport coefficient, S is membrane sieving coefficient, j_V is fluid flow between blood and dialysate, C_B and C_D are solute concentrations in blood and dialysate, respectively, and F is a weighing factor for the mean concentration (Waniewski 2001). In order to compare both approaches, one may derive fro distributed model the following expression for solute flow from the peritoneal cavity to the tissue at the steady state (Waniewski 2001):

$$J_S^{perit} = memKBD_S\left(C_D - \kappa C_B\right) + s^T J_V\left(\left(1-f\right)C_D + f\kappa C_B\right). \tag{25}$$

where $memKBD_S = \sqrt{D^T(k^T + q_L)}$ is the effective diffusive transport parameter (see previous section), $\kappa = k^{cap} / \left(k^T + q_L\right)$ describes the ratio of the equilibrium concentration of solute in the tissue over its concentration in blood (see previous section), $f = 0.5 - \alpha$, $\alpha = \sqrt{1 + Pe^2/4} - 1/Pe$, and $Pe = s^T J_V / memKBD_S$ (Waniewski 2001).

4.2.1 Effective sieving coefficient for macromolecules

The important difference between phenomenological versus distributed approach (equations (24) and (25)) is the presence of coefficient κ in equation (25). As it was discussed in previous section, this parameter is typically close to 1 for small and middle molecules, whereas its values remain substantially lower than 1 for macromolecules (c.f. Table 3). In consequence, the concentration of macromolecules in dialysate equilibrates with their concentration in the tissue equal to κC_B, instead of that in blood.

Equation (25) indicates relationship between effective sieving coefficient for macromolecules and fluid flow direction, which is not present in the membrane model. In general, the sieving coefficient may be measured directly if convective transport is prevailing, i.e. with very high fluid flow, or in isochratic conditions, i.e. during diffusive equilibrium at both sides of the membrane. If the measurement is done using solute concentration in blood as the reference, then the obtained value depends on the direction of fluid flow.

Remark 1. For $j_V^{perit} > 0$ (i.e. in the direction from peritoneal cavity to the tissue) and $Pe >> 1$ (i.e. with convective transport prevailing over diffusive one), then the measured value of sieving coefficient is equal to the sieving coefficient of solute in the tissue, s^T, whereas for fluid flux across the tissue in the opposite direction (i.e. $j_V^{perit} < 0$) and $Pe << -1$ this value is equal to κC.

4.2.2 Diffusive vs. convective penetration depth

Let us consider the combine diffusive and convective solute transport at the steady state. It can be shown that the solute penetration depth can be calculated in this case as (Waniewski 2001):

$$\Lambda = \frac{\Lambda_{Dif}{}^2}{\sqrt{\Lambda_{Dif}{}^2 + \Lambda_{Conv}{}^2 / 4} - \Lambda_{Dif} / 2} \tag{26}$$

where Λ_{Dif} is diffusive penetration depth, equation (22). The convective penetration depth for purely convective solute transport across the tissue, Λ_{Conv}, is defined as:

$$\Lambda_{Conv} = s^T j_V / \left(k^T + q_L\right) \tag{27}$$

The comparison between the overall penetration depth Λ, and its diffusive and convective components, Λ_{Dif} and Λ_{Conv}, calculated for $J_V^{perit} = 1$ ml/min is presented in Table 5. $J_V^{perit} = 1$ ml/min is a typical value for the rate of fluid absorption from the peritoneal cavity.

Remark 1. For small molecules with prevailing diffusive transport (i.e. $\left|\Lambda_{Conv} / \Lambda_{Dif}\right| << 1$) the overall solute formula for the penetration depth can be simplified to $\Lambda \approx \Lambda_{Dif} + \Lambda_{Conv} / 2$ (Waniewski 2001).

Remark 2. In the case of solutes that are transported mainly by convection $\Lambda \approx \Lambda_{Conv}$ (for $\Lambda_{Conv} / \Lambda_{Dif} >> 1$) or, if they cannot penetrate the tissue, $\Lambda \approx 0$ (for $\Lambda_{Conv} / \Lambda_{Dif} << -1$).

Remark 3. That penetration depth for small solutes (creatinine) is dominated by the process of diffusion, for middle molecules (inulin, β_2-microglobulin) both processes contribute to the depth of solute penetration, and for macromolecules (albumin, IgM) the convective transport prevails, see Table 5.

Solute	Λ_{Dif}, mm	Λ_{Conv}, mm	Λ, mm
Creatinine	0.25	0.03	0.26
Inulin	0.29	0.19	0.40
β_2-microglobulin	0.60	0.85	1.15
Albumin	0.71	2.63	2.81
IgM	0.44	3.40	3.46

Table 5. Penetration depth for different transport processes and for different solutes for $J_V^{perit} = 1$ ml/min (Waniewski 2001).

5. Kinetics of peritoneal dialysis

The phenomenological models of the peritoneal transport such as the three-pore model or the membrane model, describe the kinetic of solute and fluid in the peritoneal cavity (Stachowska-Pietka 2010; Waniewski 2006). Complementary to them, the distributed approach allows for modeling the changes in the tissue, such as space distribution of interstitial hydrostatic pressure, tissue hydration and solute concentration in the tissue (Flessner, Dedrick, and Schultz 1985; Stachowska-Pietka et al. 2006; Waniewski, Stachowska-Pietka, and Flessner 2009; Flessner 2001). However, due to the complexity of the peritoneal phenomena as well as its high nonlinearity, distributed models are solved numerically for most applications. For example, numerical simulations of a peritoneal distributed model can be performed for a single exchange with hypertonic glucose solution 3.86%, see Figure 5 (Stachowska-Pietka and Waniewski 2011). The infusion of hypertonic solution induces water inflow into adjacent tissue. In consequence, increase of interstitial hydrostatic pressure and tissue hydration (as assessed by fluid void volume) can be observed in the tissue layer close to the peritoneal cavity (about 2.5 mm from the peritoneal surface, Figure 5, left panel) during next minutes and hours whereas the hydration of deeper tissue layers remains unchanged. Glucose diffuses from the peritoneal cavity into the tissue causing increase of glucose concentration in a thin layer of the tissue close to the peritoneal cavity (less than 0.01 cm width), c.f. Figure 5, right panel.

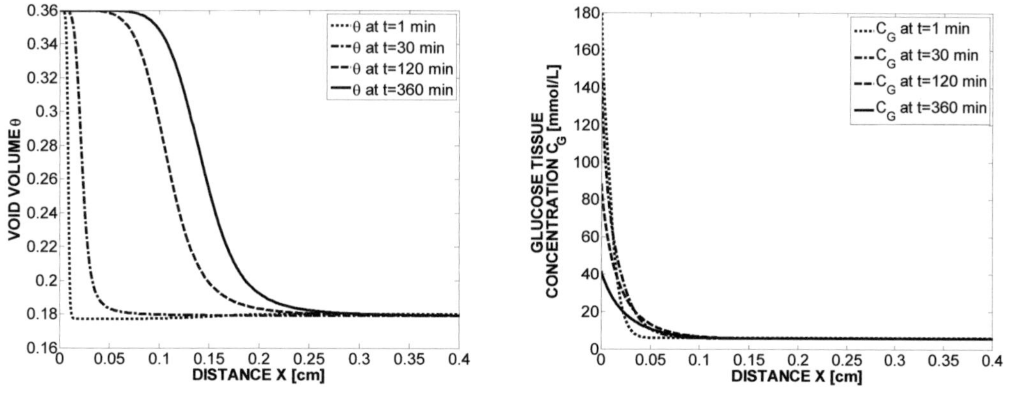

Fig. 5. Interstitial fluid void volume ratio, θ (left panel), and glucose concentration in interstitial fluid, C_G (right panel) at t=1, 60, 120, and 360 min. as a function of distance from the peritoneal cavity, X (Stachowska-Pietka and Waniewski 2011).

Concomitantly to the changes in the tissue hydration and solute concentration, the intraperitoneal fluid volume and glucose concentration change with dwell time, Figure 6 (Stachowska-Pietka and Waniewski 2011). The fluid absorption from the peritoneal cavity and ultrafiltration to the cavity results in the changes of intraperitoneal volume, as observed in clinical studies (Figure 6, left panel). Moreover, due to glucose diffusion into adjacent tissue, its intraperitoneal concentration decreases during the dwell time (Figure 6, right panel). Other results on the kinetics of dialysis according to distributed approach can be found elsewhere (Seames, Moncrief, and Popovich 1990; Flessner, Dedrick, and Schultz 1985, 1984; Flessner 2001; Stachowska-Pietka 2010; Stachowska-Pietka et al. 2005; Stachowska-Pietka, Waniewski, and Lindholm 2010, 2010).

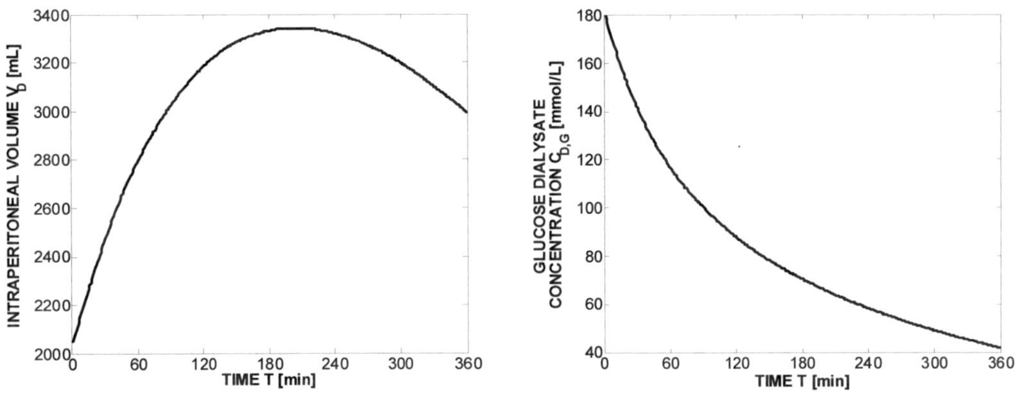

Fig. 6. Intraperitoneal volume, V_D, (left panel), and glucose concentration in dialysis fluid, C_D, (right panel) as function of dwell time T (Stachowska-Pietka and Waniewski 2011).

6. Conclusions

Distributed modeling allows for a detailed description of the peritoneal transport system with its real geometry and different characteristics for the main transport barriers of the capillary wall and the tissue (for most solutes of interest: the interstitium). Lymphatic absorption from the tissue, so important for the protein turnover, can also be taken into account. The models are based on the macroscopic approach with continuous distribution of the capillary and lymphatic vessels in the tissue instead of the real discrete system of these vessels. However, they can adequately describe the available data about solute concentrations and hydrostatic pressure inside the tissue during experimental studies on peritoneal dialysis (Stachowska-Pietka et al. 2006; Waniewski, Stachowska-Pietka, and Flessner 2009; Flessner 2001).

The distributed approach yields important relationships between the measurable transport parameters that are defined by the membrane models, as the diffusive mass transport parameter, hydraulic conductivity, sieving coefficient, etc., for the description of the net transport between blood and dialysis fluid in the peritoneal cavity, and the fundamental parameters for the description of the transport across the capillary wall, the tissue and lymphatic absorption from the tissue, see Figure 7. These basic local transport parameters are subject to interpatient variability and they can change with time on dialysis that may result in serious complications in the treatment. Unfortunately, these local transport characteristics cannot be directly measured in clinical setting and one has to derive their values using mathematical models and the information from animal studies. Some of the basic questions about peritoneal transport, as the width of the tissue layer involved in the exchange of fluid and solutes during peritoneal dialysis and rate of the blood flow that participates in this exchange can be correctly answered only if the local transport coefficients are known. The formulas for the effective transport parameters, penetration depth, effective blood flow, etc., are derived from the model for the steady state transport assuming spatial homogeneity of the transport system, and therefore their application for the real dialysis may be limited for some solutes and dialysis conditions.

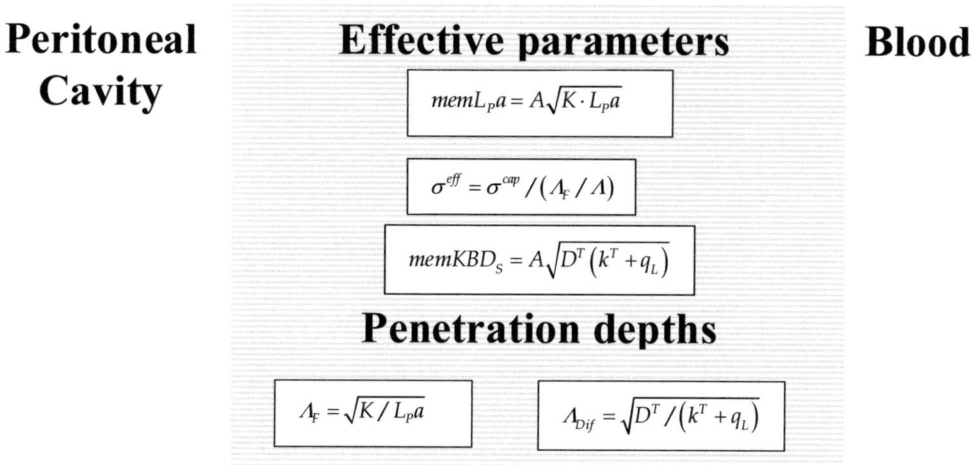

Fig. 7. Simple relationships between the effective peritoneal transport parameters and penetration depths and the local tissue and capillary wall transport parameters: $memL_pa$ - effective hydraulic conductivity, A – effective peritoneal surface area, K – tissue hydraulic conductivity, L_pa - capillary wall hydraulic conductance, σ^{eff} - effective reflection coefficient, σ^{cap} - capillary wall reflection coefficient. Λ_F - fluid penetration depth, Λ - solute penetration depth, $memKBD_S$ - effective diffusive transport parameters, D^T - solute diffusivity in the tissue, k^T - a unidirectional clearance for transport from tissue to blood, q_L - tissue lymphatic absorption.

Any realistic description of peritoneal dialysis must take into account that the conditions in the peritoneal cavity and in the tissue continuously change with dwell time due to, for example, vasodilatation induced by hyperosmolality of dialysis fluid and overhydration of the tissue induced by increased hydrostatic pressure in the peritoneal cavity. Therefore, computer modeling is necessary for such a theory as shown in Section 5, see also (Stachowska-Pietka 2010).

The distributed modeling can be applied for many problems of clinical and experimental interest, and further extensions are possible. For example, the contribution of a cellular compartment in the tissue to the transport of small ions (sodium, potassium) should be taken into account (Coester et al. 2007), and a more detailed structure of the interstitium need to be proposed to solve the problems with bidirectional transport of macromolecules (Stachowska-Pietka 2010). Nevertheless, the current understanding and quantification of the peritoneal transport obtained using the distributed approach is already a helpful tool in clinical and experimental research.

7. Acknowledgment

J. Stachowska-Pietka was supported by a grant N N518 417736 from the Polish Ministry of Science and Higher Education.

8. Nomenclature

Symbols	Parameter
A	effective peritoneal surface area, cm^2
C or C_S	solute concentration in the tissue, mmol/l
C_B or $C_{B,S}$	solute concentration in blood, mmol/l
C_D or $C_{D,S}$	solute concentration in dialysate, mmol/l
D^T or $D_S{}^T$	solute diffusivity in the tissue, cm^2/min
K	tissue hydraulic conductivity, cm^2/min/mmHg
k^T	unidirectional clearance for transport from tissue to blood, 1/min
L	tissue width, cm
L_Pa	hydraulic conductance of the capillary wall, 1/min/mmHg
$memKBD_S$	effective diffusive mass transport coefficient of the PTS, mL/min
$memL_Pa$	effective hydraulic conductivity of the PTS, mL/min/mmHg
$memOsmCond$	effective osmotic conductance of PTS, (ml/min)/(mmol/l)
P	interstitial hydrostatic pressure, mmHg
P_B	blood hydrostatic pressure, mmHg
P_D	intraperitoneal hydrostatic pressure, mmHg
p_Sa	diffusive permeability of solute across the capillary wall, 1/min
q_L	tissue lymphatic absorption, 1/min
s^{cap} or $s_S{}^{cap}$	sieving coefficient for solute across the capillary wall
s^T or $s_S{}^T$	sieving coefficient of solute in the tissue
θ	interstitial fluid void volume
θ_S	solute void volume
κ	ratio of the equilibrium concentration of solute in the tissue over its concentration in blood
Λ	solute overall penetration depth, cm
Λ_{Conv}	solute convective penetration depth, cm
Λ_{Dif}	solute diffusive penetration depth, cm
Λ_F	fluid penetration depth, cm
σ^{cap} or $\sigma_S{}^{cap}$	capillary wall reflection coefficient for solute S

σ^{eff}	effective reflection coefficient for PTS
σ^{T} or $\sigma_S{}^{T}$	tissue reflection coefficient for solute S

9. References

An, K. N., and E. P. Salathe. 1976. A theory of interstitial fluid motion and its implications for capillary exchange. *Microvasc Res* 12 (2):103-19.

Baxter, L. T., and R. K. Jain. 1989. Transport of fluid and macromolecules in tumors. I. Role of interstitial pressure and convection. *Microvasc Res* 37 (1):77-104.

———. 1990. Transport of fluid and macromolecules in tumors. II. Role of heterogeneous perfusion and lymphatics. *Microvasc Res* 40 (2):246-63.

———. 1991. Transport of fluid and macromolecules in tumors. III. Role of binding and metabolism. *Microvasc Res* 41 (1):5-23.

Cherniha, R., and J. Waniewski. 2005. Exact solutions of a mathematical model fro fluid transport in peritoneal dialysis. *Ukrainian Math. Journal* 57 (8):1112-1119.

Coester, A. M., D. G. Struijk, W. Smit, D. R. de Waart, and R. T. Krediet. 2007. The cellular contribution to effluent potassium and its relation to free water transport during peritoneal dialysis. *Nephrol Dial Transplant* 22 (12):3593-600.

Collins, J. M. 1981. Inert gas exchange of subcutaneous and intraperitoneal gas pockets in piglets. *Respir Physiol* 46 (3):391-404.

Collins, J. M., R. L. Dedrick, M. F. Flessner, and A. M. Guarino. 1982. Concentration-dependent disappearance of fluorouracil from peritoneal fluid in the rat: experimental observations and distributed modeling. *J Pharm Sci* 71 (7):735-8.

Dedrick, R. L., M. F. Flessner, J. M. Collins, and J. S. Schultz. 1982. Is the peritoneum a membrane? *ASAIO J* 5:1-8.

Flessner, M. F. 1994. Osmotic barrier of the parietal peritoneum. *Am J Physiol* 267 (5 Pt 2):F861-70.

———. 2001. Transport of protein in the abdominal wall during intraperitoneal therapy. I. Theoretical approach. *Am J Physiol Gastrointest Liver Physiol* 281 (2):G424-37.

———. 2005. The transport barrier in intraperitoneal therapy. *Am J Physiol Renal Physiol* 288 (3):F433-42.

———. 2009. Intraperitoneal Chemotherapy. In *Nolph and Gokal's textbook of peritoneal dialysis*, edited by R. Khanna and R. T. Krediet. USA: Springer.

Flessner, M. F., J. Choi, H. Vanpelt, Z. He, K. Credit, J. Henegar, and M. Hughson. 2006. Correlating structure with solute and water transport in a chronic model of peritoneal inflammation. *Am J Physiol Renal Physiol* 290 (1):F232-40.

Flessner, M. F., R. L. Dedrick, and J. S. Schultz. 1984. A distributed model of peritoneal-plasma transport: theoretical considerations. *Am J Physiol* 246 (4 Pt 2):R597-607.

———. 1985. A distributed model of peritoneal-plasma transport: analysis of experimental data in the rat. *Am J Physiol* 248 (3 Pt 2):F413-24.

———. 1985. Exchange of macromolecules between peritoneal cavity and plasma. *Am J Physiol* 248 (1 Pt 2):H15-25.

Flessner, M. F., J. D. Fenstermacher, R. L. Dedrick, and R. G. Blasberg. 1985. A distributed model of peritoneal-plasma transport: tissue concentration gradients. *Am J Physiol* 248 (3 Pt 2):F425-35.

Flessner, M. F., J. Lofthouse, and R. Zakaria el. 1997. In vivo diffusion of immunoglobulin G in muscle: effects of binding, solute exclusion, and lymphatic removal. *Am J Physiol* 273 (6 Pt 2):H2783-93.

Flessner, M., J. Henegar, S. Bigler, and L. Genous. 2003. Is the peritoneum a significant transport barrier in peritoneal dialysis? *Perit Dial Int* 23 (6):542-9.

Gupta, E., M. G. Wientjes, and J. L. Au. 1995. Penetration kinetics of 2',3'-dideoxyinosine in dermis is described by the distributed model. *Pharm Res* 12 (1):108-12.

Imholz, A. L., G. C. Koomen, D. G. Struijk, L. Arisz, and R. T. Krediet. 1993. Effect of dialysate osmolarity on the transport of low-molecular weight solutes and proteins during CAPD. *Kidney Int* 43 (6):1339-46.

Kagan, A., Y. Bar-Khayim, Z. Schafer, and M. Fainaru. 1990. Kinetics of peritoneal protein loss during CAPD: I. Different characteristics for low and high molecular weight proteins. *Kidney Int* 37 (3):971-9.

Leypoldt, J. K. 1993. Interpreting peritoneal membrane osmotic reflection coefficients using a distributed model of peritoneal transport. *Adv Perit Dial* 9:3-7.

Leypoldt, J. K., and L. W. Henderson. 1992. The effect of convection on bidirectional peritoneal solute transport: predictions from a distributed model. *Ann Biomed Eng* 20 (4):463-80.

Nolph, K. D., F. Miller, J. Rubin, and R. Popovich. 1980. New directions in peritoneal dialysis concepts and applications. *Kidney Int Suppl* 10:S111-6.

Nolph, K. D., and Z. J. Twardowski. 1989. The peritoneal dialysis system. In *Peritoneal Dialysis*, edited by K. D. Nolph. Dordrecht: Kluwer.

Pannekeet, M. M., A. L. Imholz, D. G. Struijk, G. C. Koomen, M. J. Langedijk, N. Schouten, R. de Waart, J. Hiralall, and R. T. Krediet. 1995. The standard peritoneal permeability analysis: a tool for the assessment of peritoneal permeability characteristics in CAPD patients. *Kidney Int* 48 (3):866-75.

Patlak, C. S., and J. D. Fenstermacher. 1975. Measurements of dog blood-brain transfer constants by ventriculocisternal perfusion. *Am J Physiol* 229 (4):877-84.

Perl, W. 1962. Heat and matter distribution in body tissues and the determination of tissue blood flow by local clearance methods. *J Theor Biol* 2:201-235.

———. 1963. An extension of the diffusion equation to include clearance by capillary blood flow. *Ann N Y Acad Sci* 108:92-105.

Piiper, J., R. E. Canfield, and H. Rahn. 1962. Absorption of various inert gases from subcutaneous gas pockets in rats. *J Appl Physiol* 17:268-74.

Rippe, B., and G. Stelin. 1989. Simulations of peritoneal solute transport during CAPD. Application of two-pore formalism. *Kidney Int* 35 (5):1234-44.

Rubin, J., T. Adair, Q. Jones, and E. Klein. 1985. Inhibition of peritoneal protein losses during peritoneal dialysis in dogs. *ASAIO J* 8:234-237.

Seames, E. L., J. W. Moncrief, and R. P. Popovich. 1990. A distributed model of fluid and mass transfer in peritoneal dialysis. *Am J Physiol* 258 (4 Pt 2):R958-72.

Stachowska-Pietka, J. 2010. Mathematical modeling of ultrafiltration and fluid absorption during peritoneal dialysis. PhD Thesis, Institute of Biocybernetics and Biomedical Engineering Polish Academy of Sciences, Warsaw.

Stachowska-Pietka, J., and J. Waniewski. 2011. Distributed modeling of glucose induced osmotic fluid flow during single exchange with hypertonic glucose solution. *Biocybernetics and Biomedical Engineering* 31 (1):39-50.

Stachowska-Pietka, J., J. Waniewski, M. F. Flessner, and B. Lindholm. 2006. Distributed model of peritoneal fluid absorption. *Am J Physiol Heart Circ Physiol* 291 (4):H1862-74.

———. 2007. A distributed model of bidirectional protein transport during peritoneal fluid absorption. *Adv Perit Dial* 23:23-7.

Stachowska-Pietka, J., J. Waniewski, M. Flessner, and B. Lindholm. 2005. A mathematical model of peritoneal fluid absorption in the tissue. *Adv Perit Dial* 21:9-12.

Stachowska-Pietka, J., J. Waniewski, and B. Lindholm. 2010. Bidirectional transport of fluid and protein during peritoneal dialysis assessed by distributed model with structured interstitium. *Perit Dial Int* 30 (Suppl. 2):S44.

———. 2010. Integrated distributed model of fluid and solute transport during peritoneal dialysis. *Perit Dial Int* 30 (Suppl. 1):S20.

Taylor, D. G., J. L. Bert, and B. D. Bowen. 1990. A mathematical model of interstitial transport. I. Theory. *Microvasc Res* 39 (3):253-78.

Van Liew, H. D. 1968. Coupling of diffusion and perfusion in gas exit from subcutaneous pocket in rats. *Am J Physiol* 214 (5):1176-85.

Venturoli, D., and B. Rippe. 2001. Transport asymmetry in peritoneal dialysis: application of a serial heteroporous peritoneal membrane model. *Am J Physiol Renal Physiol* 280 (4):F599-606.

Waniewski, J. 2001. Physiological interpretation of solute transport parameters for peritoneal dialysis. *J Theor Med* 3:177-190.

———. 2002. Distributed modeling of diffusive solute transport in peritoneal dialysis. *Ann Biomed Eng* 30 (9):1181-95.

———. 2006. Mathematical modeling of fluid and solute transport in hemodialysis and peritoneal dialysis. *J Mem Sci* 274:24-37.

Waniewski, J., V. Dutka, J. Stachowska-Pietka, and R. Cherniha. 2007. Distributed modeling of glucose-induced osmotic flow. *Adv Perit Dial* 23:2-6.

Waniewski, J., J. Stachowska-Pietka, and M. F. Flessner. 2009. Distributed modeling of osmotically driven fluid transport in peritoneal dialysis: theoretical and computational investigations. *Am J Physiol Heart Circ Physiol* 296 (6):H1960-8.

Waniewski, J., A. Werynski, and B. Lindholm. 1999. Effect of blood perfusion on diffusive transport in peritoneal dialysis. *Kidney Int* 56 (2):707-13.

Wientjes, M. G., R. A. Badalament, R. C. Wang, F. Hassan, and J. L. Au. 1993. Penetration of mitomycin C in human bladder. *Cancer Res* 53 (14):3314-20.

Wientjes, M. G., J. T. Dalton, R. A. Badalament, J. R. Drago, and J. L. Au. 1991. Bladder wall penetration of intravesical mitomycin C in dogs. *Cancer Res* 51 (16):4347-54.

Wiig, H., M. DeCarlo, L. Sibley, and E. M. Renkin. 1992. Interstitial exclusion of albumin in rat tissues measured by a continuous infusion method. *Am J Physiol* 263 (4 Pt 2):H1222-33.

Zakaria, E. R., J. Lofthouse, and M. F. Flessner. 1999. In vivo effects of hydrostatic pressure on interstitium of abdominal wall muscle. *Am J Physiol* 276 (2 Pt 2):H517-29.

———. 2000. Effect of intraperitoneal pressures on tissue water of the abdominal muscle. *Am J Physiol Renal Physiol* 278 (6):F875-85.

3

Membrane Biology During Peritoneal Dialysis

Kar Neng Lai[1] and Joseph C.K. Leung[2]
[1]*Nephrology Centre, Hong Kong Sanatorium and Hospital,*
[2]*Division of Nephrology, Department of Medicine, Queen Mary Hospital, University of Hong Kong, Hong Kong*

1. Introduction

Peritoneal dialysis (PD) is a life-supporting renal replacement therapy used by 10-15% of patients with end-stage renal failure worldwide. The success of long-term PD depends entirely on the longevity and integrity of the peritoneal membrane. The peritoneum is covered by a mesothelial monolayer beneath which is a basement membrane and submesothelial layer that contains collagen, fibroblasts, adipose tissue, blood vessels and lymphatics. During PD, peritoneal cells are repeatedly exposed to a non-physiological hypertonic environment with high glucose content and low pH. Mesothelial cells (MCs) play an important role in regulating the inflammatory response in the peritoneal cavity: they produce pro-inflammatory cytokines and chemoattractants. By secreting these chemokines or cytokines, MCs contribute to the recruitment of leukocytes following the expression of adhesion molecules. Chronic changes in the peritoneum with fibrosis develop after years of peritoneal dialysis. The most marked changes are in cases of severe and recurrent peritonitis. Others have made similar observations that long-term exposure to peritoneal dialysis solutions appears to increase fibrosis and the probability of ultrafiltration failure. Encapsulating peritoneal sclerosis represents the most severe and fatal complication of membrane failure.

Conventional peritoneal dialysis fluids (PDFs) make use of the osmotic gradient generated by glucose. Years of exposure to PDFs compounded with peritonitis result in the formation of an avascular layer of interstitial matrix and plasma proteins in the sub-mesothelial compact zone and an epithelial-to-mesenchymal transition (EMT) of mesothelial cells [1]. The fibrotic process in the peritoneal membrane is developed following acute and chronic release of inflammatory mediators related to PD. Independent extrinsic and intrinsic events (Table 1) contribute to chronic inflammation in patients on PD leading to complications including peritoneal membrane ultrafiltration failure, fluid overload, protein energy wasting and even atherosclerosis.

2. Extrinsic factors

2.1 Uremia

It has been shown that the peritoneum of uremic and current hemodialysis patients who have never exposed to PD is abnormal as well; this finding implies that uremia induces inflammation in the peritoneum [2]. There is a marked increase in vasculopathy below the compact zone.

Extrinsic Factors
• Uremia • PDFs • Infections – especially peritonitis
Intrinsic Factors
• Mesothelium • Sub-mesothelial compact zone • Sub-mesothelial blood vessels • Epithelial-to-mesenchymal transition (EMT) • Receptors for GDPs and AGE • Macrophages • Peritoneal adipocytes

Table 1. Events promoting chronic inflammation in PD

2.2 Peritoneal Dialysis Fluids (PDFs)

D-glucose is a reactive compound that exerts effect on the mesothelial cells directly by up-regulating the synthesis of transforming growth factor-β (TGF-β) and connective tissue growth factor by MCs or through its degradation pathway into glucose degradation products (GDPs) and formation of advanced glycation end-products (AGEs). Exposure to GDPs leads to enhanced cytotoxic damage and pro-inflammatory response in MCs stimulating the production of vascular endothelial growth factor (VEGF) that enhances vascular permeability and angiogenesis. GDPs also down-regulate the expression of intercellular tight junction proteins like ZO-1, occludine and claudin-1 in MCs, again via VEGF [3].

Factors such as the buffer, glucose or GDPs formed during heat sterilization, are critical in determining the biocompatibility of different PDFs. Mesothelial cell repair (remesothelialization) after exposure to GDPs is impaired, independent of D-glucose concentration. After exposure of mesenchymal cells to PDFs, the expression of cytokeratin 18 and E-cadherin is reduced while the expression of α-SMA and vimentin as a sign of EMT is increased [4]. Expression of intercellular tight junction proteins is down-regulated after incubation with PDFs.

2.3 Infection

Bacterial peritonitis is associated with a sharp increase in total cell and neutrophil counts (400-fold) in PDFs up to 2-3 weeks after peritonitis despite clinical remission [5]. There was a progressive increase in the percentage of mesothelial cells or dead cells in the total cell population in PDFs. Dialysate levels of interleukin-1β (IL-1β), interleukin-6 (IL-6), tumor necrosis factor-α (TNF–α) and TGF-β increased markedly on day 1 before their levels decreased gradually [5,6]. This active release of pro-inflammatory cytokines and sclerogenic growth factors may continue some time despite clinical remission of peritonitis. The peritoneal cytokine networks after peritonitis may potentially affect the physiological properties of the peritoneal membrane [5].

3. Intrinsic factors

3.1 Mesothelium

Peritoneal mesothelial cells are biologically active and play distinctive biological roles other than local host defense [3]. The MCs are sensitive to the effect of pH despite the conventional PDFs are usually buffered from pH of 5.2–7.4 in 15–30 min in clinical studies while TGF-β production by MCs is less with bicarbonate-buffered PDF. Glucose in the PDF can bring about major changes in the environment of the mesothelial cells as well as that of the cells underlying the mesothelium and the production of various cytokines are increased as a result of this exposure (Table 2). The peritoneal membrane also synthesizes prosteoglycans, expresses AGE receptors and produces aquaporins [3,7]. It is noteworthy that glucose may exert little effect on the synthesis of specific mediators, such as VEGF yet its synthesis is greatly enhanced by GDPs or AGE. Serial peritoneal biopsy study shows denudation of the mesothelial monolayer as early as six months after maintenance PD.

- Synthesis of chemokines: MCP-1, RANTES, Interferon-γ-inducible protein-10
- Synthesis of fibrogenic cytokines - TGF-β, bFGF
- Synthesis of prosteoglycans
- Induction of angiogenesis - VEGF
- Expression of AGE receptors

Table 2. Biological role of peritoneal mesothelium

3.2 Sub-mesothelial compact zone

After years of continuous peritoneal dialysis, a good percentage of patients would have marked increase in the thickness of the submesothelial compact zone. The layer resembles scar tissue with a relatively amorphous, avascular appearance. Animal studies reveal that a spotty inflammation is detected at different places of the peritoneum in the first few weeks of exposure to PDF. With time, these areas of inflammation and sclerosis gradually coalesce and become more uniform to cover much of the peritoneum that is in contact with the PDF. As the fibrosis becomes more uniform, the patient will gradually lose ultrafiltration.

3.3 Sub-mesothelial blood vessels

In parallel with fibrosis, the peritoneum shows a progressive increase in capillary number (angiogenesis) and vasculopathy, which are involved in both the elevation of small solute transport across the peritoneal membrane and ultrafiltration failure. GDPs stimulate VEGF production by MCs [8]. Local production of VEGF during PD appears to play a central role in the processes leading to peritoneal neo-angiogenesis and functional decline. The changes in the structure of the peritoneal function over time on PD as found in functional tests has been confirmed in biopsy studies performed on patients [2]. These show both neo-angiogenesis and fibrosis as the underlying morphological changes contributing to these phenomena. As mentioned previously, uptake of the glucose by sub-mesothelial blood vessels will be quite rapid following increased permeability due to abnormal angiogenic vessels and the increased surface area of the microvasculature. This results in dissipation of the osmotic driving force through increased area and solute transport. In addition, disruption of intercellular tight junction in MCs may occur following down-regulation of ZO-1 expression in which VEGF plays an important role [3,8].

3.4 Epithelial-to-mesenchymal transition (EMT)

Chronic exposure of the mesothelium to sterile PDFs may result in an EMT. Local inflammation and oxidative stress, which results from the continuous peritoneal injury, accelerate the EMT of peritoneal mesothelial cells resulting in peritoneal fibrosis and ultrafiltration failure. EMT is a process by which the MCs undergo a progressive loss of epithelial phenotype and acquire fibroblast-like characteristics, which allows these cells to invade the mesothelial stroma contributing to angiogenesis, fibrosis and ultrafiltration failure. Yanez-Mo *et al.* [9] recovered and cultured human MCs from the spent dialysate of 54 stable patients. Eighty-five percent of these patients had no previous peritonitis. Omental fibroblasts were separated from three of omental MCs samples from 39 CAPD patients. There was a transition from an epithelial type of mesothelial cell to a fibroblast-like cell with loss of normal markers of the mesothelium and phenotypic changes following progressive and continuous exposure to PDFs. For patients who were exposed to dialysate for more than 12 months, their mesothelial cells changed from 75% cobblestone phenotype to less than 30% with thc remainder being fibroblast-like. In some patients they observed that in less than 9 months there was loss of cytokeratin in the mesothelial cell layer. These findings suggest chronic exposure to the peritoneum to the current glucose-based PDFs could lead to morphologic and phenotypic changes in the mesothelium with 24 months.

Transforming growth factor-β, more specifically TGF-β1, is one of the main mediators of the PD solutions' profibrotic effects through the Smads 2 and 3 pathways. These effects include fibroblast activation, collagen deposition, inhibition of fibrinolysis, maintenance of fibrosis and neoangiogenesis [3]. Acting through the Smad pathway, TGF-β induces β-catenin formation which in conjunction with Activator Protein-1 activates matrix metalloproteinase-9 expression facilitating the invasion of the extracellular matrix [10]. Interestingly, angiotensin II inhibitors (which are TGF-β activity suppressors) have recently been shown to reduce peritoneal fibrosis and neoangiogenesis, as well as to prevent the increase of small solute transport in long-term PD patients [11]. Non-viral microbubble-delivery of Smad7 transgene markedly abolishes the peritoneal fibrosis induced by glucose-containing PDF [12]. Neutrophil gelatinase-associated lipocalin (NGAL) is specifically induced in human peritoneal MCs by interleukin-1β. Leung *et al.* [13] demonstrated that incubation of human peritoneal MCs with recombinant NGAL reversed the TGF- β-induced up-regulation of Snail and vimentin but rescued the down-regulation of E-cadherin. Their *in vitro* data suggest that NGAL may exert a protective effect in modulating the EMT activated following peritonitis.

Lately, Bajo *et al.* [14] demonstrated a clear association between GDPs present in conventional heat-sterilized PDFs and the induction of EMT in the peritoneal membrane. To date, no study has investigated the direct correlation between the inflammatory environment created as a consequence of recurrent peritonitis episodes and EMT, but many of the inflammatory cytokines known to be involved in driving EMT such as IL-1β, tumor necrosis factor-α (TNF-α) and TGF-β are present at high concentrations within the peritoneal membrane during peritonitis, and more importantly perhaps, the levels of these cytokines may remain elevated after the acute inflammatory response has subsided [5]. Clearly, the constant exposure of the mesothelial cells to increased levels of inflammatory cytokines and growth factors that have a known role to play in driving EMT could significantly increase the process of EMT-driven membrane fibrosis. In their study, Bajo et al. [14] reported no correlation between number of previous peritonitis episodes and mesothelial cell EMT observed in these patients; however, their results do suggest that the severity and duration of the peritonitis episode may supersede the protective effects of the low-GDP PDFs.

3.5 Receptors for GDPs and AGE

AGEs have been detected immunohistochemically in the peritoneum of PD patients. Receptor for advanced glycation end-products (RAGE) is the best characterized signal transduction receptor for AGEs. Primarily binding of AGEs to their receptor was regarded as a scavenger receptor involved in AGE removal and AGE clearance. However, ligand binding to RAGE results in an activation of key signal transduction pathways, such as NF-κB and multiple cellular signaling cascades like activation of MAP kinase. Local interaction between RAGE and AGEs/GDPs leads to the development of peritoneal inflammation, neo-angiogenesis and, finally, fibrosis. Anti-RAGE antibody partially prevents the development of submesothelial and interstitial fibrosis and EMT in an animal model of peritoneal fibrosis [15]. Aminoguanidine (AG) prevents formation of AGE. Supplementation of AG to PDF showed inhibitory effects on peritoneal AGE accumulation, mesothelial denudation, submesothelial monocyte infiltration, peritoneal permeability and ultrafiltration, and preserved the functional capacity of peritoneal macrophages in the rat. PDF-induced fibrosis was significantly reduced by AG [16]. The use of AG in human is limited by its pH and toxicity.

It is now evident that RAGE is much more than a single receptor for AGEs or a scavenger receptor; it has a broad repertoire of ligands. The key pathophysiological step seems to be GDP-dependent AGE formation in the uremic milieu, through which an enhanced expression of RAGE in the peritoneum could be observed. Recently, other AGE receptors, including AGE-R-1 (p 60), AGE-R-2 (p 90) and AGE-R-3 (gallectin-3) are also found to be expressed on MCs [17]. Different GDPs exert differential regulation on the regulation and expression of these receptors on human peritoneal MCs [17]. However, the functional significance of these various forms has not yet been completely delineated.

3.6 Macrophages

Resident macrophages increase markedly with bacterial peritonitis and are able to enhance the release of peroxide and pro-inflammatory cytokines including interleukin-1β and TNF-α. TGF-β complementary DNA (cDNA) molecules per macrophage are significantly greater than those of macrophages in non-infective PDFs throughout the peritonitis period [5]. There was no significant correlation between PDFs levels of TGF-β and TGF-β cDNA molecules per macrophage, suggesting that peritoneal macrophages are not the predominant source of TGF-β in PDFs.

4. The "less recognized" inflammatory role of peritoneal adipocytes in PD

Adipose tissue is abundant in omental or mesenteric peritoneum but less so in parietal, intestinal and diaphragmatic peritoneum. Contrary to the prevailing view that adipose tissue functions only as an energy storage depot, compelling evidence reveals that adipocytes can mediate various physiological processes through secretion of an array of mediators and adipokines that include leptin, adiponectin, resistin, TNF-α, IL-6, TGF-β, VEGF and other growth factors [18]. Moreover, adipocytes express receptors for leptin, insulin growth factor-1 (IGF-1), TNF-α, IL-6, TGF-β and may form a network of local autocrine, paracrine and endocrine signals [19]. All of these adipokines exert important endocrine functions in chronic kidney diseases and may also contribute to systemic inflammation in these patients. This is of special significance in patients undergoing PD as the initiation of treatment is often associated with an increase in fat mass that could be associated with the genetic effect on energy metabolism in addition to glucose absorption from the PDFs [20]. A recent study indicates that an increased fat mass in PD, like in other patient groups, may indeed have adverse metabolic consequences with increased systemic inflammation and worst survival [21]. Interestingly, there is a difference in the release of growth factors between visceral and subcutaneous adipose tissue [22]. The omental adipose tissue, most affected by PD, releases IL-6 two to three folds higher than the subcutaneous fat tissue [23]. The visceral (truncal) fat mass correlates significantly with circulating IL-6 levels but not for non-truncal fat mass [24].

Ultrastructural study reveals that a portion of omental adipocytes protrude from the mesothelial surface, thus may come into direct contact with dialysate [25]. In addition, dialysate may also reach the parietal adipose tissue when the mesothelial monolayer is damaged. It is therefore logical to postulate that with repeated exposure to PDFs and the continuous change in peritoneal physiology during PD, peritoneal adipocytes will inevitably be "activated". Although much work has focused on peritoneal mesothelial cells, scant attention has been paid to the role of peritoneal adipocytes during PD.

5. Crosstalk between peritoneal cells and adipocytes

Leptin is a peptide hormone mainly derived from adipocytes and is cleared principally by the kidney. The serum leptin concentration is increased in patients with chronic renal failure or undergoing dialysis [26,27] and the serum leptin increases by 189% within a month after the initiation of PD treatment [28]. Leptin is also elevated during acute infection, in response to proinflammatory cytokines including IL-1β and TNF-α [26]. In the kidney, leptin stimulates cell proliferation and synthesis of collagen IV and TGF-β in glomerular endothelial cells. In glomerular mesangial cells, leptin increases the glucose transport, up-regulates the expression of TGF-β type II receptor and the synthesis of collagen I through phosphatidylinositol-3-kinase related pathway [26]. Available data suggests that leptin triggers a paracrine interaction between glomerular endothelial and mesangial cells through the increased synthesis of TGF-β in glomerular endothelial cells and upregulated TGF-β receptor expression in mesangial cells. Whether such paracrine interaction is operating between peritoneal adipocytes and MCs remains to be explored. To the best of our knowledge, there is only one previous study on the effect of PDF on adipocytes that demonstrates increased leptin synthesis in a murine adipocyte cell line (3T3-L1) by glucose-containing PDFs [29]. It is likely that proinflammatory mediators released by MCs upon exposure to PDF could induce functional alteration of adjacent adipocytes. The likely candidates are IL-1β and TNF-α, TGF-β, VEGF and IL-6. Indeed, a recent *in vitro* study has shown that IL-6 modulates leptin production and lipid metabolism in human adipose tissue [30]. Using MC and adipocyte cell cultures established in our laboratory, we have shown that high glucose content in dialysate fluid is one of the major culprits that causes structural and functional abnormalities in peritoneal cells during PD [8,31,32]. Glucose significantly increases the protein synthesis of leptin by adipocytes in a dose-dependent manner and up-regulates the expression of leptin receptor, Ob-Rb, in MCs [31]. The increased leptin production by adipocytes and enhanced Ob-Rb expression in MC following exposure to glucose suggest the existence of a cross-talk mechanism between adipocytes and MCs that may be relevant in peritoneal membrane dysfunction developed during peritoneal dialysis.

6. Persistent release of proinflammatory mediators in patients under maintenance PD or after an episode of peritonitis

Patients on maintenance PD have increased intra-peritoneal levels of hyaluronan and cytokines including IL-1β, IL-6 and TGF-β [33,34]. Chronic inflammation remains an important cause of morbidity in patients with end-stage renal failure. The main causes for inflammation in PD patients are PD-related peritonitis, continuous exposure to dialysis solutions and exit site infection [35]. Patients on PD with peritonitis may experience prolonged inflammation even when clinical evaluation suggests resolution of PD-related peritonitis [5]. The highly sensitive C-reactive protein remains significantly higher than baseline even by day 42 after an episode of peritonitis [36].

A longitudinal study conducted in patients treated for PD-related peritonitis also revealed elevation of serum leptin levels during acute peritonitis. The rise was contributed to anorexia in the earlier stage. In contrast, the serum adiponectin levels fell showing an inverse correlation between these two adipokines during acute peritonitis. Furthermore, the protracted course of inflammation even after bacterial cure of peritonitis was likely to cause the loss of lean body mass and to increase mortality [36].

7. Clinical syndrome of chronic inflammation in PD

The above-mentioned dialysis risk factors and certain PD-specific characteristics are associated with the inflammatory burden possibly linking inflammation, increased peritoneal solute transport rate and declined residual renal function to poor outcome. Both local (intra-peritoneal) and systemic inflammation may additively be the cause and consequence of peritoneal membrane failure, and are important prognosticators of mortality in PD patients. Several factors deserve special emphasis. It has been shown that even with apparent clinical remission of PD-related peritonitis, dialysis patients, after an episode of peritonitis, may still be affected by prolonged systemic chronic inflammation. The significantly prolonged inflammation contributed to a poorer nutritional status and higher mortality [36]. The finding is consistent with our previous study that the level of cytokines in the peritoneal effluent remained higher than that in non-infective effluent throughout the 6-week post-peritonitis period in parallel with elevated serum C reactive protein (CRP), despite clinical remission [5]. One-sixth of these patients with prolonged elevation of serum CRP died of a cardiovascular event over a median period of 17 months [37]. Therefore, the prolonged inflammation is likely to potentiate atherogenesis and increase the risk of cardiovascular events.

Other than persistent low-grade inflammation, subclinical malnutrition may be another factor for the high mortality in these patients. Chronic inflammation with atherosclerosis is closely related to malnutrition, forming the malnutrition–inflammation–atherosclerosis (MIA) syndrome [37]. The underlying mechanism for malnourishment is likely to be multifactorial. Possible contributory factors include protein loss in the dialysate, the feeling of fullness due to PDF in abdomen, uremia-associated cachexia caused by leptin signaling through the hypothalamic melanocortin receptor [38], and protein energy wasting. The complications of membrane failure and fluid overload further enhance a higher incidence of cardiovascular events. Our proposal of a hypothetical mechanism of chronic inflammation in PD is shown in Figure 1.

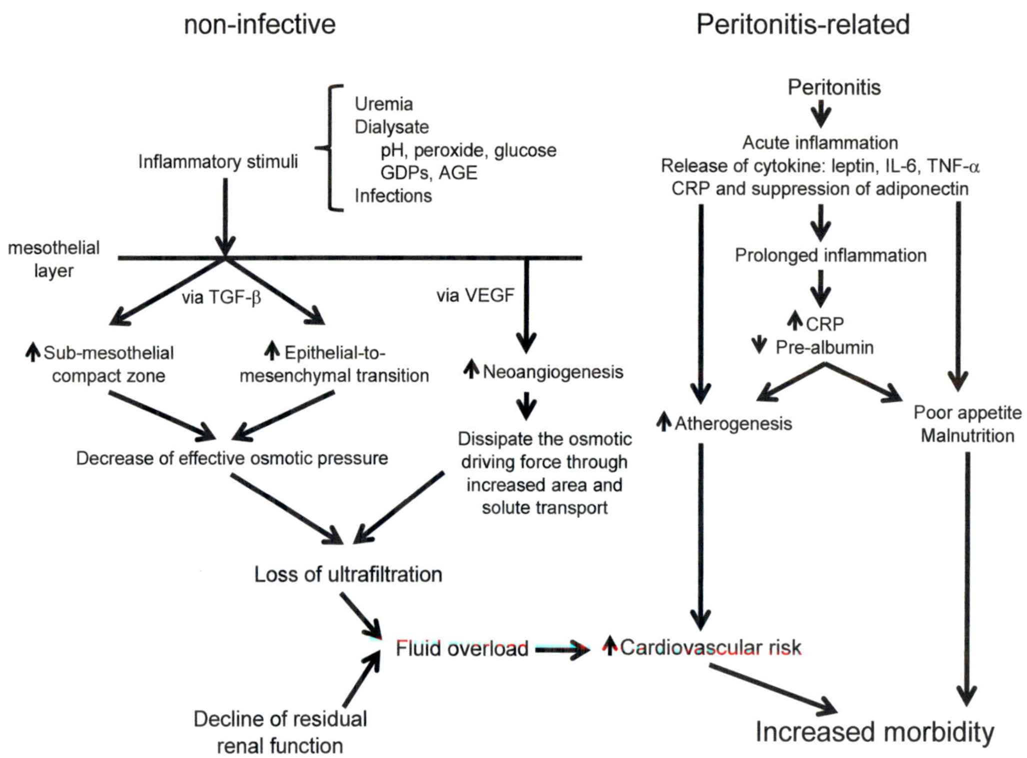

Fig. 1. Interactions between peritonitis-related and non-infective factors leading to chronic inflammation and increased morbidity in peritoneal dialysis patients

8. Newer osmotic agents in PDFs

Low-GDP PDFs clearly have an advantage over high GDP solutions [14,39]. But the continued presence of glucose remains a significant problem for the cells. Alternative hypertonic agents with additive that may prevent chronic inflammation will continue to be a subject of research.

9. Conclusion

During long-term maintenance PD, the peritoneal biology changes with chronic exposure to dialysate. Meticulous attention for chronic inflammation should be practiced in peritoneal dialysis patients, especially following peritonitis. Adequate nutritional support and screening for persistent inflammation are warranted such that the vicious circle like malnutrition–inflammation–atherosclerosis syndrome can be abolished.

10. Acknowledgement

Part of the work described in this paper was supported by the Baxter Extramural Grant and L & T Charitable Foundation & the House of INDOCAFE

11. References

[1] McLoughlin RM, Toply N. Switching on EMT in the peritoneal membrane: considering the evidence. *Nephrol Dialy Transplant* 2011; 26: 12-15.

[2] Williams JD, Craig KJ, Topley N, Von Ruhland C, Fallon M, Newman GR, Mackenzie RK, Williams GT. Peritoneal Biopsy Study Group: Morphologic changes in the peritoneal membrane of patients with renal disease. *J Am Soc Nephrol* 2002; 13: 470–479.

[3] Lai KN, Tang SC, Leung JC. Mediators of inflammation and fibrosis. *Perit Dial Int* 2007; Suppl 2: S65-71.

[4] Oh EJ, Ryu HM, Choi SY, Yook JM, Kim CD, Park SH, Chung HY, Kim IS, Yu MA, Kang DH, Kim YL. Impact of low glucose degradation product bicarbonate/lactate-buffered dialysis solution on the epithelial-mesenchymal transition of peritoneum. Am J Nephrol. 2010; 31:58-67.

[5] Lai KN, Lai KB, Chan TM, Lam CW, Li FK, Leung JCK. Changes of cytokine profile during peritonitis in patients on continuous ambulatory peritoneal dialysis. *Am J Kidney Dis 2000; 35: 644-652.*

[6] Zemel D, Koomen GCM, Hart, AAM, TenBerge RJM, Struijk DG, Krediet RT. Relationship of TNFalpha, interleukin-6, and prostaglandins to peritoneal permeability for macromolecules during longitudinal follow-up of peritonitis in continuous ambulatory peritoneal dialysis. J Lab Clin Med 1993;122:686-696

[7] Lai KN, Lam MF, Leung JC. Peritoneal function: the role of aquaporins. *Perit Dial Int* 2003; Suppl 2: S20-25.

[8] Leung JC, Chan LY, Li FF, Tang SC, Chan KW, Chan TM, Lam MF, Wieslander A, Lai KN. Glucose degradation products downregulate ZO-1 expression in human peritoneal mesothelial cells: the role of VEGF. *Nephrol Dial Transplant* 2005; 20: 1336-1349.

[9] Yanez-Mo M, Lara-Pezzi E, Selgas R, Ramirez-Huesca M, Dominguez-Jimenez C, Jimenez-Heffernan JA, Aguilera A, Sánchez-Tomero JA, Bajo MA, Alvarez V, Castro MA, del Peso G, Cirujeda A, Gamallo C, Sánchez-Madrid F, López-Cabrera M. Peritoneal dialysis and epithelialto-mesenchymal transition of mesothelial cells. *N Engl J Med* 2003; 348:403–413.

[10] Selgas R, Bajo A, Jiménez-Heffernan JA, Sánchez-Tomero JA, Del Peso G, Aguilera A, López-Cabrera M. Epithelial-to-mesenchymal transition of the mesothelial cell—its role in the response of the peritoneum to dialysis. *Nephrol Dial Transplant.* 2006; 21 (Suppl 2): S2-S7.

[11] Kolesnyk I, Noordzij M, Dekker FW, Boeschoten EW, Krediet RT. A positive effect of AII inhibitors on peritoneal membrane function in long-term PD patients. *Nephrol Dial Transplant* 2009; 24:272-277.

[12] Guo H, Leung JC, Lam MF, Chan LY, Tsang AW, Lan HY, Lai KN. Smad7 transgene attenuates peritoneal fibrosis in uremic rats treated with peritoneal dialysis. *J Am Soc Nephrol* 2007; 18: 2689-2703.

[13] Leung JC, Lam MF, Tang SC, Chan LY, Tam KY, Yip TP, Lai KN. Roles of neutrophil gelatinase-associated lipocalin in continuous ambulatory peritoneal dialysis-related peritonitis. *J Clin Immunol* 2009; 29:365-378

[14] Bajo MA, Pérez-Lozano ML, Albar-Vizcaino P, del Peso G, Castro MJ, Gonzalez-Mateo G, Fernández-Perpén A, Aguilera A, Sánchez-Villanueva R, Sánchez-Tomero JA, López-Cabrera M, Peter ME, Passlick-Deetjen J, Selgas R. Low GDP peritoneal dialysis fluid ('balance') has less impact in vitro and ex vivo on epithelial-to-mesenchymal transition (EMT) of mesothelial cells than a standard fluid. *Nephrol Dial Transplant* 2011; 26:282-291.

[15] De Vriese AS, Tilton RG, Mortier S, Lameire NH. Myofibroblast transdifferentiation of mesothelial cells is mediated by RAGE and contributes to peritoneal fibrosis in uraemia. *Nephrol Dial Transplant* 2006 21: 2549-2555.

[16] Zareie M, Tangelder GJ, ter Wee PM, Hekking LH, van Lambalgen AA, Keuning ED, Schadee-Eestermans IL, Schalkwijk CG, Beelen RH, van den Born J. Beneficial effects of aminoguanidine on peritoneal microcirculation and tissue remodelling in a rat model of PD. *Nephrol Dial Transplant* 2005; 20:2783-2792.

[17] Lai KN, Leung JC, Chan LY, Li FF, Tang SC, Lam MF, Lam MF, Tse KC, Yip TP, Chan TM, Wieslander A, Vlassara H. Differential expression of receptors for advanced glycation end-products in peritoneal mesothelial cells exposed to glucose degradation products. *Clin Exp Immunol* 2004 138: 466-475

[18] Friedman JM. Obesity in the new millennium. *Nature* 2000; 404:632-634.

[19] Myers MG, Jr. Leptin receptor signaling and the regulation of mammalian physiology. *Recent Prog Horm Res* 2004; 59:287-304.

[20] Nordfors L, Heimburger O, Lonnqvist F, *et al.* Fat tissue accumulation during peritoneal dialysis is associated with a polymorphism in uncoupling protein 2. *Kidney Int* 2000; 57:1713-1719

[21] Araujo IC, Kamimura MA, Draibe SA, *et al.* Nutritional parameters and mortality in incident hemodialysis patients. *J Ren Nutr* 2006; 16:27-35

[22] Fain JN, Madan AK, Hiler ML, Cheema P, Bahouth SW. Comparison of the release of adipokines by adipose tissue, adipose tissue matrix, and adipocytes from visceral and subcutaneous abdominal adipose tissues of obese humans. *Endocrinology* 2004; 145:2273-2282

[23] Mohamed-Ali V, Goodrick S, Rawesh A, *et al.* Subcutaneous adipose tissue releases interleukin-6, but not tumor necrosis factor-alpha, in vivo. *J Clin Endocrinol Metab* 1997; 82:4196-4200

[24] Axelsson J, Rashid Qureshi A, Suliman ME, *et al.* Truncal fat mass as a contributor to inflammation in end-stage renal disease. *Am J Clin Nutr* 2004; 80:1222-1229.

[25] Di Paolo N, Sacchi G. Atlas of peritoneal histology. *Perit Dial Int* 2000; 20 Suppl 3:S5-96

[26] Wolf G, Chen S, Han DC, Ziyadeh FN. Leptin and renal disease. *Am J Kidney Dis* 2002; 39:1-11

[27] Fruhbeck G, Gomez-Ambrosi J, Muruzabal FJ, Burrell MA. The adipocyte: a model for integration of endocrine and metabolic signaling in energy metabolism regulation. *Am J Physiol Endocrinol Metab* 2001; 280:E827-847

[28] Kim DJ, Oh DJ, Kim B, *et al.* The effect of continuous ambulatory peritoneal dialysis on change in serum leptin. *Perit Dial Int* 1999; 19 Suppl 2:S172-175

[29] Teta D, Tedjani A, Burnier M, Bevington A, Brown J, Harris K. Glucose-containing peritoneal dialysis fluids regulate leptin secretion from 3T3-L1 adipocytes. *Nephrol Dial Transplant* 2005; 20:1329-1335

[30] Trujillo ME, Sullivan S, Harten I, Schneider SH, Greenberg AS, Fried SK. Interleukin-6 regulates human adipose tissue lipid metabolism and leptin production in vitro. *J Clin Endocrinol Metab* 2004; 89:5577-5582

[31] Leung JC, Chan LY, Tang SC, Chu KM, Lai KN. Leptin induces TGF-beta synthesis through functional leptin receptor expressed by human peritoneal mesothelial cell. *Kidney Int* 2006; 69:2078-2086

[32] Leung JC, Chan LY, Tam KY, *et al.* Regulation of CCN2/CTGF and related cytokines in cultured peritoneal cells under conditions simulating peritoneal dialysis. *Nephrol Dial Transplant* 2009; 24:458-469.

[33] Lai KN, Szeto CC, Lai KB, Lam CW, Chan DT, Leung JC. Increased production of hyaluronan by peritoneal cells and its significance in patients on CAPD. *Am J Kidney Dis* 1999; 33:318-324

[34] Lai KN, Lai KB, Szeto CC, Lam CW, Leung JC. Growth factors in continuous ambulatory peritoneal dialysis effluent. Their relation with peritoneal transport of small solutes. *Am J Nephrol* 1999; 19:416-422

[35] Pecoits-Filho R, Stenvinkel P, Wang AY, Heimburger O, Lindholm B. Chronic inflammation in peritoneal dialysis: the search for the holy grail? *Perit Dial Int* 2004; 24:327-339.

[36] Lam MF, Leung JC, Lo WK. Tam S, Mong MC, Lui SL, Tse KC, Chan TM, Lai KN. Hyperleptinaemia and chronic inflammation after peritonitis predicts poor nutritional status and mortality in patients on peritoneal dialysis. *Nephrol Dial Transplant* 2007; 22:1445-1450.

[37] Stenvinkel P, Heimburger O, Lindholm B, Kaysen GA, Bergstrom J. Are there two types of malnutrition in chronic renal failure? Evidence for relationships between malnutrition, inflammation and atherosclerosis (MIA syndrome). *Nephrol Dial Transplant* 2000; 15:953–960.

[38] Cheung W, Yu PX, Little BM, Cone RD, Marks DL, Mak RH. Role of leptin and melanocortin signaling in uremia-associated cachexia. *J Clin Invest* 2005; 115:1659–1665.

[39] Flessner MF. Sterile solutions and peritoneal inflammation. *Contrib Nephrol* 2006; 150: 156-165.

4

Angiogenic Activity of the Peritoneal Mesothelium: Implications for Peritoneal Dialysis

Janusz Witowski[1,2] and Achim Jörres[2]
[1]*Department of Pathophysiology, Poznań University of Medical Sciences, Poznań*
[2]*Department of Nephrology and Medical Intensive Care, Charité Universitätsmedizin Berlin, Campus Virchow-Klinikum, Berlin*
[1]*Poland*
[2]*Germany*

1. Introduction

Functional deterioration of the peritoneum as a dialyzing organ is a leading cause of peritoneal dialysis (PD) failure. The problem usually develops 2-4 years after the initiation of therapy (Davies et al., 1996; Struijk et al., 1994) and may affect as many as 50% of all PD patients (Kawaguchi et al., 1997). The alterations that develop in the peritoneal membrane over time include submesothelial thickening, fibrosis, angiogenesis, and vascular degeneration (Honda et al., 2008; Mateijsen et al., 1999; Williams et al., 2002; Williams et al., 2003). These changes are associated with an increase in peritoneal solute transport with resultant dissipation of the osmotic gradient and loss of ultrafiltration. Indeed, it has been estimated that up to 75% of patients with ultrafiltration failure will have increased vascular area (Heimburger et al., 1990; Ho-Dac-Pannekeet et al., 1997). Pathological angiogenesis not only increases vascular surface area of the peritoneum but is also a key step in the progression of fibrosis (Wynn, 2007). Therefore, it is essential to understand how PD environment impacts on peritoneal vasculature.

2. Vascular endothelial growth factor

The process of angiogenesis requires tight coordination of cell proliferation, differentiation, migration, and cell-matrix interactions. The most important molecules that control blood vessel growth and permeability are vascular endothelial growth factors (VEGFs). VEGF-A (also designated and further referred to as VEGF) is the founding member of the VEGF family and was originally discovered by its ability to enhance vascular permeability (Nagy et al., 2007). In mammals, other VEGF family members include VEGF-B, -C, and -D, as well as placenta growth factor (PlGF). Structurally, the VEGFs are related to the family of platelet-derived growth factors (PDGF) (Olsson et al., 2006). VEGF is a highly conserved, disulfide-bonded dimeric glycoprotein, encoded by a single gene. The human *Vegf* gene is located on the short arm of chromosome 6 and alternative RNA splicing gives rise to peptide isoforms of 121, 145, 165, 189, and 206 amino acids. VEGF exerts its biologic effects mainly through cell-surface tyrosine kinase receptors VEGFR-2, and - to lesser extent - VEGFR-1 (Nagy et al., 2007). Although VEGF isoforms display similar basic activities, their bio-availability may be modulated by proteolytic processing and differences in binding to co-receptors such as heparan sulphate proteoglycans and neuropilins (Olsson et al., 2006).

VEGF is an extremely potent and rapid inducer of vascular permeability (Olsson et al., 2006). This effect depends on the production of nitric oxide (NO) by endothelial NO synthase (eNOS). Consequently, targeted deletion of eNOS abrogates VEGF-induced permeability (Fukumura et al., 2001). Other biological effects of VEGF include vasodilation, endothelial cell proliferation, migration and tube formation. It also delays senescence of endothelial cells, promotes their survival, and mobilizes endothelial cell precursors (Nagy et al., 2007; Otrock et al., 2007). Inactivation of a single *Vegf* allele in mice results in early embryonic lethality caused by impaired development of endothelial cells and blood vessels (Carmeliet et al., 1996; Ferrara et al., 1996). In turn, an increase in VEGF expression is commonly associated with pathological angiogenesis observed in malignancies, inflammation, and wound healing (Nagy et al., 2007).

2.1 VEGF in the peritoneal cavity

Given its role in controlling vascular permeability and proliferation, VEGF became an obvious target in research efforts to define the mechanism of peritoneal membrane failure. VEGF was promptly detected in the effluent dialysate (Zweers et al., 1999) in concentrations higher than could be expected on the basis of simple diffusion from the circulation (Selgas et al., 2001; Zweers et al., 1999). This pointed to the local production of VEGF in the peritoneum. Moreover, the rate of VEGF appearance in the dialysate was found to increase with time on PD (Cho et al., 2010) and to be elevated in patients with high peritoneal transport status (Pecoits-Filho et al., 2002; Rodrigues et al., 2007). Further analyses showed that the dialysate appearance of VEGF correlated also with that of cancer antigen 125 (CA125) (Cho et al., 2010; Rodrigues et al., 2004; Rodrigues et al., 2007). CA125 is thought to reflect the mass of peritoneal mesothelial cells (Krediet, 2001), therefore the mesothelium was considered to be the main source of intraperitoneal VEGF. Indeed, immunochemical staining of peritoneal biopsies showed that VEGF expression was confined mainly to the mesothelial monolayer (Aroeira et al., 2005; Combet et al., 2000). The mesothelial origin of peritoneal VEGF was ultimately confirmed in an elegant study, during which various cell types were isolated from the peritoneal lavage and the omentum, and analysed by several techniques for the ability to generate VEGF (Gerber et al., 2006). It transpired that omental mesothelial cells were responsible for the majority of peritoneal VEGF produced. These results were corroborated by the demonstration of constitutive VEGF secretion by mesothelial cells isolated either from the dialysate effluent (Selgas et al., 2000) or from the omentum (Mandl-Weber et al., 2002). Moreover, VEGF released by mesothelial cells was shown to exhibit biologic activity (Boulanger et al., 2007). The formation of capillary tubes by endothelial cells in vitro was found to increase either in the presence of peritoneal mesothelial cells or after the addition of conditioned medium from mesothelial cell cultures. These effects could be abolished by anti-VEGF antibodies (Boulanger et al., 2007).

3. Mesothelial cell VEGF expression during PD

The above data have given support to a long held belief that although the mesothelium forms only a single-cell layer over the peritoneum, it may significantly impact on the dialytic function of the whole peritoneal membrane by producing powerful mediators that act on the peritoneal interstitium and vasculature. Immunochemical analysis of peritoneal biopsies revealed only weak mesothelial expression of VEGF in control subjects, but extensive VEGF staining in patients undergoing PD (Aroeira et al., 2005; Combet et al., 2000). In an interesting experimental model mesothelial cells were isolated from dialysate effluent of PD patients, propagated ex vivo and analysed for the ability to release VEGF (Aroeira et al., 2005). It turned out that mesothelial cells isolated from patients with high peritoneal permeability secreted more VEGF compared to cells from patients with lower peritoneal transport properties.

Several factors have been implicated in the pathogenesis of increased peritoneal permeability in PD. They include the state of uraemia, episodes of peritonitis, and chronic exposure to dialysis fluids (Margetts & Churchill, 2002). Increasing evidence indicate that such conditions may modulate the release of VEGF by mesothelial cells. It is therefore essential to delineate mesothelial cell responses to these challenges.

3.1 Peritonitis

An increase in vascular permeability is a hallmark of inflammation. As a result, when acute peritonitis occurs during PD, it leads to rapid absorption of instilled glucose and a decrease in osmotic gradient-driven ultrafiltration. Modelling of PD-associated peritonitis in mice revealed significant increases in vascular density, the relative endothelial area, and the diameter of peritoneal vessels (Ni et al., 2003). These alterations were evident several days after bacterial infection and were accompanied by a huge increase in the dialysate VEGF concentration.

The inflammatory response is orchestrated by a coordinated release of cytokines with interleukin-1β (IL-1β) and tumour necrosis factor-α (TNFα) acting as crucial promoters of the reaction. The concentrations of IL-1β and TNFα in PD effluent increase very early and dramatically in the course of peritonitis (Brauner et al., 1996; Moutabarrik et al., 1995; Zemel et al., 1994). Transient, adenovirus-mediated over-expression of either IL-1β or TNFα in the rat peritoneum was found to increase the expression of VEGF in the peritoneal tissue and fluid (Margetts et al., 2002). This effect was followed by extensive angiogenesis, increased peritoneal permeability, and impaired ultrafiltration. In keeping with these results, it has been demonstrated that either IL-1β or TNFα were capable of inducing time- and dose-dependent VEGF production in mesothelial cells in vitro (Mandl-Weber et al., 2002). Moreover, in vitro exposure of mesothelial cells to dialysate effluent drained during peritonitis resulted in a significantly increased VEGF release compared to when cells were maintained in the non-infected dialysate (Witowski & Jörres, personal observations).

3.2 Exposure to dialysis fluids

The observation that the ultrafiltration capacity of the peritoneum decreases with time on PD (Davies et al., 1996; Heimburger et al., 1999) suggested that long-term exposure to bioincompatible PD fluids might have a deleterious impact on the peritoneal membrane. Early experiments pointed to low pH, high concentrations of lactate and glucose, and the presence of glucose degradation products (GDPs) as the elements curtailing biocompatibility of standard PD solutions (Wieslander et al., 1991). In recent years particular attention has been paid to GDPs. They are reactive carbonyl derivatives of glucose (such as formaldehyde, methylglyoxal or 3-deoxyglucosone), which are formed predominantly during heat sterilization of PD fluids. It has been demonstrated that conventional PD fluids with high GDPs content recruited capillaries and induced vasodilation of mesenteric arteries in the rat peritoneum (Mortier et al., 2002). Moreover, the peritonea of rats injected intraperitoneally for several days with methylglyoxal were found to display increased vascularization (Nakayama et al., 2003) and VEGF expression (Inagi et al., 1999). Subsequent experiments confirmed that extensive peritoneal expression of VEGF in rats receiving methylglyoxal-containing PD fluids was associated with neoangiogenesis and increased permeability (Hirahara et al., 2006). Furthermore, it has been demonstrated that direct in vitro exposure of mesothelial cells to several GDPs (methylglyoxal, 3,4-dideoxy-glucosone-3-ene, 2-furaldehyde) resulted in an increased VEGF expression (Inagi et al., 1999; Lai et al., 2004; Leung et al., 2005).

The adverse effects of GDPs on the peritoneal membrane can also be mediated through advanced glycation-end products (AGEs). GDPs react with amino groups of proteins to form AGEs and it has been demonstrated that PD fluids with high GDP levels significantly promote the generation of AGEs (Tauer et al., 2001). Animal experiments showed that intraperitoneal infusion of GDP-containing solutions led to the accumulation in the peritoneal membrane of both methylglyoxal and AGEs (Mortier et al., 2004). The presence of AGE deposits was associated with increased expression of VEGF, increased vascular density, and lower ultrafiltration. These observations were in line with earlier data showing that the intensity of peritoneal AGE accumulation in PD patients correlated with changes in peritoneal transport and ultrafiltration (Honda et al., 1999; Nakayama et al., 1997). Moreover, mesothelial cells were found to bear a receptor for AGEs (RAGE) and to up-regulate its expression following exposure to GDP in either in vitro (Lai et al., 2004) or in vivo setting (Mortier et al., 2004). In turn, incubation of mesothelial cells with AGEs led to a dose-dependent increase in VEGF production (Boulanger et al., 2007; Mandl-Weber et al., 2002). Interestingly, GDP-induced VEGF release by mesothelial cells could be reduced by aminoguanidine, an inhibitor of AGE formation (Lai et al., 2004). Also, a rise in peritoneal VEGF expression and vascular density that was induced in wild-type mice by chronic exposure to GDP-containing fluids, did not occur in RAGE-deficient animals (Schwenger et al., 2006). Correspondingly, the promoting effect of AGE-treated mesothelial cells on capillary tube formation could be substantially diminished by the blockade of RAGE with specific antibodies (Boulanger et al., 2007). These data indicate that GDPs exert their effect by inducing glycation of proteins that subsequently activate RAGE on mesothelial cells and stimulate them to release angiogenic VEGF (Fig. 1).

3.3 Uraemia

After analysing peritoneal specimens from a large cohort of individuals, the Peritoneal Biopsy Study Group concluded that in many patients with uraemia some changes in the peritoneum occurred even before the commencement of PD (Williams et al., 2002). Compared to healthy individuals, such patients often had significant thickening of the submesothelial compact zone and extensive vasculopathy. These changes are generally attributed to the build-up of uraemic toxins, however, their exact nature remains poorly defined. The peritonea of rats made uraemic by subtotal nephrectomy were found to have increased permeability and showed focal areas of vascular proliferation, up-regulation of VEGF and accumulation of AGEs (Combet et al., 2001). Furthermore, there was the evidence of mesothelial cell conversion into myofibroblasts (De Vriese et al., 2006). A more recent study in humans confirmed the presence of submesothelial thickening, focal fibrosis, and increased vascularization in the uraemic peritoneum (Kihm et al., 2008). These alterations were accompanied by increased peritoneal expression of methylglyoxal-induced AGEs, RAGE, VEGF, as well as of nuclear factor-κB (NF-κB) and interleukin-6 (IL-6). The peritoneal accumulation of AGEs and RAGE in uraemia may be not so surprising, since it is now well recognized that the uraemic state is associated with increased generation of glucose-derived dicarbonyl compounds (such as glyoxal, methylglyoxal, or 3-deoxyglucosone), which are strong inducers of AGEs (Miyata et al., 1999; Miyata et al., 2001) (Fig. 1). In turn, binding of AGEs to RAGE on mesothelial cells can activate NF-κB and increase the production of NF-κB-controlled inflammatory cytokines, including IL-6 (Nevado et al., 2005).

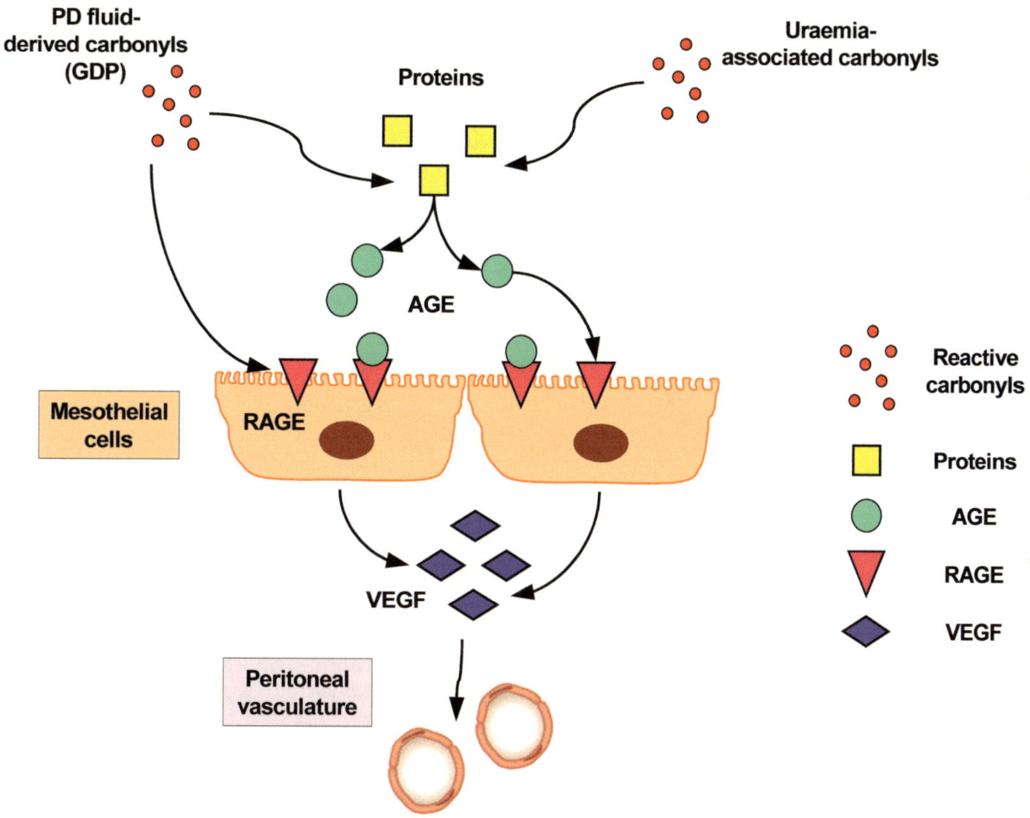

Fig. 1. Effect of reactive carbonyls and advanced glycation end-products on VEGF release by mesothelial cells.

4. Mesothelial cell phenotype and VEGF expression

It is now clear that mesothelial cells may undergo some phenotypic changes both in vitro and in vivo. These changes are related to distinct biological programmes activated by cells exposed to environmental challenges. The exact context at which certain stimuli trigger a given cellular response is not fully understood. Nevertheless, increasing evidence suggest that such reactions may occur also in the milieu of PD. Interestingly, transforming growth factor-β (TGF-β) has emerged as a mediator being critically involved at several steps of these pathways.

4.1 Epithelial-to-mesenchymal transition

During epithelial-to-mesenchymal transition (EMT) epithelial cells adapt a fibroblast-like phenotype. It includes the loss of distinctive apical-basal cell polarity, disassembly of tight intercellular junctions, and the acquirement of ability to migrate and shape extracellular matrix. Mounting evidence indicate that during PD mesothelial cells differentiate into submesothelial fibroblasts and impact on the underlying stroma and vasculature (Aroeira et al., 2007). Mesothelial cells isolated from dialysate effluent of PD patients were found to exhibit phenotypes ranging from the typical epithelial cobblestone-like appearance to the fibroblast spindle-like morphology (Yanez-Mo et al., 2003). The occurrence of fibroblast-like mesothelial cells increased with time on PD (Yanez-Mo et al., 2003) and was greater in patients who exhibited increased peritoneal permeability (Aroeira et al., 2005) or received PD solutions with high GDP concentrations (Aroeira et al., 2009; Bajo et al., 2011). The role of mesothelial cell phenotypic conversion in inducing functional alterations in peritoneal transport could be linked to the augmented VEGF and TGF-β1 release. Mesothelial cells with fibroblast-like morphology were found to release significantly more TGF-β1 and VEGF when propagated ex vivo compared to cells with classic epithelioid appearance (Aroeira et al., 2005; Bajo et al., 2011). A precise study with the use of immunofluorescence-aided laser capture microdissection confirmed that phenotypic changes in rat mesothelial cells occurred after adenoviral over-expression of TGF-β1 in the peritoneum and were associated with increased VEGF expression (Zhang et al., 2008). The process was largely mediated through Smad3, a crucial element of the TGF-β signalling pathway (Patel et al., 2010a). These data indicate that the gradual accumulation of transdifferentiated mesothelial cells in the peritoneum of PD patients may favour the development of excessive peritoneal vascularization and/or permeability.

Studies on the molecular mechanisms coordinating EMT identified TGF-β1 and bone morphogenetic protein-7 (BMP-7) as the key mediators (Zavadil & Bottinger, 2005; Zeisberg et al., 2003). As in other cell types, TGF-β1 was shown to induce EMT in mesothelial cells both in vitro (Yang et al., 2003) and in vivo (Margetts et al., 2005; Patel et al., 2010a; Zhang et al., 2008). In contrast, BMP-7 was found to act as an inhibitor of EMT and blocked the mesothelial cell conversion (Loureiro et al., 2010; Vargha et al., 2006; Yu et al., 2009). Interestingly, it has recently been demonstrated that PD fluids with high GDP content induced EMT in mesothelial cells either during short-term direct in vitro exposure or following chronic PD regimen (Bajo et al., 2011). This finding was in line with earlier observations of EMT in the peritoneal membrane of rats treated with chronic intraperitoneal administration of methylglyoxal (Hirahara et al., 2009). The process was associated with increased peritoneal expression of TGF-β and RAGE. Interestingly, in uraemic rats the inhibition of signalling from RAGE decreased the extent of mesothelial EMT and TGF-β expression (De Vriese et al., 2006). Moreover, PD fluid-induced EMT of mesothelial cells in rats could be substantially reduced by peritoneal rest (Yu et al., 2009), which has long been advocated as a means of restoring ultrafiltration in patients with the hyperpermeable peritoneum (de Alvaro et al., 1993; Rodrigues et al., 2002). It has also been demonstrated that PD fluid-induced EMT was associated with increased signalling from Notch receptors in mesothelial cells and the process was mediated through TGF-β1 (Zhu et al., 2010). Notch receptors are involved in the determination of cell fate, differentiation, and maintenance. The inhibition of Notch signalling resulted in the attenuation of both TGF-β1-induced EMT in vitro and PD fluid-induced EMT and peritoneal fibrosis in vivo (Zhu et al., 2010). Importantly, in both processes, the blockade of Notch led to a decrease in mesothelial cell VEGF expression. In a recent intriguing study (Patel et al., 2010b), platelet derived growth factor B (PDGF-B) was found to induce some, but not all, features of EMT in mesothelial cells. They included, however, increased VEGF expression.

4.2 Cell senescence

Gradual senescence of cells, which can easily be seen in vitro, has been believed to reflect the process of organismal aging. Extensive studies over the past decade have revealed, however, that cellular senescence is a more general phenomenon. It appears to be a cellular stress response set off by factors that may put the integrity of the genome in danger (Campisi, 2010). They include DNA breaks, dysfunctional telomeres and mitochondria, oxidative stress, disrupted chromatin, or excessive mitogenic stimulation. The hallmark of cellular senescence is an essentially irreversible growth arrest. As this prevents the transmission of potentially oncogenic mutations to daughter cells, the senescence response is thought to have evolved as a powerful cancer suppression mechanism. Other features of senescence include an enlarged morphology, the expression of senescence-associated β-galactosidase (SA-β-gal), and the up-regulation of p16, a cyclin-dependent cell cycle inhibitor.

Human peritoneal mesothelial cells in vitro enter the senescent state relatively quickly (Ksiazek et al., 2006). The process does not result from critical telomere shorthening (Ksiazek et al., 2007c), but is associated with extensive accumulation of DNA double-strand breaks in non-telomeric DNA regions. The damages are most likely caused by oxidative stress (Ksiazek et al., 2008b), which is viewed as one of the main triggers of premature senescence. As increased generation of reactive oxygen species occurs in hyperglycaemia (Bashan et al., 2009), it was logical to examine how glucose impacted on senescence of mesothelial cells. It turned out that chronic exposure to high glucose accelerated the development of senescent features in mesothelial cells, and the effect could be largely prevented by antioxidants (Ksiazek et al., 2007a). Interestingly, a further downstream mediator of the process appeared to be TGF-β1, since some features of the high glucose-induced senescent phenotype could be abolished by anti-TGF-β antibodies or reproduced by exogenous TGF-β1 (Ksiazek et al., 2007b).

The presence of senescent mesothelial cells in vivo is only scarcely documented. Cells expressing SA-β-Gal were found in freshly explanted human omenta (Ksiazek et al., 2008b), in mesothelial cell imprints from mice exposed to PD fluids (Gotloib et al., 2003) or in mesothelial cell derived from PD effluents (Gotloib et al., 2007). The detection of senescent cells following in vivo exposure to PD fluids or after in vitro exposure to high glucose rises an interesting question of whether dialysate glucose and/or glucose derivatives promote the senescence of mesothelial cells. Some date indicate that direct exposure to GDP-containing PD fluid may, indeed, result in increased expression of SA-β-Gal in mesothelial cells (Witowski et al., 2008).

The potential significance of such a change in the mesothelial cell phenotype is that senescent cells display an altered pattern of secretion of various cytokines, growth factors, proteases, and matrix components. The senescence-associated secretory phenotype may contribute to tissue dysfunction and pave the way for other pathologies (Coppe et al., 2010). VEGF has been identified as one of the mediators released at increased levels by senescent cells (Coppe et al., 2006). As a matter of fact, senescent mesothelial were also found to release significantly more VEGF than their pre-senescent counterparts (Witowski et al., 2008). Moreover, media obtained from cultures of senescent mesothelial cells promoted endothelial cell growth to a greater degree compared with young cells (Ksiazek et al., 2008a). The increase in VEGF secretion by senescent mesothelial cells could be partly related to the senescence-associated oxidative stress, since the antioxidant precursors of glutathione were found to decrease VEGF release (Witowski et al., 2008). It could also be mediated by the augmented activity of TGF-β1 observed in senescence (Ksiazek et al., 2007b). In this respect TGF-β1 has been shown to induce VEGF in many cell types, including mesothelial cells (Szeto et al., 2005).

An interesting aspect of the process delineated above is the involvement of TGF-β1 in both EMT and cellular senescence. Intriguingly enough, TGF-β1 may also act as a mediator of apoptosis (Siegel & Massague, 2003). Indeed, TGF-β1 was found to increase the rate of apoptosis in mesothelial cells, probably by down-regulating the expression of an anti-apoptotic gene *bcl-2l* (Szeto et al., 2006). Therefore, it remains to be elucidated how cells read TGF-β1 signals so that the response proceeds along a given pathway. Furthermore, it is not clear whether there is some relationship between the resulting processes. It has been suggested that the senescence-associated secretory phenotype may promote EMT in neighbouring cells (Coppe et al., 2008).

5. VEGF polymorphism

The *Vegf* gene is a highly polymorphic gene with several variations identified in a 5′-promotor region of the gene (Brogan et al., 1999). Such polymorphisms are thought to bear functional significance and may, for example, affect VEGF production by mononuclear leukocytes (Watson et al., 2000) or malignant cells (Schneider et al., 2009). Several known *Vegf* polymorphisms were analysed in the context of PD. They were found to have no association with baseline permeability of the peritoneal membrane at the start of PD (Gillerot et al., 2005; Maruyama et al., 2007; Szeto et al., 2004). Interestingly, however, patients with the A allele at -2578 position of the *Vegf* gene had higher mRNA VEGF expression in the sediment of effluent cells compared to the individuals with the C allele (Szeto et al., 2004). Moreover, this genotype was associated with a gradual increase in peritoneal transport over time and with greater patient mortality. The data suggest that certain genotypes may predispose to increased local VEGF release in response to PD environment and thus impact on peritoneal membrane function. Since mesothelial cell EMT or senescence are associated with increased secretion of VEGF, it would be interesting to know whether certain genotypes have an effect on the incidence of such changes in PD patients.

6. Conclusions

The mesothelium is the main source of peritoneal VEGF. By secreting VEGF, mesothelial cells impact on peritoneal vasculature. In PD patients the exposure of mesothelial cells to uraemic environment, bioincompatible dialysis fluids, and the bouts of infection may change the secretory phenotype of mesothelial cells so that they release more VEGF. In some patients (possibly with a certain genetic background), VEGF secretion may become excessive, and mediate pathological angiogenesis. On the other hand, however, VEGF-induced neoangiogenesis cannot be viewed as the sole culprit of the peritoneal membrane dysfunction. Computer simulations suggest that an increase in peritoneal exchange surface area alone will not account for a massive decrease in drained volumes (Rippe et al., 1991). One has to bear in mind, however, there exists a tight link between angiogenesis and fibrosis (Wynn, 2007). In fact, detailed studies of peritoneal biopsies showed that the degree of peritoneal fibrosis correlated with greater vascular density and, conversely, fibrosis occurred infrequently in the absence of vasculopathy (Williams et al., 2002). Thus, the contribution of mesothelial cell-derived VEGF to the peritoneal membrane dysfunction is probably multifactorial, and is related both to a direct increase in peritoneal permeability and the involvement in peritoneal fibrosis (Fig. 2).

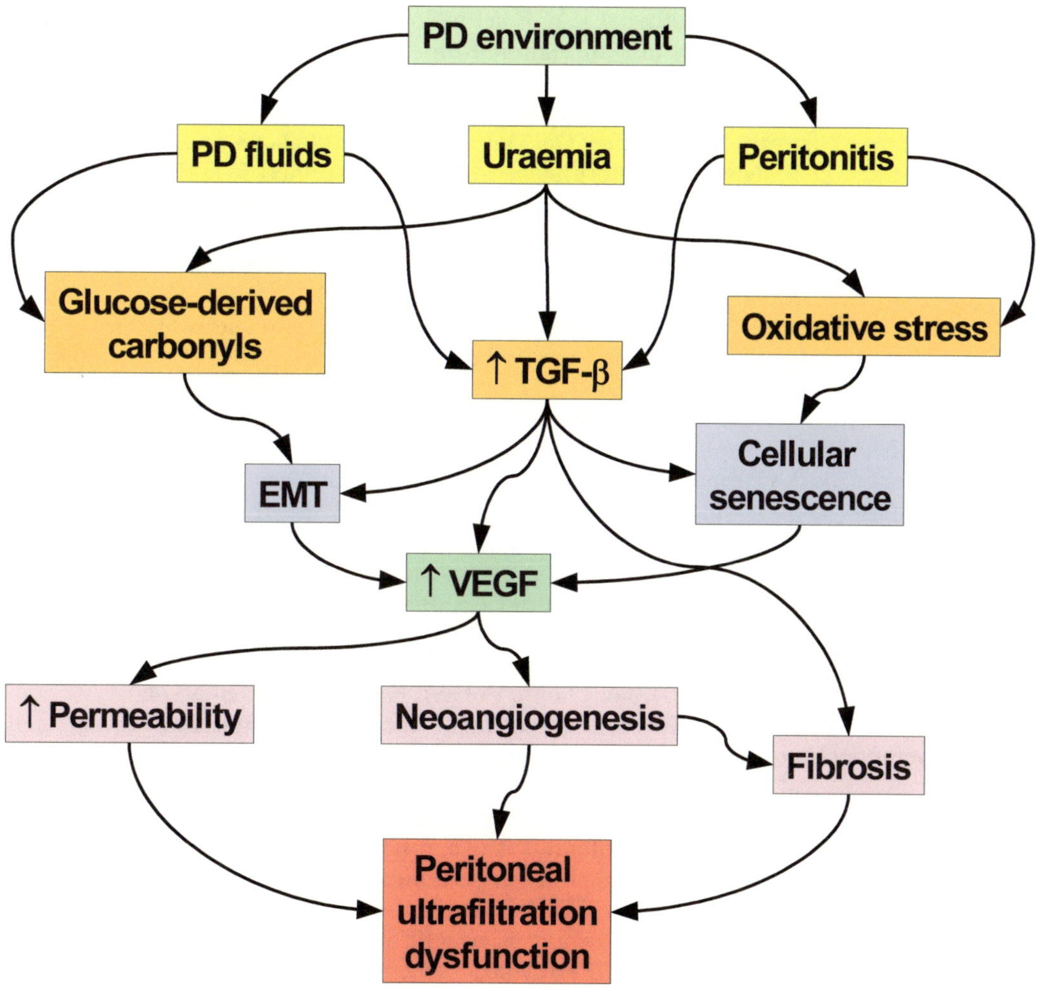

Fig. 2. Possible impact of PD environment on mesothelial cell VEGF expression and peritoneal membrane dysfunction.

7. References

Aroeira, L.S. et al. (2007). Epithelial to mesenchymal transition and peritoneal membrane failure in peritoneal dialysis patients: pathologic significance and potential therapeutic interventions. J.Am.Soc.Nephrol., Vol.18, No.7, pp. 2004-2013.

Aroeira, L.S. et al. (2005). Mesenchymal conversion of mesothelial cells as a mechanism responsible for high solute transport rate in peritoneal dialysis: role of vascular endothelial growth factor. Am.J.Kidney Dis., Vol.46, No.5, pp. 938-948.

Aroeira, L.S. et al. (2009). Cyclooxygenase-2 mediates dialysate-induced alterations of the peritoneal membrane. J.Am.Soc.Nephrol., Vol.20, No.3, pp. 582-592.

Bajo, M.A. et al. (2011). Low-GDP peritoneal dialysis fluid ('balance') has less impact in vitro and ex vivo on epithelial-to-mesenchymal transition (EMT) of mesothelial cells than a standard fluid. Nephrol.Dial.Transplant., Vol.26, No.1, pp. 282-291.

Bashan, N. et al. (2009). Positive and negative regulation of insulin signaling by reactive oxygen and nitrogen species. Physiol.Rev., Vol.89, No.1, pp. 27-71.

Boulanger, E. et al. (2007). Mesothelial RAGE activation by AGEs enhances VEGF release and potentiates capillary tube formation. Kidney Int., Vol.71, No.2, pp. 126-133.

Brauner, A. et al. (1996). Tumor necrosis factor-alpha, interleukin-1 beta, and interleukin-1 receptor antagonist in dialysate and serum from patients on continuous ambulatory peritoneal dialysis. Am.J.Kidney Dis., Vol.27, No.3, pp. 402-408.

Brogan, I.J. et al. (1999). Novel polymorphisms in the promoter and 5' UTR regions of the human vascular endothelial growth factor gene. Hum.Immunol., Vol.60, No.12, pp. 1245-1249.

Campisi, J. (2011). Cellular senescence: putting the paradoxes in perspective. Curr.Opin.Genet.Dev., Vol.21, No.1, pp.107-112.

Carmeliet, P. et al. (1996). Abnormal blood vessel development and lethality in embryos lacking a single VEGF allele. Nature, Vol.380, No.6573, pp. 435-439.

Cho, J.H. et al. (2010). Impact of systemic and local peritoneal inflammation on peritoneal solute transport rate in new peritoneal dialysis patients: a 1-year prospective study. Nephrol.Dial.Transplant., Vol.25, No.6, pp. 1964-1973.

Combet, S. et al. (2001). Chronic uremia induces permeability changes, increased nitric oxide synthase expression, and structural modifications in the peritoneum. J.Am Soc.Nephrol., Vol.12, No.10, pp. 2146-2157.

Combet, S. et al. (2000). Vascular proliferation and enhanced expression of endothelial nitric oxide synthase in human peritoneum exposed to long-term peritoneal dialysis. J.Am Soc.Nephrol., Vol.11, No.4, pp. 717-728.

Coppe, J.P. et al. (2006). Secretion of vascular endothelial growth factor by primary human fibroblasts at senescence. J.Biol.Chem., Vol.281, No.40, pp. 29568-29574.

Coppe, J.P. et al. (2008). Senescence-associated secretory phenotypes reveal cell-nonautonomous functions of oncogenic RAS and the p53 tumor suppressor. PLoS.Biol., Vol.6, No.12, pp. 2853-2868.

Coppe, J.P. et al. (2010). The senescence-associated secretory phenotype: the dark side of tumor suppression. Annu.Rev.Pathol., Vol.5, pp. 99-118.

Davies, S.J. et al. (1996). Longitudinal changes in peritoneal kinetics: the effects of peritoneal dialysis and peritonitis. Nephrol.Dial.Transplant., Vol.11, No.3, pp. 498-506.

de Alvaro, F. et al. (1993). Peritoneal resting is beneficial in peritoneal hyperpermeability and ultrafiltration failure. Adv.Perit.Dial., Vol.9, pp. 56-61.

De Vriese, A.S. et al. (2006). Myofibroblast transdifferentiation of mesothelial cells is mediated by RAGE and contributes to peritoneal fibrosis in uraemia. Nephrol.Dial.Transplant., Vol.21, No.9, pp. 2549-2555.

Ferrara, N. et al. (1996). Heterozygous embryonic lethality induced by targeted inactivation of the VEGF gene. Nature, Vol.380, No.6573, pp. 439-442.

Fukumura, D. et al. (2001). Predominant role of endothelial nitric oxide synthase in vascular endothelial growth factor-induced angiogenesis and vascular permeability. Proc.Natl.Acad.Sci.U.S.A, Vol.98, No.5, pp. 2604-2609.

Gerber, S.A. et al. (2006). Preferential attachment of peritoneal tumor metastases to omental immune aggregates and possible role of a unique vascular microenvironment in metastatic survival and growth. Am.J.Pathol., Vol.169, No.5, pp. 1739-1752.

Gillerot, G. et al. (2005). Genetic and clinical factors influence the baseline permeability of the peritoneal membrane. Kidney Int., Vol.67, No.6, pp. 2477-2487.

Gotloib, L. et al. (2003). Icodextrin-induced lipid peroxidation disrupts the mesothelial cell cycle engine. Free Radic.Biol.Med., Vol.34, No.4, pp. 419-428.

Gotloib, L. et al. (2007). The use of peritoneal mesothelium as a potential source of adult stem cells. Int.J.Artif.Organs, Vol.30, No.6, pp. 501-512.

Heimburger, O. et al. (1990). Peritoneal transport in CAPD patients with permanent loss of ultrafiltration capacity. Kidney Int., Vol.38, No.3, pp. 495-506.

Heimburger, O. et al. (1999). Alterations in water and solute transport with time on peritoneal dialysis. Perit.Dial.Int., Vol.19 Suppl 2, pp. S83-S90.

Hirahara, I. et al. (2006). Peritoneal injury by methylglyoxal in peritoneal dialysis. Perit.Dial.Int., Vol.26, No.3, pp. 380-392.

Hirahara, I. et al. (2009). Methylglyoxal induces peritoneal thickening by mesenchymal-like mesothelial cells in rats. Nephrol.Dial.Transplant., Vol.24, No.2, pp. 437-447.

Ho-Dac-Pannekeet, M.M. et al. (1997). Analysis of ultrafiltration failure in peritoneal dialysis patients by means of standard peritoneal permeability analysis. Perit.Dial.Int., Vol.17, No.2, pp. 144-150.

Honda, K. et al. (1999). Accumulation of advanced glycation end products in the peritoneal vasculature of continuous ambulatory peritoneal dialysis patients with low ultra-filtration. Nephrol.Dial.Transplant., Vol.14, No.6, pp. 1541-1549.

Honda, K. et al. (2008). Impact of uremia, diabetes, and peritoneal dialysis itself on the pathogenesis of peritoneal sclerosis: a quantitative study of peritoneal membrane morphology. Clin.J.Am.Soc.Nephrol., Vol.3, No.3, pp. 720-728.

Inagi, R. et al. (1999). Glucose degradation product methylglyoxal enhances the production of vascular endothelial growth factor in peritoneal cells: role in the functional and morphological alterations of peritoneal membranes in peritoneal dialysis. FEBS Lett., Vol.463, No.3, pp. 260-264.

Kawaguchi, Y. et al. (1997). Issues affecting the longevity of the continuous peritoneal dialysis therapy. Kidney Int.Suppl, Vol.62, pp. S105-S107.

Kihm, L.P. et al. (2008). RAGE expression in the human peritoneal membrane. Nephrol.Dial.Transplant., Vol.23, No.10, pp. 3302-3306.

Krediet, R.T. (2001). Dialysate cancer antigen 125 concentration as marker of peritoneal membrane status in patients treated with chronic peritoneal dialysis. Perit.Dial.Int., Vol.21, No.6, pp. 560-567.

Ksiazek, K. et al. (2006). Early loss of proliferative potential of human peritoneal mesothelial cells in culture: the role of p16INK4a-mediated premature senescence. J.Appl.Physiol, Vol.100, No.3, pp. 988-995.

Ksiazek, K. et al. (2007a). Oxidative stress contributes to accelerated development of the senescent phenotype in human peritoneal mesothelial cells exposed to high glucose. Free Radic.Biol.Med., Vol.42, No.5, pp. 636-641.

Ksiazek, K. et al. (2007b). Accelerated senescence of human peritoneal mesothelial cells exposed to high glucose: the role of TGF-beta1. Lab.Invest, Vol.87, No.4, pp. 345-356.

Ksiazek, K. et al. (2007c). Premature senescence of mesothelial cells is associated with non-telomeric DNA damage. Biochem.Biophys.Res.Commun., Vol.362, No.3, pp. 707-711.

Ksiazek, K. et al. (2008a). Senescence induces a proangiogenic switch in human peritoneal mesothelial cells. Rejuvenation Res., Vol.11, No.3, pp. 681-683.

Ksiazek, K. et al. (2008b). Oxidative stress-mediated early senescence contributes to the short replicative life span of human peritoneal mesothelial cells. Free Radic.Biol.Med., Vol.45, pp. 460-467.

Lai, K.N. et al. (2004). Differential expression of receptors for advanced glycation end-products in peritoneal mesothelial cells exposed to glucose degradation products. Clin.Exp.Immunol., Vol.138, No.3, pp. 466-475.

Leung, J.C. et al. (2005). Glucose degradation products downregulate ZO-1 expression in human peritoneal mesothelial cells: the role of VEGF. Nephrol.Dial.Transplant., Vol.20, No.7, pp. 1336-1349.

Loureiro, J. et al. (2010). BMP-7 blocks mesenchymal conversion of mesothelial cells and prevents peritoneal damage induced by dialysis fluid exposure. Nephrol.Dial.Transplant., Vol.25, No.4, pp. 1098-1108.

Mandl-Weber, S. et al. (2002). Vascular endothelial growth factor production and regulation in human peritoneal mesothelial cells. Kidney Int., Vol.61, No.2, pp. 570-578.

Margetts, P.J. & Churchill, D.N. (2002). Acquired ultrafiltration dysfunction in peritoneal dialysis patients. J.Am.Soc.Nephrol., Vol.13, No.11, pp. 2787-2794.

Margetts, P.J. et al. (2002). Inflammatory cytokines, angiogenesis, and fibrosis in the rat peritoneum. Am.J.Pathol., Vol.160, No.6, pp. 2285-2294.

Margetts, P.J. et al. (2005). Transient overexpression of TGF-{beta}1 induces epithelial mesenchymal transition in the rodent peritoneum. J.Am.Soc.Nephrol., Vol.16, No.2, pp. 425-436.

Maruyama, Y. et al. (2007). Relationship between the -374T/A receptor of advanced glycation end products gene polymorphism and peritoneal solute transport status at the initiation of peritoneal dialysis. Ther.Apher.Dial., Vol.11, No.4, pp. 301-305.

Mateijsen, M.A. et al. (1999). Vascular and interstitial changes in the peritoneum of CAPD patients with peritoneal sclerosis. Perit.Dial.Int., Vol.19, No.6, pp. 517-525.

Miyata, T. et al. (1999). Alterations in nonenzymatic biochemistry in uremia: origin and significance of "carbonyl stress" in long-term uremic complications. Kidney Int., Vol.55, No.2, pp. 389-399.

Miyata, T. et al. (2001). Reactive carbonyl compounds related uremic toxicity ("carbonyl stress"). Kidney Int.Suppl, Vol.78, pp. S25-S31.

Mortier, S. et al. (2002). Hemodynamic effects of peritoneal dialysis solutions on the rat peritoneal membrane: role of acidity, buffer choice, glucose concentration, and glucose degradation products. J.Am.Soc.Nephrol., Vol.13, No.2, pp. 480-489.

Mortier, S. et al. (2004). Long-term exposure to new peritoneal dialysis solutions: Effects on the peritoneal membrane. Kidney Int., Vol.66, No.3, pp. 1257-1265.

Moutabarrik, A. et al. (1995). Interleukin-1 and its naturally occurring antagonist in peritoneal dialysis patients. Clin.Nephrol., Vol.43, No.4, pp. 243-248.

Nagy, J.A. et al. (2007). VEGF-A and the induction of pathological angiogenesis. Annu.Rev.Pathol., Vol.2, pp. 251-275.

Nakayama, M. et al. (1997). Immunohistochemical detection of advanced glycosylation end-products in the peritoneum and its possible pathophysiological role in CAPD. Kidney Int., Vol.51, No.1, pp. 182-186.

Nakayama, M. et al. (2003). Hyper-vascular change and formation of advanced glycation endproducts in the peritoneum caused by methylglyoxal and the effect of an anti-oxidant, sodium sulfite. Am.J.Nephrol., Vol.23, No.6, pp. 390-394.

Nevado, J. et al. (2005). Amadori adducts activate nuclear factor-kappaB-related proinflammatory genes in cultured human peritoneal mesothelial cells. Br.J.Pharmacol., Vol.146, No.2, pp. 268-279.

Ni, J. et al. (2003). Mice that lack endothelial nitric oxide synthase are protected against functional and structural modifications induced by acute peritonitis. J.Am.Soc.Nephrol., Vol.14, No.12, pp. 3205-3216.

Olsson, A.K. et al. (2006). VEGF receptor signalling - in control of vascular function. Nat.Rev.Mol.Cell Biol, Vol.7, No.5, pp. 359-371.

Otrock, Z.K. et al. (2007). Vascular endothelial growth factor family of ligands and receptors: review. Blood Cells Mol.Dis., Vol.38, No.3, pp. 258-268.

Patel, P. et al. (2010a). Smad3-dependent and -independent pathways are involved in peritoneal membrane injury. Kidney Int., Vol.77, No.4, pp. 319-328.

Patel, P. et al. (2010b). Platelet derived growth factor B and epithelial mesenchymal transition of peritoneal mesothelial cells. Matrix Biol., Vol.29, No.2, pp. 97-106.

Pecoits-Filho, R. et al. (2002). Plasma and dialysate IL-6 and VEGF concentrations are associated with high peritoneal solute transport rate. Nephrol.Dial.Transplant., Vol.17, No.8, pp. 1480-1486.

Rippe, B. et al. (1991). Computer simulations of peritoneal fluid transport in CAPD. Kidney Int., Vol.40, No.2, pp. 315-325.

Rodrigues, A. et al. (2002). Peritoneal rest may successfully recover ultrafiltration in patients who develop peritoneal hyperpermeability with time on continuous ambulatory peritoneal dialysis. Adv.Perit.Dial., Vol.18, pp. 78-80.

Rodrigues, A. et al. (2004). Evaluation of effluent markers cancer antigen 125, vascular endothelial growth factor, and interleukin-6: relationship with peritoneal transport. Adv.Perit.Dial., Vol.20, pp. 8-12.

Rodrigues, A. et al. (2007). Evaluation of peritoneal transport and membrane status in peritoneal dialysis: focus on incident fast transporters. Am.J.Nephrol., Vol.27, No.1, pp. 84-91.

Schneider, B.P. et al. (2009). The role of vascular endothelial growth factor genetic variability in cancer. Clin.Cancer Res., Vol.15, No.17, pp. 5297-5302.

Schwenger, V. et al. (2006). Damage to the peritoneal membrane by glucose degradation products is mediated by the receptor for advanced glycation end-products. J.Am.Soc.Nephrol., Vol.17, No.1, pp. 199-207.

Selgas, R. et al. (2000). Spontaneous VEGF production by cultured peritoneal mesothelial cells from patients on peritoneal dialysis. Perit.Dial.Int., Vol.20, No.6, pp. 798-801.

Selgas, R. et al. (2001). Vascular endothelial growth factor (VEGF) levels in peritoneal dialysis effluent. J.Nephrol., Vol.14, No.4, pp. 270-274.

Siegel, P.M. & Massague, J. (2003). Cytostatic and apoptotic actions of TGF-beta in homeostasis and cancer. Nat.Rev.Cancer, Vol.3, No.11, pp. 807-821.

Struijk, D.G. et al. (1994). A prospective study of peritoneal transport in CAPD patients. Kidney Int., Vol.45, No.6, pp. 1739-1744.

Szeto, C.C. et al. (2004). Genetic polymorphism of VEGF: Impact on longitudinal change of peritoneal transport and survival of peritoneal dialysis patients. Kidney Int., Vol.65, No.5, pp. 1947-1955.

Szeto, C.C. et al. (2005). Differential effects of transforming growth factor-beta on the synthesis of connective tissue growth factor and vascular endothelial growth factor by peritoneal mesothelial cell. Nephron Exp.Nephrol., Vol.99, No.4, pp. e95-e104.

Szeto, C.C. et al. (2006). Connective tissue growth factor is responsible for transforming growth factor-beta-induced peritoneal mesothelial cell apoptosis. Nephron Exp.Nephrol., Vol.103, No.4, pp. e166-e174.

Tauer, A. et al. (2001). In vitro formation of N(epsilon)-(carboxymethyl)lysine and imidazolones under conditions similar to continuous ambulatory peritoneal dialysis. Biochem.Biophys.Res.Commun., Vol.280, No.5, pp. 1408-1414.

Vargha, R. et al. (2006). Ex vivo reversal of in vivo transdifferentiation in mesothelial cells grown from peritoneal dialysate effluents. Nephrol.Dial.Transplant., Vol.21, No.10, pp. 2943-2947.

Watson, C.J. et al. (2000). Identification of polymorphisms within the vascular endothelial growth factor (VEGF) gene: correlation with variation in VEGF protein production. Cytokine, Vol.12, No.8, pp. 1232-1235.

Wieslander, A.P. et al. (1991). Toxicity of peritoneal dialysis fluids on cultured fibroblasts, L-929. Kidney Int., Vol.40, No.1, pp. 77-79.

Williams, J.D. et al. (2002). Morphologic changes in the peritoneal membrane of patients with renal disease. J.Am.Soc.Nephrol., Vol.13, No.2, pp. 470-479.

Williams, J.D. et al. (2003). The natural course of peritoneal membrane biology during peritoneal dialysis. Kidney Int.Suppl., No.88, pp. S43-S49.

Witowski, J. et al. (2008). Glucose-induced mesothelial cell senescence and peritoneal neoangiogenesis and fibrosis. Perit.Dial.Int., Vol.28 Suppl.5, pp. S34-S37.

Wynn, T.A. (2007). Common and unique mechanisms regulate fibrosis in various fibroproliferative diseases. J.Clin.Invest, Vol.117, No.3, pp. 524-529.

Yanez-Mo, M. et al. (2003). Peritoneal dialysis and epithelial-to-mesenchymal transition of mesothelial cells. N.Engl.J.Med., Vol.348, No.5, pp. 403-413.

Yang, A.H. et al. (2003). Myofibroblastic conversion of mesothelial cells. Kidney Int., Vol.63, No.4, pp. 1530-1539.

Yu, M.A. et al. (2009). HGF and BMP-7 ameliorate high glucose-induced epithelial-to-mesenchymal transition of peritoneal mesothelium. J.Am.Soc.Nephrol., Vol.20, No.3, pp. 567-581.

Zavadil, J. & Bottinger, E.P. (2005). TGF-beta and epithelial-to-mesenchymal transitions. Oncogene, Vol.24, No.37, pp. 5764-5774.

Zeisberg, M. et al. (2003). BMP-7 counteracts TGF-beta1-induced epithelial-to-mesenchymal transition and reverses chronic renal injury. Nat.Med., Vol.9, No.7, pp. 964-968.

Zemel, D. et al. (1994). Appearance of tumor necrosis factor-alpha and soluble TNF-receptors I and II in peritoneal effluent of CAPD. Kidney Int., Vol.46, No.5, pp. 1422-1430.

Zhang, J. et al. (2008). Vascular endothelial growth factor expression in peritoneal mesothelial cells undergoing transdifferentiation. Perit.Dial.Int., Vol.28, No.5, pp. 497-504.

Zhu, F. et al. (2010). Preventive effect of Notch signaling inhibition by a gamma-secretase inhibitor on peritoneal dialysis fluid-induced peritoneal fibrosis in rats. Am.J.Pathol., Vol.176, No.2, pp. 650-659.

Zweers, M.M. et al. (1999). Growth factors VEGF and TGF-beta1 in peritoneal dialysis. J.Lab.Clin.Med., Vol.134, No.2, pp. 124-132.

5

Matrix Metalloproteinases Cause Peritoneal Injury in Peritoneal Dialysis

Ichiro Hirahara, Tetsu Akimoto, Yoshiyuki Morishita,
Makoto Inoue, Osamu Saito, Shigeaki Muto and Eiji Kusano
*Division of Nephrology, Department of Internal Medicine, Jichi Medical University
Japan*

1. Introduction

Long-term peritoneal dialysis (PD) leads to peritoneal injury with functional decline, such as ultrafiltration loss. Peritoneal injury is often accompanied by histological changes, such as peritoneal fibrosis and sclerosis. These complications involve evident diffuse fibrous thickening and/or edema of the peritoneum, and chronic inflammation (epithelial to mesenchymal transition of mesothelial cells as well as migration and proliferation of polynuclear leucocytes, macrophages, and mesenchymal cells in the peritoneum). At worst, peritoneal injury leads to encapsulating peritoneal sclerosis (EPS), a serious complication of PD [1-6]. At early stage of EPS (preEPS stage), peritoneal effluent with signs of inflammation is often observed [2]. At advanced stages of EPS, the small intestine adheres and is encapsulated within a collagen rich thick peritoneum to form a cocoon-like mass. As a result, EPS is associated with clinical symptoms, such as loss of appetite, nausea, vomiting, and emaciation due to malnutrition, as well as symptoms of intestinal obstruction that include abdominal pain, diarrhea, constipation, or lowered peristaltic bowel sounds. The incidence of EPS is not high: it occurs in about 0.4%–3.3% of patients who undergo PD. However, EPS has a high mortality rate, about half of the patients with EPS die [2-5]. The causes of functional disorders of the peritoneum are believed to be fibrosis, sclerosis, inflammation, angiogenesis, and vasculopathy. Peritoneal injury is probably caused by multiple factors, such as infection with bacteria or fungi resulting in peritonitis [2, 5, 6]; antiseptics [7-11]; exogenous materials like particulates and plasticizers [7]; and continuous exposure to nonphysiological PD solutions having high concentrations of glucose and glucose degradation products (GDPs), low pH, and high osmolarity [2, 12, 13]. Administration of corticosteroids, tamoxifen, immunosuppressive agents, and total parenteral nutrition are effective in the early stage of EPS development [2-4, 6]. However, for advanced EPS, in which bowel adhesions have formed, the only effective therapeutic method is surgical dissection of the encapsulated peritoneum; this must be performed by skilled surgeons using specialized techniques [2-5, 7]. It is important to monitor peritoneal injury, and develop methods for an early diagnosis of EPS. At present, major diagnostic methods for EPS include abdominal palpation (for identification of a mass) and finding clinical symptoms of bowel obstruction, like those found in the ileus [2]. However, these are not objective criteria and it is not rare that no typical symptoms are found even in advanced cases of EPS. Some physicians utilize diagnostic imaging methods for detection of EPS, such as X-ray, computed tomography, and ultrasonography; however, these methods are not suitable for early diagnosis because they can detect only EPS in an advanced stage [2, 3, 6]. C-reactive protein (CRP) and interleukin-6 (IL-6) are often used as biochemical markers for inflammation [2, 6, 14, 15]. However, since their levels also increase during infectious peritonitis, they are inadequate to be used as definitive diagnostic markers that can differentiate EPS from infectious peritonitis [14]. As mentioned previously, corticosteroids and immunosuppressive agents have been employed as effective initial therapies for EPS [2-4, 6]; however these drugs, compromise the immune system with the risk of aggravating symptoms when administered to patients with infectious peritonitis. Therefore, a method can differentiate EPS from infectious peritonitis is required for the early diagnosis of EPS. To perform PD safely, it is important to monitor peritoneal injury that may progress to EPS and diagnose EPS at an early stage; it is then necessary to prevent peritoneal injury from developing into severe EPS.

During tissue injury, such as sclerosis or fibrosis, tissue destruction and excessive remodeling occur. In such events, matrix metalloproteinases (MMPs) degrade components of the extracellular matrix (ECM) and play significant roles in regulating angiogenesis, epithelial to mesenchymal transition, and migration of cells that promote fibroplasias or inflammation. MMP-1, an interstitial collagenase, degrades types I, II, III, VII, and X collagen. MMP-2, a gelatinase, degrades gelatin, type IV collagen, fibronectin, laminin, proteoglycan, and elastin. MMP-3, a stromelysin, degrades proteoglycan, gelatin, fibronectin, laminin, elastin, and type IV collagen. MMP-9, a gelatinase, degrades gelatin, type IV collagen, proteoglycans, elastin, and entactin. Membrane-type MMP-1 (MT1-MMP) contains a C-terminal transmembrane domain that anchors to the plasma membrane and cleaves proMMP-2 to produce its active form on the cell surface. Tissue inhibitors of MMP (TIMPs) inhibit ECM degradation by MMPs and play important roles in the proteolytic/antiproteolytic balance. TIMP-2 inhibits the activity of MT-MMPs, but TIMP-1 does not. MMP expression is enhanced in various tissues during inflammation, fibrosis and sclerosis. Increased serum levels of MMP-1 and MMP-3 in rheumatoid arthritis [16], MMP-1, MMP-8, and MMP-9 in cystic fibrosis [17], MMP-9 in chronic obstructive pulmonary disease [18], MMP-2, MMP-9, and TIMP-1 in acute coronary syndrome [19], MMP-9 and TIMP-1 in aortic sclerosis [20], MMP-2 in liver cirrhosis [21], MMP-2 and TIMP-1 in hepatic fibrosis [22], and MMP-2 in chronic kidney disease [23, 24] suggest a relationship between MMP levels and pathology of tissue injury.

2. Production of MMP-2 in animal models of peritoneal injury

MMP-2 production increases in animal models of peritoneal injury induced by stimuli such as antiseptics, exogenous materials, and GDPs.

In rodent models of peritoneal injury, the development of EPS was analyzed by injecting the antiseptic chlorhexidine gluconate into the peritoneal cavity to induce inflammation [7-11]. In this model, MMP-2 levels in the peritoneal effluent and MMP-2 gene expression in the peritoneum correlated with changes in thickness of the peritoneum, inflammation, D/D0 glucose levels, and net ultrafiltration. In another model, peritoneal injury was induced by injecting talc, an exogenous material, into the peritoneal cavity. MMP-2 levels in the peritoneal effluent and MMP-2 gene expression in the peritoneum increased with the development of peritoneal injury [7]. GDPs are generated in PD solutions during heat sterilization and storage, and contribute to the bioincompatibility of conventional PD solutions. MMP-2 levels in the peritoneal effluent increased in models of peritoneal injury induced by methylglyoxal (MGO) or formaldehyde, both extremely toxic GDPs [12, 13]. In models of peritoneal injury induced by chlorhexidine gluconate and MGO, abdominal cocoons were often formed, while in models induced by talc and formaldehyde, adhesions of the peritoneum were observed [7-9, 11, 12]. In many animal models of peritoneal injury, MMP-2 levels in the peritoneal effluent correlated with changes in inflammation, thickness of the peritoneum, D/D0 glucose levels, and net ultrafiltration. Thus, peritoneal injury is caused by increased MMP-2 induced by various stimuli, such as antiseptics, exogenous materials, and GDPs in the PD solution. Therefore, MMP-2 may play an important role in the development of peritoneal injury leading to EPS.

3. MMPs as peritoneal injury markers in clinical diagnosis

Results of the peritoneal equilibration test (PET) performed clinically have shown that MMP-2, -3, and TIMP-1 levels in the peritoneal effluent correlate with peritoneal injury (Figure 1) [25, 26]. PET is the method most frequently used to estimate PD efficiency and peritoneal injury [2, 27]. MMP-3 levels are influenced by gender and etiology of end-stage renal disease [26] and TIMP-1 expression is known to be induced by various factors, such as IL-1, tumor necrosis factor-α, and transforming growth factor-β [23]; however, MMP-2 is usually expressed constitutively. MMP-3 and TIMP-1 may therefore be more easily affected by various factors than MMP-2. The measured D/S ratios of MMP-3 were nearly equal to the predicted D/S ratios when MMP-3 was transported only from the circulation [26]. This result suggests that most MMP-3 in the peritoneal effluent may be transported from the circulation. In contrast, the measured D/S ratios of MMP-2 and TIMP-1 were significantly higher than those predicted [26]. In addition, the correlation coefficient between the drainage levels of MMP-2 and TIMP-1 was higher than that between the drainage levels of MMP-2 and MMP-3 [26]. The difference between the measured D/S ratio and the predicted ratio may be attributable to the local production of MMP-2 and TIMP-1 in the peritoneal tissue along with their transport from the circulation [28]. In addition, MMP-1 and TIMP-2 were not detected in the peritoneal effluent of most patients. Therefore, MMP-1 and TIMP-2 are unsuitable as markers for determining the extent of peritoneal injury. These results suggest that MMP-2 may be a more useful marker of peritoneal injury with increased solute transport than other MMPs or TIMPs.

IL-6, hyaluronic acid, and cancer antigen (CA) 125 are often used as markers of peritoneal injury [2, 29]. In the study by Kaku et al., although the sample size was not sufficient for a statistically significant relationship, the correlation coefficient between the peritoneal solute transport rate and MMP-2 levels was higher than that for IL-6, hyaluronic acid, or CA125 [15].

MMP-2 and/or MMP-9 degrade the endothelial basal lamina and increase vascular permeability [30]. Swann et al. have also reported that an increase in the permeability of the blood-brain barrier is associated with an increase in MMP levels, which digests the endothelial basal lamina that forms the barrier [31]. In PD, the microvascular wall and probably the interstitial tissue are the main barriers for peritoneal fluid and solute transport. MMP-2 digests type IV collagen and laminin, which are the main basement membrane components of the microvascular wall and the mesothelial layer. Thus, injury to the basement membrane by MMP-2 may result in fast solute transport rates. Giebel et al. have reported that elevated MMP-2 or MMP-9 expression in the retina may facilitate an increase in vascular permeability by degrading occludin, the tight junction protein of endothelial or epithelial cells [32]. Osada et al. have reported that MMP-2 was mainly observed around

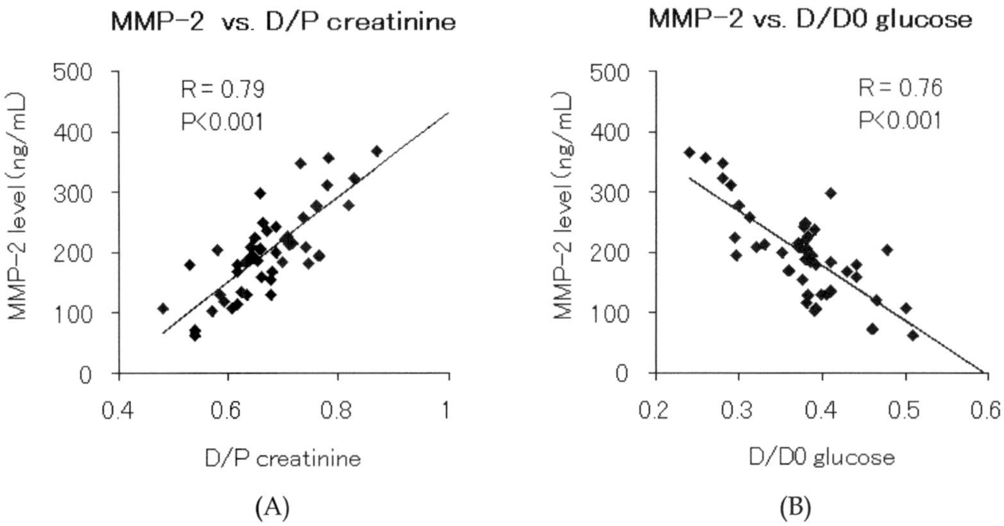

Fig. 1. Relationship between the peritoneal solute transport rate and MMP-2 levels in the peritoneal effluent.
The peritoneal solute transport rate was assessed using PET. MMP-2 levels in the peritoneal effluent obtained from PET were analyzed by enzyme-linked immunosorbent assay. (A) D/P creatinine ratios versus MMP-2 levels. (B) D/D0 glucose ratios versus MMP-2 levels.

the blood vessels in the peritoneal tissues from long-term PD patients [33]. In PD, destruction of the tight junction of endothelial cells by MMP-2 may result in hyperpermeability of the peritoneum. From these studies, it is apparent that MMP-2 may directly increase the permeability of the peritoneum by destruction of the basement membrane and tight junction of endothelial cells.

A multi-center clinical study and a case report revealed markedly increased MMP-2 levels in peritoneal effluents of patients with moderate peritoneal injury with ascites [2, 25, 34]. In addition, EPS was shown to develop in more than half the patients having MMP-2 levels of more than 600 ng/ml, although half of the patients had been treated with steroids [26]. On the other hand, MMP-2 levels in the effluents of patients with EPS tended to be lower than those of patients with moderate peritoneal injury [26]. In advance-stage of EPS, the inflammation is weak and then MMP-2 levels in the effluents may be decreased. These findings suggest that a change in MMP-2 levels may be used as indicator of peritoneal injury or progression to EPS.

MMP-9 is hardly detected in the peritoneal effluent of patients without infectious peritonitis. However, in patients with infectious peritonitis, MMP-9 levels in the peritoneal effluent increased markedly with a slight increase in MMP-2 levels [25, 35, 36]. These findings suggest that peritoneal injury that may lead to EPS can be clearly distinguished from infectious peritonitis by analyzing MMP-2 and MMP-9 levels in the peritoneal effluent (Figure 2). Many biomarkers, such as IL-6 and CRP, increase during peritoneal injury and infectious peritonitis. Therefore, MMP-2 may be a useful indicator for peritoneal injury that can differentiate from infectious peritonitis.

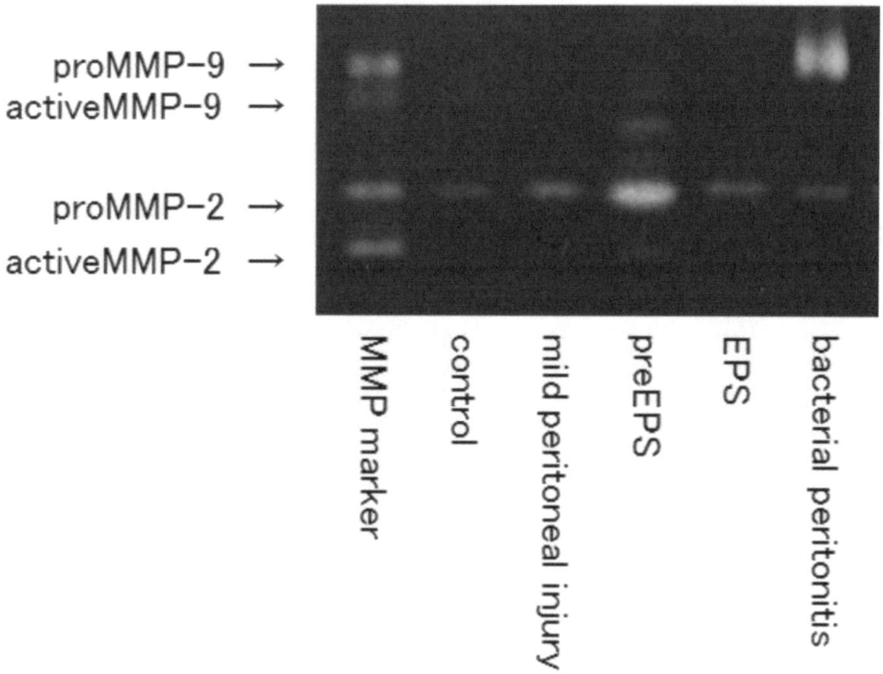

Fig. 2. Analysis of the peritoneal effluent with gelatin zymography.
Gelatinases in the peritoneal effluent were analyzed by gelatin zymography. Gelatinases were detected as unstained proteolytic bands in gel stained with Coomassie Brilliant Blue. Lane 1: MMP marker (Chemicon International, Inc., Temecula, CA, USA). Lane 2: Control patient. Lane 3: Patient with mild peritoneal injury. Lane 4: Patient with moderate peritoneal injury (preEPS). Lane 5: Patient with severe peritoneal injury (EPS). Lane 6: Patient with bacterial peritonitis.

Minami et al. investigated the correlations between β_2-microglobulin (β_2MG) and peritoneal injury biomarkers (e.g. hyaluronic acid, IL-6, MMP-2) in the peritoneal effluent obtained from a 7.5% icodextrin-based PD solution (ICO effluent) [37]. β_2MG, hyaluronic acid, and MMP-2 levels in the ICO effluent were significantly higher than those in the 2.27% glucose-based PD solution effluent. There was a trend toward higher IL-6 levels in the ICO effluent, although no significant differences were seen. There were positive correlations between the levels of various biomarkers and β_2MG. Those authors proposed that subclinical injury of the peritoneum by ICO treatment may accelerate peritoneal permeability to increase β_2MG in the effluent.

Nishina et al. have reported that MMP-2 levels decreased in the peritoneal effluent and peritoneal function improved when conventional solutions (acidic pH and containing high levels of GDPs) were replaced with new PD solutions (neutral pH and containing low levels of GDPs) in high-transporter patients undergoing PD [38].

Thus MMPs are possible markers of peritoneal injury that can differentiate from infectious peritonitis. A diagnostic method using peritoneal effluents enables easy sampling, is non-invasive, and is not painful for patients. An MMP-9 test kit has been developed to diagnose infectious peritonitis. This kit consists of an anti-MMP-9 antibody conjugated to a colloidal dye designed to detect MMP-9 in a nitrocellulose membrane dipstick assay based on immunochromatography [36, 39]. The diagnosis can be successfully completed within 10 min. If such a test kit were developed for MMP-2, peritoneal injury could be monitored easily and rapidly at home.

4. Production of MMP-2 in the peritoneum

MMP-2 in the peritoneal tissue and effluent is considered to be primarily derived from activated cells in the peritoneum.

Gene expression analysis and/or immunohistochemistry analysis revealed that MMP-2, MT1-MMP, and TIMP-2 are produced in the peritoneal tissue [7-13, 25]. MMP-2 is produced by peritoneal cells, such as macrophages, mesenchymal cells, endothelial cells, and mesothelial cells (Figures 3 and 4, Table). These peritoneal cells are activated by various stimuli, such as infectious peritonitis; exogenous materials like particulates; antiseptics; advanced glycation products; and GDPs and also the pH of the PD solution. These activated cells produce various cytokines, growth factors, and other mediators that induce peritoneal injury. Macrophages may infiltrate or migrate into the peritoneum while ECM is being degraded by MMP-2 produced by these cells [8, 12]. In cultured human mesothelial cells, the production of MMP-2 is upregulated by transforming growth factor-β and is decreased by thrombin [40-42]. Activated mesothelial cells transform to mesenchymal cells and then the epithelial-to-mesenchymal transition of mesothelial cells subsequently induces MMP-2 production [13, 43]. Transformed mesothelial cells may invade the peritoneum while ECM is being digested by MMP-2 and upregulates the production of vascular endothelial growth factor that enhances angiogenesis, nitric oxide synthesis, and vascular permeability [25, 26].

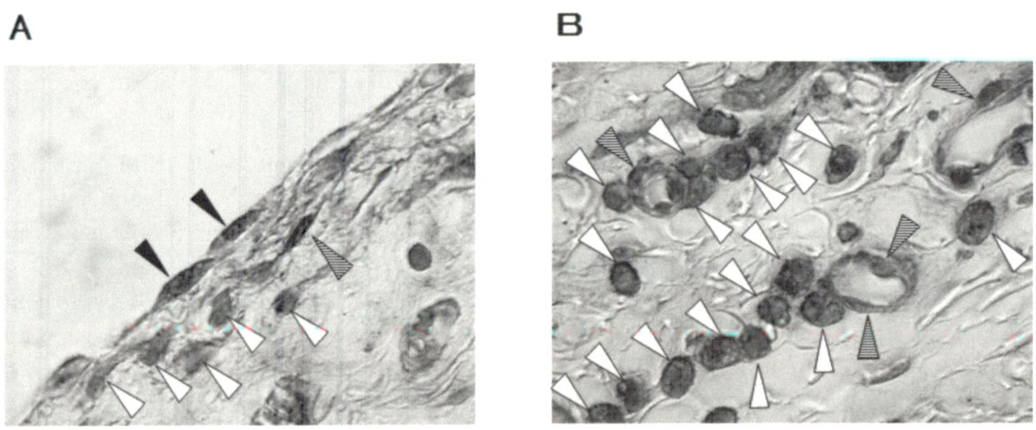

Fig. 3. MMP-2 production in the peritoneum of rat models of peritoneal injury.
MMP-2 production in the parietal peritoneum was immunohistologically analyzed using an anti-MMP-2 antibody. (A) The histological image of the parietal peritoneum of the talc-treated rats. Mesenchymal cells, macrophages, and peritoneal mesothelial cells that produce MMP-2 are shown by shaded arrow heads, open arrow heads, and closed arrow heads, respectively. (B) The histological image of the parietal peritoneum of the chlorhexidine gluconate-treated rats. Macrophages and vascular endothelial cells are shown by open arrow heads and shaded arrow heads, respectively.

MMP-2-producing cells	target of MMP-2	histological change
macrophages	ECM	inflammation
mesenchymal cells (fibroblasts)	ECM	fibrosis, inflammation
mesothelial cells	ECM, BM	EMT
endothelial cell	ECM, BM	angiogenesis

ECM: extracellular matrix, BM: basement membrane, EMT: epithelial-to-mesenchymal transition

Table 1. Tissue destruction by MMP-2 in the peritoneum

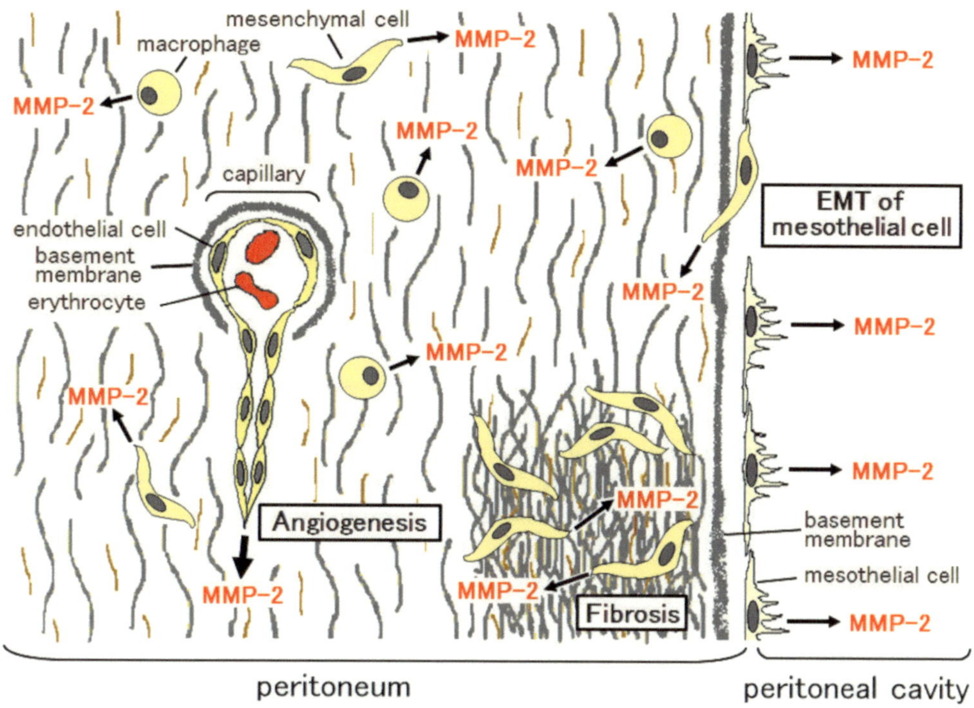

Fig. 4. Tissue destruction by MMP-2 in the peritoneum.
MMP-2 is assumed to destroy peritoneal tissue. Macrophages may infiltrate or migrate into the peritoneum while ECM is being degraded by the MMP-2 produced by these cells. Mesothelial cells may transform to mesenchymal cells (epithelial to mesenchymal transition: EMT) and infiltrate or migrate into the peritoneum, which is being digested by MMP-2. Activated mesenchymal cells synthesize ECM proteins that lead to peritoneal fibrosis or migrate during the disassemble of ECM of the peritoneum by MMP-2. Angiogenesis of capillaries may occur while ECM is being degraded by MMP-2 produced by activated endothelial cells.

Del Peso et al. have reported that the transition of mesothelial cells to mesenchymal cells is an early event during PD and is associated with fast peritoneal transport [44], which may explain why drainage levels of MMP-2 reflects the peritoneal transport ratio. Activated mesenchymal cells, such as myofibroblasts or fibroblasts, synthesize ECM proteins or migrate during the disassemble of ECM of the peritoneum by MMP-2 or other proteinases [8-12, 33]. Presence of excessive ECM proteins, such as collagen, leads to peritoneal fibrosis

with peritoneal thickening and promotes the production of MMP-2 by myofibroblasts [9]. In addition, neomicrovascularization may occur while ECM is being degraded by MMP-2 produced by activated endothelial cells in the microvasculature [10, 12, 33].
According to the results of D/S ratio analysis, most MMP-2 in the peritoneal effluent is not transported from the circulation [26]. The measured D/S ratios of MMP-2 were higher than those predicted when MMP-2 was transported from the circulation only by diffusion.
In summary, MMP-2 is produced by various peritoneal cells activated by a variety of stimuli. Because MMP-2 is produced primarily in the peritoneum, its drainage levels may indicate the condition of peritoneal injury.

5. Protection from peritoneal injury by inhibition of MMP-2

Peritoneal injury may be avoided by drugs that inhibit MMP-2 activity. Ro et al. have reported that the MMP inhibitor ONO-4817 controlled angiogenesis, infiltration of macrophage, and peritoneal fibrosis in rat models of peritoneal sclerosis [10], which suggests the possibility of protection from peritoneal injury by inhibition of MMP-2 activities.
Angiotensin-converting enzyme (ACE) inhibitors have been shown to have inhibitory effects on MMP-2 activity [45, 46]. Yamamoto et al. have proposed a mechanism for the inhibitory specificity of ACE inhibitors against MMP-2 using three-dimensional models of the MMP-2-ACE inhibitor complex. Furthermore, these authors showed that ACE inhibitors directly inhibited MMP-2 activity in the peritoneal effluent from patients on PD [47]. In experimental animal models, use of ACE inhibitors protected the animals from peritoneal injury with fibrosis thickening and functional decline, such as increased solute transport [48-50]. Sampimon et al. have reported the clinical possibility of a protective effect of ACE inhibitors on the development of EPS although it did not achieve statistical significance [51].
Thus, randomized controlled trials are needed to determine the level of protection gained against peritoneal injury using drugs, such as ACE inhibitors, that have an inhibitory effect on MMP-2 activity.

6. Conclusions

MMPs play critical roles in peritoneal injury. To perform PD safely, it is important to clarify the mechanisms by which MMPs cause peritoneal injury. MMP levels in the peritoneal effluent may be used as markers of peritoneal injury that can differentiate early EPS from infectious peritonitis. In addition, patients undergoing PD may be protected against peritoneal injury by controlling MMP activities. Future studies should examine the changes in MMP-2 levels with regard to progression of peritoneal injury to EPS and confirm the effects of MMPs inhibitors in controlling peritoneal injury

7. References

[1] Gandhi VC, Humayun HM, Ing TS, Daugirdas JT, Geis WP, Hano JE. Sclerotic thickening of the peritoneal membrane in maintenance peritoneal dialysis patients. Arch Intern Med 1980; 140: 1201-1203.

[2] Kawanishi H, Moriishi M, Ide K, Dohi K. Recommendation of the surgical option for treatment of encapsulating peritoneal sclerosis. Perit Dial Int 2008; 28 Suppl 3: S205-210.

[3] Balasubramaniam G, Brown EA, Davenport A, Cairns H, Cooper B, Fan SL, Farrington K, Gallagher H, Harnett P, Krausze S, Steddon S. The Pan-Thames EPS study: treatment and outcomes of encapsulating peritoneal sclerosis. Nephrol Dial Transplant 2009; 24, 3209-3215.
[4] Brown MC, Simpson K, Kerssens JJ, Mactier RA; Scottish Renal Registry. Encapsulating peritoneal sclerosis in the new millennium: a national cohort study. Clin J Am Soc Nephrol 2009; 4:1222-1229.
[5] Johnson DW, Cho Y, Livingston BE, Hawley CM, McDonald SP, Brown FG, Rosman JB, Bannister KM, Wiggins KJ. Encapsulating peritoneal sclerosis: incidence, predictors, and outcomes. Kidney Int 2010; 77: 904-912.
[6] Brown EA, Van Biesen W, Finkelstein FO, Hurst H, Johnson DW, Kawanishi H, Pecoits-Filho R, Woodrow G; ISPD Working Party. Length of time on peritoneal dialysis and encapsulating peritoneal sclerosis: position paper for ISPD. Perit Dial Int 2009; 29: 595-600.
[7] Hirahara I, Umeyama K, Urakami K, Kusano E, Masunaga Y, Asano Y. Serial analysis of matrix metalloproteinase-2 in dialysate of rat sclerosing peritonitis models. Clin Exp Nephrol 2001; 5:103-108.
[8] Hirahara I, Umeyama K, Shofuda K, Kusano E, Masunaga Y, Honma S, Asano Y. Increase of matrix metalloproteinase-2 in dialysate of rat sclerosing encapsulating peritonitis model. Nephrology 2002; 7: 161-169.
[9] Hirahara I, Ogawa Y, Kusano E, Asano Y. Activation of matrix metalloproteinase-2 causes peritoneal injury during peritoneal dialysis in rats. Nephrol Dial Transplant 2004; 19: 1732-1741.
[10] Ro Y, Hamada C, Inaba M, Io H, Kaneko K, Tomino Y. Inhibitory effects of matrix metalloproteinase inhibitor ONO-4817 on morphological alterations in chlorhexidine gluconate-induced peritoneal sclerosis rats. Nephrol Dial Transplant 2007; 22: 2838-2848.
[11] Kurata K, Maruyama S, Kato S, Sato W, Yamamoto J, Ozaki T, Nitta A, Nabeshima T, Morita Y, Mizuno M, Ito Y, Yuzawa Y, Matsuo S. Tissue-type plasminogen activator deficiency attenuates peritoneal fibrosis in mice. Am J Physiol Renal Physiol 2009; 297: F1510-1517.
[12] Hirahara I, Kusano E, Yanagiba S, Miyata Y, Ando Y, Muto S, Asano Y. Peritoneal injury by methylglyoxal in peritoneal dialysis. Perit Dial Int 2006; 26: 380-392.
[13] Hirahara I, Ishibashi Y, Kaname S, Kusano E, Fujita T. Methylglyoxal induces peritoneal thickening by mesenchymal-like mesothelial cells in rats. Nephrol Dial Transplant 2009; 24: 437-447.
[14] Hind CR, Thomson SP, Winearls CG, Pepys MB. Serum C-reactive protein concentration in the management of infection in patients treated by continuous ambulatory peritoneal dialysis. J Clin Pathol 1985; 38: 459-463.
[15] Kaku Y, Nohara K, Tsutsumi Y, Kanemitsu S, Hara T, Yoshimura H, Hirahara I, Kusano E. The relationship among the markers of peritoneal function such as PET, MMP-2, IL-6 etc, in pediatric and adolescent PD patients. Jin To Touseki 2004; 57 (Suppl): 296-298.
[16] Green MJ, Gough AK, Devlin J, et al. Serum MMP-3 and MMP-1 and progression of joint damage in early rheumatoid arthritis. Rheumatology 2003; 42: 83-88.

[17] Roderfeld M, Rath T, Schulz R, Seeger W, Tschuschner A, Graf J, Roeb E. Serum matrix metalloproteinases in adult CF patients: Relation to pulmonary exacerbation. J Cyst Fibros 2009; 8: 338-347.

[18] Brajer B, Batura-Gabryel H, Nowicka A, Kuznar-Kaminska B, Szczepanik A. Concentration of matrix metalloproteinase-9 in serum of patients with chronic obstructive pulmonary disease and a degree of airway obstruction and disease progression. J Physiol Pharmacol 2008; 59 Suppl 6: 145-152.

[19] Tziakas DN, Chalikias GK, Parissis JT, Hatzinikolaou EI, Papadopoulos ED, Tripsiannis GA, Papadopoulou EG, Tentes IK, Karas SM, Chatseras DI. Serum profiles of matrix metalloproteinases and their tissue inhibitor in patients with acute coronary syndromes. The effects of short-term atorvastatin administration. Int J Cardiol 2004; 94: 269-277.

[20] Rugina M, Caras I, Jurcut R, Jurcut C, Serbanescu F, Salageanu A, Apetrei E. Systemic inflammatory markers in patients with aortic sclerosis. Roum Arch Microbiol Immunol 2007; 66: 10-16.

[21] Murawaki Y, Yamada S, Ikuta Y, Kawasaki H. Clinical usefulness of serum matrix metalloproteinase-2 concentration in patients with chronic viral liver disease. J Hepatol 1999; 30: 1090-1098.

[22] Kasahara A, Hayashi N, Mochizuki K, Oshita M, Katayama K, Kato M, Masuzawa M, Yoshihara H, Naito M, Miyamoto T, Inoue A, Asai A, Hijioka T, Fusamoto H, Kamada T. Circulating matrix metalloproteinase-2 and tissue inhibitor of metalloproteinase-1 as serum markers of fibrosis in patients with chronic hepatitis C. Relationship to interferon response. J Hepatol 1997; 26: 574-583.

[23] Jones CL. Matrix degradation in renal disease. Nephrology 1996; 2: 13-23.

[24] Nagano M, Fukami K, Yamagishi S, Ueda S, Kaida Y, Matsumoto T, Yoshimura J, Hazama T, Takamiya Y, Kusumoto T, Gohara S, Tanaka H, Adachi H, Okuda S. Circulating matrix metalloproteinase-2 is an independent correlate of proteinuria in patients with chronic kidney disease. Am J Nephrol 2009; 29: 109-115.

[25] Hirahara I, Inoue M, Okuda K, Ando Y, Muto S, Kusano E. The potential of matrix metalloproteinase-2 as a marker of peritoneal injury, increased solute transport, or progression to encapsulating peritoneal sclerosis during peritoneal dialysis--a multicentre study in Japan. Nephrol Dial Transplant 2007; 22: 560-567.

[26] Hirahara I, Inoue M, Umino T, Saito O, Muto S, Kusano E. Matrix metalloproteinase levels in the drained dialysate reflect the peritoneal solute transport rate: A multicenter study in Japan. Nephrol Dial Transplant 2011; 26: 1695-1701.

[27] Twardowski ZJ, Nolph KD, Khanna R, et al. Peritoneal equilibration test. Perit Dial Bull 1987; 7: 138-147.

[28] Zweers MM, de Waart DR, Smit W, Struijk DG, Krediet RT. Growth factors VEGF and TGF-beta1 in peritoneal dialysis. J Lab Clin Med 1999; 134: 124-132.

[29] Coester AM, Smit W, Struijk DG, Krediet RT. Peritoneal function in clinical practice: the importance of follow-up and its measurement in patients. Recommendations for patient information and measurement of peritoneal function. Nephrol Dial Transplant Plus 2009; 2: 104-110.

[30] Soccal PM, Gasche Y, Pache JC, et al. Matrix metalloproteinases correlate with alveolar-capillary permeability alteration in lung ischemia-reperfusion injury. Transplantation 2000; 70: 998-1005.

[31] Swann K, Berger J, Sprague SM, et al. Peripheral thermal injury causes blood-brain barrier dysfunction and matrix metalloproteinase (MMP) expression in rat. Brain Res 2007; 1129: 26-33.

[32] Giebel SJ, Menicucci G, McGuire PG, Das A. Matrix metalloproteinases in early diabetic retinopathy and their role in alteration of the blood-retinal barrier. Lab Invest 2005; 85: 597-607.

[33] Osada S, Hamada C, Shimaoka T, Kaneko K, Horikoshi S, Tomino Y. Alterations in proteoglycan components and histopathology of the peritoneum in uraemic and peritoneal dialysis (PD) patients. Nephrol Dial Transplant 2009; 24: 3504-3512.

[34] Masunaga Y, Hirahara I, Shimano Y, Kurosu M, Iimura O, Miyata Y, Amemiya M, Homma S, Kusano E, Asano Y. A case of encapsulating peritoneal sclerosis at the clinical early stage with high concentration of matrix metalloproteinase-2 in peritoneal effluent. Clin Exp Nephrol 2005; 9: 85-89.

[35] Fukudome K, Fujimoto S, Sato Y, Hisanaga S, Eto T. Peritonitis increases MMP-9 activity in peritoneal effluent from CAPD patients. Nephron 2001; 87: 35-41.

[36] Ro Y, Hamada C, Io H, Hayashi K, Hirahara I, Tomino Y. Rapid, simple, and reliable method for the diagnosis of CAPD peritonitis using the new MMP-9 test kit. J Clin Lab Anal 2004; 18: 224-230.

[37] Minami S, Hora K, Kamijo Y, Higuchi M. Relationship between effluent levels of beta(2)-microglobulin and peritoneal injury markers in 7.5% icodextrin-based peritoneal dialysis solution. Ther Apher Dial 2007; 11: 296-300.

[38] Nishina M, Endoh M, Suzuki D, et al. Neutral-pH peritoneal dialysis solution improves peritoneal function and decreases matrix metalloproteinase-2 (MMP-2) in patients undergoing continuous ambulatory peritoneal dialysis (CAPD). Clin Exp Nephrol 2004; 8: 339-343.

[39] Ro Y, Hamada C, Io H, Hayashi K, Inoue S, Hirahara I, Tomino Y. Early diagnosis of CAPD peritonitis using a new test kit for detection of matrix metalloproteinase (MMP)-9. Perit Dial Int 2004; 24: 90-91.

[40] Martin J, Yung S, Robson RL, Steadman R, Davies M. Production and regulation of matrix metalloproteinases and their inhibitors by human peritoneal mesothelial cells. Perit Dial Int 2000; 20: 524-533.

[41] Naiki Y, Matsuo K, Matsuoka T, Maeda Y. Possible role of hepatocyte growth factor in regeneration of human peritoneal mesothelial cells. Int J Artif Organs 2005; 28: 141-149.

[42] Haslinger B, Mandl-Weber S, Sitter T. Thrombin suppresses matrix metalloproteinase 2 activity and increases tissue inhibitor of metalloproteinase 1 synthesis in cultured human peritoneal mesothelial cells. Perit Dial Int 2000; 20: 778-783.

[43] Margetts PJ, Bonniaud P, Liu L, et al. Transient overexpression of TGF-{beta}1 induces epithelial mesenchymal transition in the rodent peritoneum. J Am Soc Nephrol 2005; 16: 425-436.

[44] Del Peso G, Jiménez-Heffernan JA, Bajo MA, et al. Epithelial-to-mesenchymal transition of mesothelial cells is an early event during peritoneal dialysis and is associated with high peritoneal transport. Kidney Int 2008; 108 (Suppl): S26-33.

[45] Lods N, Ferrari P, Frey FJ, Kappeler A, Berthier C, Vogt B, Marti HP. Angiotensin-converting enzyme inhibition but not angiotensin II receptor blockade regulates

matrix metalloproteinase activity in patients with glomerulonephritis. J Am Soc Nephrol 2003; 14: 2861-2872.

[46] Williams RN, Parsons SL, Morris TM, Rowlands BJ, Watson SA. Inhibition of matrix metalloproteinase activity and growth of gastric adenocarcinoma cells by an angiotensin converting enzyme inhibitor in in vitro and murine models. Eur J Surg Oncol 2005; 31: 1042-1050.

[47] Yamamoto D, Takai S, Hirahara I, Kusano E. Captopril directly inhibits matrix metalloproteinase-2 activity in continuous ambulatory peritoneal dialysis therapy. Clin Chim Acta 2010; 411: 762-764.

[48] Imai H, Nakamoto H, Ishida Y, Yamanouchi Y, Inoue T, Okada H, Suzuki H. Renin-angiotensin system plays an important role in the regulation of water transport in the peritoneum. Adv Perit Dial 2001; 17: 20-24.

[49] Sawada T, Ishii Y, Tojimbara T, Nakajima I, Fuchinoue S, Teraoka S. The ACE inhibitor, quinapril, ameliorates peritoneal fibrosis in an encapsulating peritoneal sclerosis model in mice. Pharmacol Res 2002; 46: 505-510.

[50] Duman S, Wieczorowska-Tobis K, Styszynski A, Kwiatkowska B, Breborowicz A, Oreopoulos DG. Intraperitoneal enalapril ameliorates morphologic changes induced by hypertonic peritoneal dialysis solutions in rat peritoneum. Adv Perit Dial 2004; 20: 31-36.

[51] Sampimon DE, Kolesnyk I, Korte MR, Fieren MW, Struijk DG, Krediet RT. Use of angiotensin ii inhibitors in patients that develop encapsulating peritoneal sclerosis. Perit Dial Int 2010; 30: 656-659.

6

Proteomics in Peritoneal Dialysis

Hsien-Yi Wang[1,2], Hsin-Yi Wu[3] and Shih-Bin Su[4,5]
[1]*Department of Nephrology, Chi-Mei Medical Center, Tainan*
[2]*Department of Sports Management, College of Leisure and Recreation Management, Chia Nan University of Pharmacy and Science, Tainan*
[3]*Institute of Chemistry, Academia Sinica, Taipei*
[4]*Department of Family Medicine, Chi-Mei Medical Center, Tainan*
[5]*Department of Biotechnology, Southern Taiwan University, Tainan*
Taiwan

1. Introduction

Relatively little is known about proteins in peritoneal effluent, that are lost or changed during peritoneal dialysis(PD) and in different diseases, leaving various unclear questions. Biomarkers that can indicate damages caused by peritoneal dialysis, like cancer antigen 125 and interleukin-6 are some exemples. Therefore, tools such as proteomic approaches that can globally identify, characterize, and quantify a set of proteins and their changes in peritoneal dialysate, could shed light to the mechanisms of peritonitis and membrane damage. The availability of fluid from dialysis for study and the potential importance of specific protein change during peritoneal dialysis making this a potentially fruitful area for further observation. Since the renal community is embracing proteomic technologies at an increasing rate, growing numbers of studies that would be carried out through this process can be envisaged. In this chapter we intend to introduce basic proteomic tools and highlight important advances in peritoneal dialysis using proteomic approaches as well as the future perspective that proteomic tools can contribute in the field of peritoneal dialysis

2. Proteomic tools

In recent years, proteomic analyses of particular biological samples or clinical samples have drawn much interest and provided much information. Proteomic tools such as two dimensional gel electrophoresis (2DE) and mass spectrometry analysis have been widely applied in the study of body fluids, e.g. cerebrospinal fluid, pleural and pericardial effusions (Liu et al. 2008; Tyan et al. 2005a; Tyan et al. 2005b), and urine (Bennett et al. 2008; Tan et al. 2008). For peritoneal dialysis, several issues have been addressed as described in the following sections. . The advantages and disadvantages of the various techniques have been reviewed previously (Fliser et al. 2007; Mischak et al. 2007).

2.1 Two dimensional gel electrophoresis (2DE)

Proteins are separated by isoelectric point and size. The protein spot can be visualized by gel staining. It is widely available and the posttranslational modification of the protein can be revealed by separation of charge forms. However, low-abundance, large, and hydrophobic proteins are difficult to be detected. 2DE is technically demanding and time-consuming. The low number of independent datasets and the high variability of the gel make the definition of biomarkers difficult or even impossible. 2DE with fluorescent labeling of proteins before separation in gel (DIGE) has been proposed to improve reproducibility. Additional expense for fluorescent dyes and three color imaging system is required.

2.2 Liquid chromatography-tandem mass spectrometry (LC-MS/MS)

Proteins are digested before separation by liquid chromatography coupled to MS instruments. MS detection is more sensitive than 2DE. It is easily automated, allowing analyzing a serious of samples. Drawback in comparison to 2DE is that information on the molecular mass of the actual biomarker as well as on any posttranslational modifications (PTM) is generally lost. This requires additional tools.

2.3 Surface-enhanced laser desorption ionization (SELDI)

Proteins are bound to affinity surface on a MALDI chip. Samples can be enriched for specific low-abundance proteins. Bound proteins are detected in a mass spectrometer. The SELDI technology draws a lot of interest because of its ease of use and its high throughput for biomarker discovery. However, the low-resolution of the mass spectrometer, the large amount of variability between labs, and its lack of reproducibility, hamper its potential clinical application (McLerran et al. 2008).

2.4 Capillary electrophoresis coupled to mass spectrometry (CE-MS)

Proteins were separated by elution time in CE and by size in MS. High reproducibility, robustness, high resolution and sensitivity make it a potential technique for biomarker discovery. Its limitation is that proteins can't be identified without additional steps and only proteins/peptides <20 kDa can be analyzed.

3. Analyses of peritoneal dialysis by proteomics tools

3.1 Preliminary proteomic studies on peritoneal dialysis effluent

A descriptive study was performed on the dialysate of nine paediatric PD children patients to obtain a representative overview of the proteome of peritoneal fluid (Raaijmakers et al. 2008). None of the patients suffered from peritonitis in the 3 months before the collection. Proteins were resolved on the SDS-PAGE and the protein spots identification was achieved by nanoLC-MS/MS. A total of 189 proteins were identified, with 88 proteins shared by all the patients. The function of these shared proteins were classified into 8 classes. As listed in Table 1, acute phase proteins, complement factors, hormones, coagulation factors, and apolipoproteins were found.

These factors were related to the number of frequently occurring proteins in the dialysate (Pecoits-Filho et al. 2004; Reddingius et al. 1995; Saku et al. 1989; van der Kamp et al. 1999). The proteome of PD fluid also reveals some interesting proteins, Gelsolin, intelectin, and parapxonase, which could possible involve in protecting the mesothelial cell damage and against infection, against parasites, and anti-atherogenic capacitities, respectively. The proteome of PD may help understand the functional mechanism of the peritoneum.

Classification	Different proteins	Mean emPAI	SD
1. Acute phase proteins	24	1435	706
(a) Antiproteases	13	84.4	18.8
(b) Transport proteins	3	1333	713
(c) Other acute phase proteins	8	18.4	4.26
2. Complement factors	18	31.9	7.9
3. Apolipoproteins	7	40.4	22.8
4. Coagulation proteins	8	6.46	1.73
5. Extracellular matrix proteins	8	6.74	2.23
6. Hormone and vitamin binding proteins	5	19.8	7.98
7. Enzymes	4	7.02	1.38
8. Others	14	25.2	9.8

Table 1. Protein classification according to function of the proteins present in all the patients, relative abundances are given with mean emPAI values [Adapted from (Raaijmakers et al. 2008)]

3.2 Dialysis-related peritonitis

Peritonitis caused by CAPD may lead to peritoneal abnormalities. To search for potential biomarkers for peritonitis, Lin et al. have compared the proteome of peritoneal dialysate from 16 patients with and without peritonitis (Lin et al. 2008). Proteins were separated on 2DE, indicating several differential expressed spots (Figure 1).

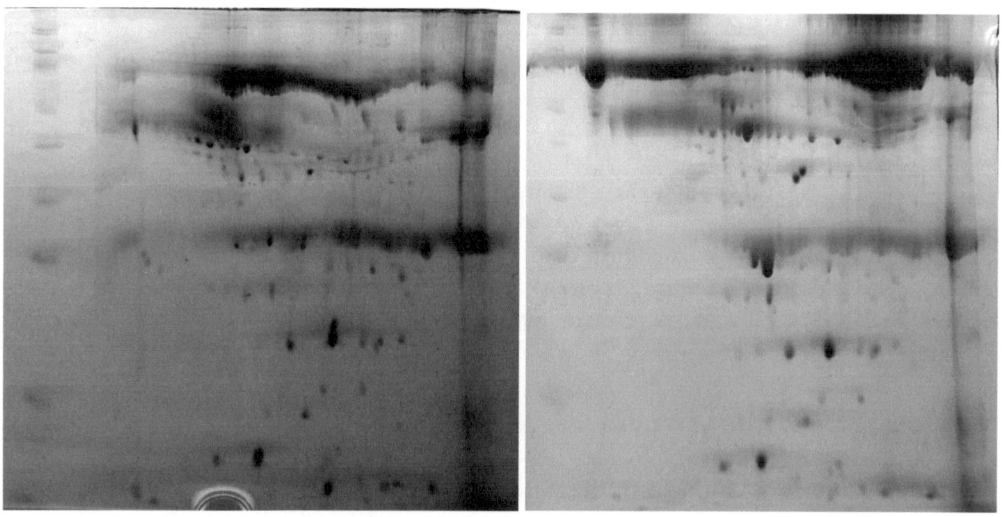

Fig. 1. Protein map, obtained by 2DE, of protein lysates prepared from CAPD dialysis effluent without (left) and with (right) peritonitis. Proteins are first separated according to their pI using iso-electric focusing and then separated according to their respective molecular weight using (10%) SDS-PAGE. [Adapted from (Lin et al. 2008)]

Samples were also analyzed by SELDI-TOF MS, revealing that signal peak at m/z of 11117.4 only appeared in the peritonitis sample. This signal was identified as β2-microglobulin by using MALDI-TOF/TOF MS. Protein β2-microglobulin has been linked to CAPD peritonitis in previous studies. In CAPD dialysate from patients with bacterial peritonitis, β2-microglobulin showed higher levels than in those without peritonitis (Carozzi et al. 1990). Minami et al. the level of β2-microglobulin in the peritoneal dialysate was correlated with peritoneal injural (Minami et al. 2007). Using the protein profile approach, this study confirmed β2-microglobulin as a biomarker for CAPD peritonitis.

3.3 Different types of peritoneal membranes

The efficacy and clinical outcome of CAPD depend on peritoneal membrane function. Peritoneal membranes can be classified as high (H), high average (HA), low average (LA), and low (L) transporters by using peritoneal equilibration test (PET). Whether there is a difference in proteins removed by different types of peritoneal membranes has been discussed in a study conducted by Sritippayawan et al. (Sritippayawan et al. 2007). They performed a proteomic analysis of peritoneal dialysate in CAPD patients with H, HA, LA, and L transport rates. Five patients were included for each group, makes up to 20 patient samples. Proteins from each sample were resolved in each 2D-gel (total 20 gels). Representative gels are shown in Figure 2. After gel visualization by staining and spot quantitation by image analysis software, the mean values of individual parameters were compared among the four different groups. Five proteins were found to show differed levels among groups. They were identified as serum albumin in a complex with myristic acid and triiodobenzoic acid, α1-antitrypsin, complement component C4A, immunoglobulin κ light chain, and apolipoprotein A-I by MALDI-Q-TOF MS and MS/MS analyses. ELISA was used to confirm the difference expression of C4A and immunoglobulin κ in a set of other 24 patients. Functional significance of differential levels of these proteins may associate with dialysis adequacy, residual renal function, risk of peritonitis, and nutritional status. The level of serum albumin in a complex with myristic acid and triiodobenzoic acid was higher in the L LA groups, implying that the modified or complexed form of albumin may be associated with peritoneal membrane transport. The level of C4A was higher in H and HA group. In peritoneal dialysate, C4A originates from vascular leakage, resulting in the lower C4A level in L group. The immunoglobulin κ light chain VLJ region, whose level was higher in H and HA groups also tended to be higher in patients with peritonitis. The higher level of immunoglobulin κ light chain VLJ region might be related to poorer function of neutrophils. Patients in H and HA group also had higher apolipoprotein A-I in peritoneal dialysate compared to L and LA groups, which may explain that high solute transporters are prone to develop atherosclerosis.

3.4 The role of glucose in peritoneal dialysis

The abdominal cavity is covered by the mesothelial cell (MC) layer. Peritoneal dialysis fluid may remove solutes and fluid from the patients due to its hypertonicity. Long period and frequent peritoneal dialysis could lead to structural and functional alterations of the MC layer, leading to a final failure of peritoneal dialysis (Davies et al. 2001; Heimburger et al. 1990; Ho-dac-Pannekeet et al. 1997; Imholz et al. 1993; Williams et al. 2002). Hperosmolarity in peritoneal dialysis effluents is generated by high concentrations of glucose which could be degraded into carbonyl compounds as various glucose degradation products (GDPs) after heat sterilization (Linden et al. 1998; Nilsson-Thorell et al. 1993; Pischetsrieder 2000; Witowski and Jorres 2000; Witowski et al. 2003). These GDPs are reported as being

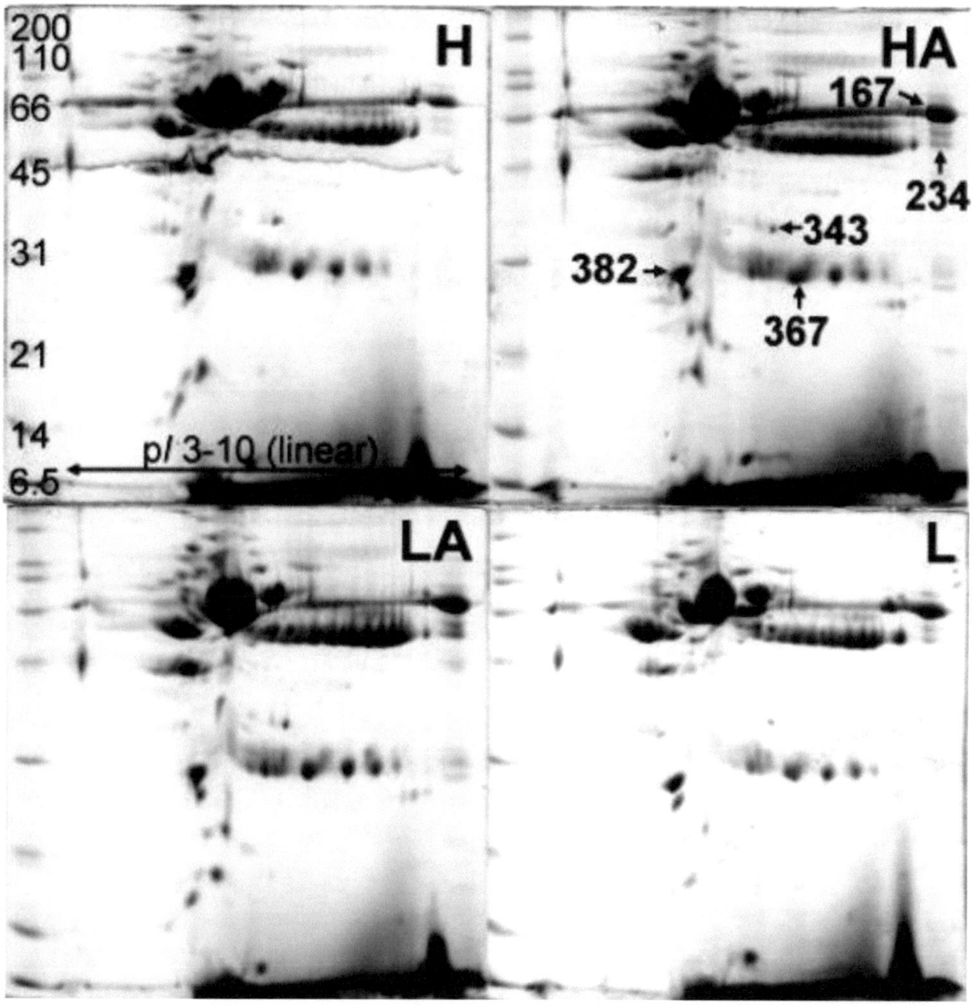

Fig. 2. Representative 2-D gel images of the PDE proteins derived from different types of peritoneal membranes. Proteins were precipitated with 75% ethanol, and an equal amount of total protein (200 íg) obtained from each patient was resolved in each 2-D gel (n) 5 gels for each group; total n) 20). The resolved protein spots were visualized by CBB-R250 stain. Quantitative intensity analysis and ANOVA with Tukey's posthoc multiple comparisons revealed five protein spots whose intensity levels significantly differed among groups (see Table 2). These protein spots (labeled with numbers) were subsequently identified by MALDI-Q-TOF MS and MS/MS analyses. [Adapted from (Sritippayawan et al. 2007)]

mitogenic and cytotoxic. Thus, peritoneal dialysis effluent is considered as a significant stressor for the MC layer (Breborowicz et al. 1995; Wieslander et al. 1991). To address this issue, a cell line derived from the MC layers was used as a model to study the glucose-related pathways induced by high concentration of glucose (Lechner et al. 2010). Using two-dimensional fluorescence-difference gel electrophoresis (DIGE), altered proteins upon glucose stress in Met-5A cell were revealed. A total of 947 spots were present in 32 gels (16 controls, 16 glucose stress). A representative gel is shown in Figure 3. Among them, 140 spots were of differential expression under full-peritoneal dialysis fluid stress consisting of high glucose concentration, pH 5.8, and the presence of GDPs, when compared to untreated cells, of which 100 proteins can be identified by MALDI-MS and MS/MS techniques. Further studies on these factors suggested that glucose exposure alone was not sufficient to explain the differential abundant of these proteins, supporting the hypothesis that stressors, pH, lactate, and GDPs, might have essential impact for activation of the glucose -related pathways. . By comparing peritoneal dialysis effluent with different glucose concentrations, four proteins were found to be under-expressed in the highest osmolar solution. All of them were considered to be involved in the inflammatory processes.

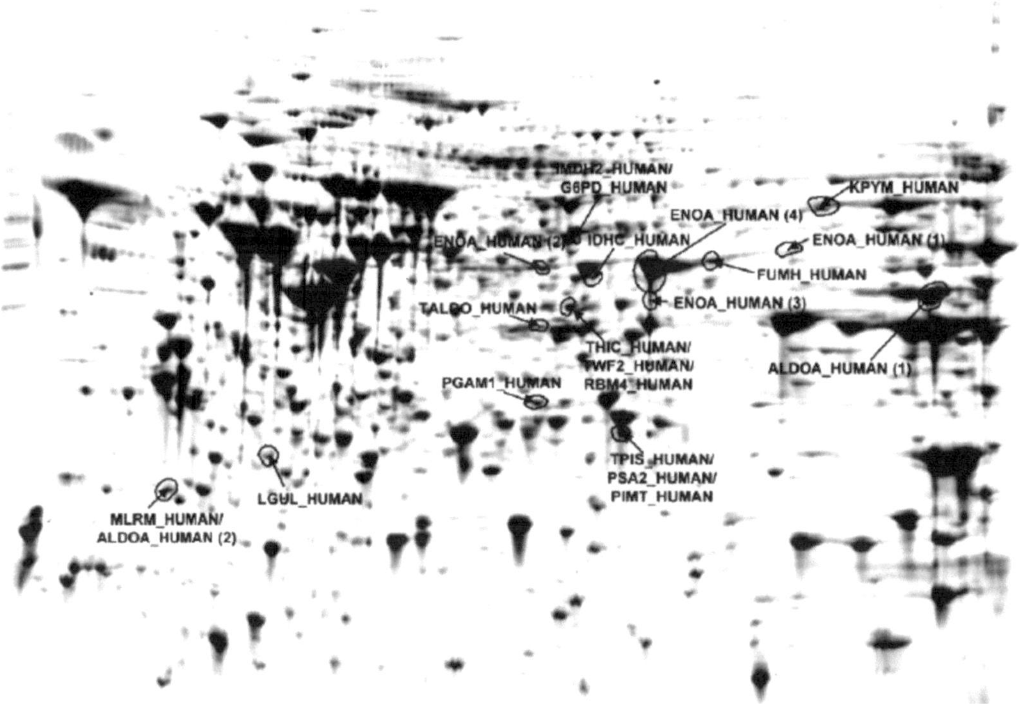

Fig. 3. CBB stained 2-DE gel of a MeT-5A cell lysate. Proteins, differently abundant after full-PDF exposure and assigned to significantly enriched glucose associated pathways, are indicated with a circle and labeled with their Swiss-Prot entry names. Protein isoforms are distinguished by numbers in brackets. [Adapted from (Lechner et al. 2010)]

Another laboratory works on analyzing the protein composition of peritoneal fluid from patients receiving peritoneal dialysis with different concentration of glucose (Cuccurullo et al. 2010). Peritoneal dialysis effluent with different glucose concentrations were revealed by 2DE. The representative gels for each group are shown in Figure 4.

Combining the data from 2DE and shotgun proteomics analysis, 151 non-redundant identifications were reached. Through the cellular component analysis, proteins related to extracellular region were over-expressed. As for the molecular function and biological process, proteins associated with protein binding and inflammatory processes were over-represented. Four proteins, Alpha-1-antitrypsin (1603), fibrinogen beta chain (4308- 5303), transthyretin (4303 and 2101), and apolipoprotein A-IV (4208) were found to be under-expressed in the highest osmolar solution. The result provides potential targets for future therapeutic implementation in preventing inflammatory processes induced by the exposure to dialysis solutions.

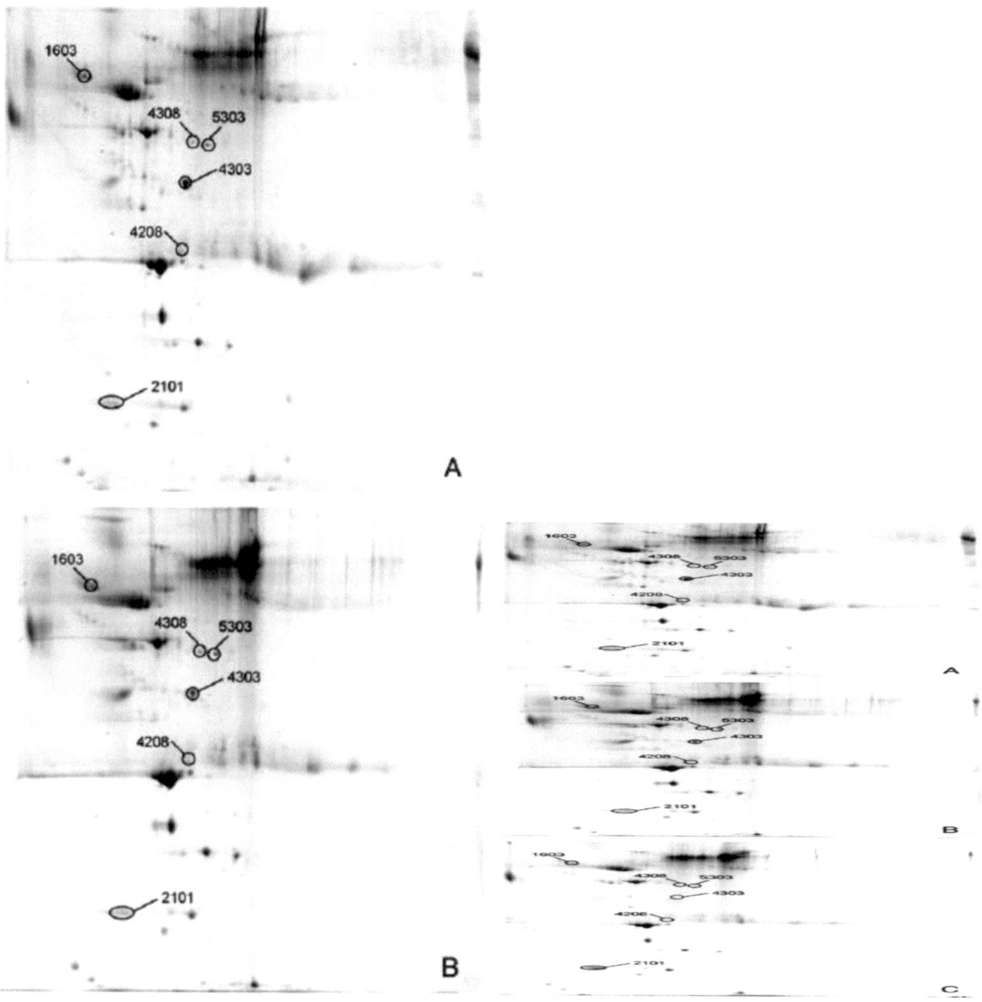

Fig. 4. Representative 2D gel images of PDE protein profiles from one (out of five) adult patient treated with peritoneal dialysis solutions differing for glucose percentages (A = glucose percentage 1.5%, B = glucose percentage 2.5%, C = glucose percentage 4.25%). Circled spots correspond to proteins whose expression undergoes quantitative changes. Alpha-1-antitrypsin (1603), fibrinogen beta chain (4308- 5303), transthyretin (4303 and 2101), apolipoprotein A-IV (4208). [Adapted from (Cuccurullo et al. 2010)]

3.5 Peritoneal dialysate from diabetic patients

Fluid overload related cardiovascular disease is one important factor to mortality in patients receiving CAPD (Brown et al. 2003). Other proposed mechanism is the glucotoxicity cause by the high concentration of glucose contained in PD fluid (Sitter and Sauter 2005).

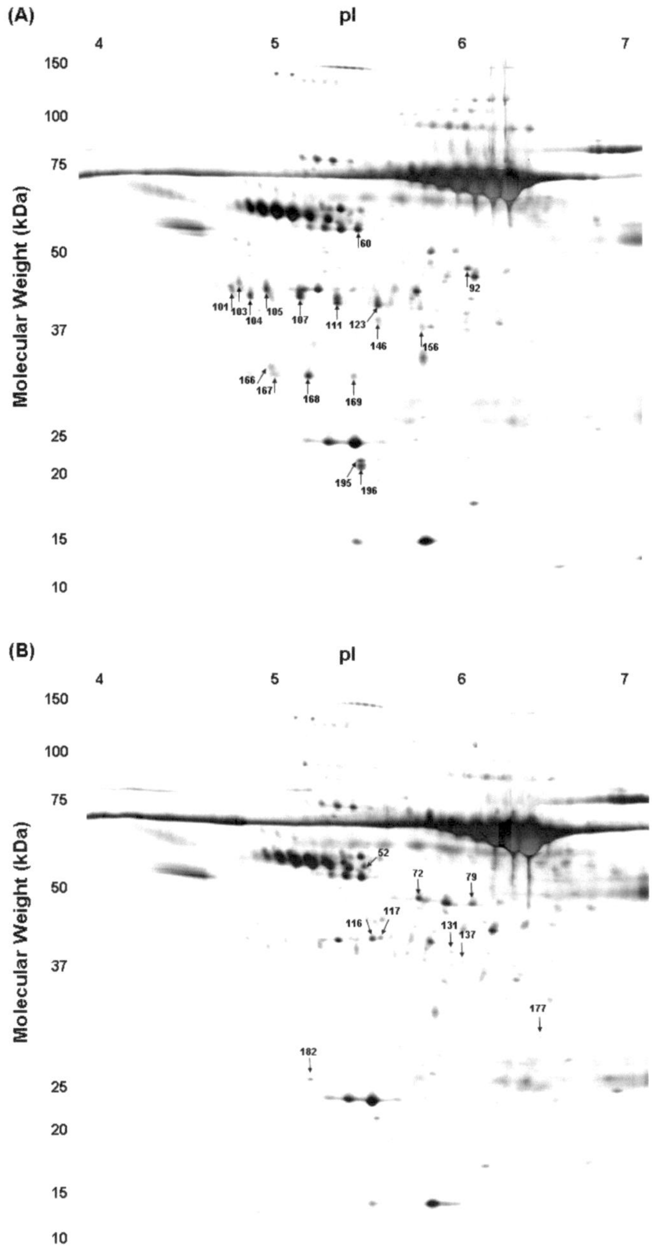

Fig. 6. Representative 2DE gels for the DM samples (A) and the non-DM (B) samples. DM samples and non-DM samples were pooled separately for 2DE analysis (pH 4-7). A total of 120 µg was used. The analysis of each group was repeated six times and two representative gels are shown. An average of 200 protein spots were detected in both gels. Among these, 17 spots were found with higher levels in the peritoneal dialysate (indicated in A by arrows) and 9 spots were found with higher levels in the control samples (indicated in B by arrows) [Adapted from (Wang et al. 2010)]

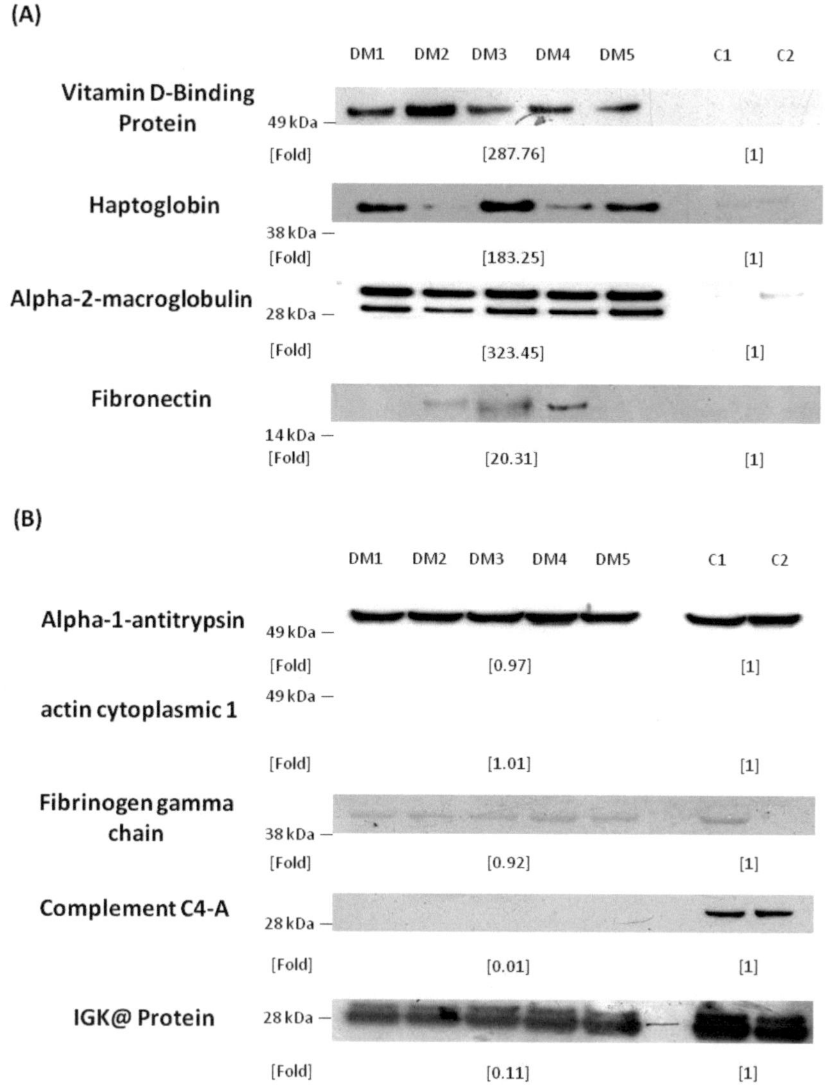

Fig. 7. Western blotting of the identified proteins in five individual DM samples and two individual control samples: the mean band density of five DM samples and two control samples were calculated and fold change between the two groups was calculated by dividing the mean band density of the DM samples by that of the control samples; the mean density of the control group was adjusted as 1, and the fold change was put in the bracket below each set of bands [(A) proteins, vitamin D-binding protein, haptoglobin and α-2-microglobulin show higher expression levels in the DM samples than in the control samples; (B) proteins, complement C4-A and IGK@ protein show higher expression levels in the two control samples than in the five DM samples].[Adapted from (Wang et al. 2010)]

However, the details of the pathogenic mechanism remain unclear. Protein changes between peritoneal dialysate from specific disease and normal peritoneal fluids may shed light to better understanding of the mechanism involved in peritoneal damage resulting from peritoneal dialysis. For clinical application, altered proteins in the peritoneum may function as biomarkers for monitoring which functions as a non-invasive way of detecting peritoneal damage. Wang et al. have compared the diabetic peritoneal dialysate versus normal peritoneal fluid (Wang et al. 2010). From the 2DE (as shown in Figure 6), 26 protein spots were considered altered between two sample groups.

According to the western confirmation results (Figure 7), vitamin D-binding protein, haptoglobin and α-2-microglobulin showed higher levels in the DM samples, while complement C4-A and IGK@ protein were of lower levels compared to the control samples. The work concluded that the loss of some specific proteins may be due to a change in the permeability of the peritoneal membrane to middle-sized proteins or leakage from peritoneal inflammation. It has been reported that PD leads to loss of DBP, and this causes loss of vitamin D. Vitamin D deficiency results in reduced insulin secretion in rats and humans, and its replacement improves B cell function and glucose tolerance (Boucher et al. 1995; Kumar et al. 1994; Norman et al. 1980; Tanaka et al. 1984). Thus the level of Vitamin D binding protein should be monitored after long-term PD. It has been suggested that haptoglobin may play a role in defending against haemoglobin toxicity, mainly renal toxicity (Lim et al. 2000). The observation of α-2-microglobulin in dialysate may be indicative of high levels of α-2-microglobulin in serum and a potential for amyloidosis. Complement activation happens in the peritoneal cavity in patients on chronic PD (Reddingius et al. 1995; Young et al. 1993), suggesting that local production of complement may be a possible inflammatory injury effectors in the initiation of chronic peritoneal damage. Lower levels of complement C4-A in dialysis effluent may indicate the beginning of peritoneal scleroses. The limited studies of the role of IGK@ protein in the peritoneum posted this protein a novel target for further investigation of its defect in dialysate, which may provide a new insight for peritoneal change or damage during PD.

4. Concluding remarks and outlook

Recent publication of potential biomarkers is only based on limited datasets in the absence of any validation. Future implementation of proteomics to the peritoneal dialysis will depend largely on establishment of generally accepted validity of the identified biomarkers. Development of standardization procedures for clinical proteomic studies is also required, including the sample collection procedures. However, these primary works suggested that proteome analysis may be a helpful tool to evaluate therapeutic effects of drugs on a molecular level. These studies may serve as a basis for the future identification of toxins and biomarkers for monitoring and improving the PD. Although it is evident that significant efforts, including larger studies are required to reach these goals, those studies also provide a possible platform for future diagnostic and therapeutic applications in the field of peritoneal dialysis and allowed the identification of potential targets to be used in preventing inflammatory processes induced by the exposure to dialysis solutions. Some reviews on this field claimed that recent findings underscore proteomic tools in defining molecules removed by the treatment modalities. Most of the studies were conducted by using 2DE which is widely used but also lacking in sensitivity and reproducibility. Thus, we can envisage that in the future, using rapidly evolved proteomic tools such as LC-MS/MS and accurate quantitative proteomic approaches such as iTRAQ and label free analyses will bring more information and novel insight into this field.

5. References

Bennett, M. R., et al. (2008), 'Using proteomics to identify preprocedural risk factors for contrast induced nephropathy', *Proteomics Clin Appl,* 2 (7-8), 1058-64.

Boucher, B. J., et al. (1995), 'Glucose intolerance and impairment of insulin secretion in relation to vitamin D deficiency in east London Asians', *Diabetologia,* 38 (10), 1239-45.

Brauner, A., et al. (2003), 'CAPD peritonitis induces the production of a novel peptide, daintain/allograft inflammatory factor-1', *Perit Dial Int,* 23 (1), 5-13.

Breborowicz, A., Martis, L., and Oreopoulos, D. G. (1995), 'Changes in biocompatibility of dialysis fluid during its dwell in the peritoneal cavity', *Perit Dial Int,* 15 (2), 152-7.

Brown, E. A., et al. (2003), 'Survival of functionally anuric patients on automated peritoneal dialysis: the European APD Outcome Study', *J Am Soc Nephrol,* 14 (11), 2948-57.

Carozzi, S., et al. (1990), 'Bacterial peritonitis and beta-2 microglobulin (B2M) production by peritoneal macrophages (PM0) in CAPD patients', *Adv Perit Dial,* 6, 106-9.

Cuccurullo, M., et al. (2010), 'Proteomic analysis of peritoneal fluid of patients treated by peritoneal dialysis: effect of glucose concentration', *Nephrol Dial Transplant.*

Davies, S. J., et al. (2001), 'Peritoneal glucose exposure and changes in membrane solute transport with time on peritoneal dialysis', *J Am Soc Nephrol,* 12 (5), 1046-51.

Fliser, D., et al. (2007), 'Advances in urinary proteome analysis and biomarker discovery', *J Am Soc Nephrol,* 18 (4), 1057-71.

Heimburger, O., et al. (1990), 'Peritoneal transport in CAPD patients with permanent loss of ultrafiltration capacity', *Kidney Int,* 38 (3), 495-506.

Ho-dac-Pannekeet, M. M., et al. (1997), 'Analysis of ultrafiltration failure in peritoneal dialysis patients by means of standard peritoneal permeability analysis', *Perit Dial Int,* 17 (2), 144-50.

Imholz, A. L., et al. (1993), 'Effect of dialysate osmolarity on the transport of low-molecular weight solutes and proteins during CAPD', *Kidney Int,* 43 (6), 1339-46.

Kumar, S., et al. (1994), 'Improvement in glucose tolerance and beta-cell function in a patient with vitamin D deficiency during treatment with vitamin D', *Postgrad Med J,* 70 (824), 440-3.

Lechner, M., et al. (2010), 'A proteomic view on the role of glucose in peritoneal dialysis', *J Proteome Res,* 9 (5), 2472-9.

Lim, Y. K., et al. (2000), 'Haptoglobin reduces renal oxidative DNA and tissue damage during phenylhydrazine-induced hemolysis', *Kidney Int,* 58 (3), 1033-44.

Lin, W. T., et al. (2008), 'Proteomic analysis of peritoneal dialysate fluid in patients with dialysis-related peritonitis', *Ren Fail,* 30 (8), 772-7.

Linden, T., et al. (1998), '3-Deoxyglucosone, a promoter of advanced glycation end products in fluids for peritoneal dialysis', *Perit Dial Int,* 18 (3), 290-3.

Liu, Y. W., et al. (2008), 'Proteomic analysis of pericardial effusion: Characteristics of tuberculosis-related proteins', *Proteomics Clin Appl,* 2 (4), 458-66.

McLerran, D., et al. (2008), 'SELDI-TOF MS whole serum proteomic profiling with IMAC surface does not reliably detect prostate cancer', *Clin Chem,* 54 (1), 53-60.

Minami, S., et al. (2007), 'Relationship between effluent levels of beta(2)-microglobulin and peritoneal injury markers in 7.5% icodextrin-based peritoneal dialysis solution', *Ther Apher Dial,* 11 (4), 296-300.

Mischak, H., Julian, B. A., and Novak, J. (2007), 'High-resolution proteome/peptidome analysis of peptides and low-molecular-weight proteins in urine', *Proteomics Clin Appl,* 1 (8), 792-804.

Nilsson-Thorell, C. B., et al. (1993), 'Heat sterilization of fluids for peritoneal dialysis gives rise to aldehydes', *Perit Dial Int,* 13 (3), 208-13.

Norman, A. W., et al. (1980), 'Vitamin D deficiency inhibits pancreatic secretion of insulin', *Science,* 209 (4458), 823-5.

Pecoits-Filho, R., et al. (2004), 'Chronic inflammation in peritoneal dialysis: the search for the holy grail?', *Perit Dial Int,* 24 (4), 327-39.

Pischetsrieder, M. (2000), 'Chemistry of glucose and biochemical pathways of biological interest', *Perit Dial Int,* 20 Suppl 2, S26-30.

Raaijmakers, R., et al. (2008), 'Proteomic profiling and identification in peritoneal fluid of children treated by peritoneal dialysis', *Nephrol Dial Transplant,* 23 (7), 2402-5.

Reddingius, R. E., et al. (1995), 'Complement in serum and dialysate in children on continuous ambulatory peritoneal dialysis', *Perit Dial Int,* 15 (1), 49-53.

Saku, K., et al. (1989), 'Lipoprotein and apolipoprotein losses during continuous ambulatory peritoneal dialysis', *Nephron,* 51 (2), 220-4.

Sitter, T. and Sauter, M. (2005), 'Impact of glucose in peritoneal dialysis: saint or sinner?', *Perit Dial Int,* 25 (5), 415-25.

Sritippayawan, S., et al. (2007), 'Proteomic analysis of peritoneal dialysate fluid in patients with different types of peritoneal membranes', *J Proteome Res,* 6 (11), 4356-62.

Tan, L. B., et al. (2008), 'Proteomic analysis for human urinary proteins associated with arsenic intoxication', *Proteomics Clin Appl,* 2 (7-8), 1087-98.

Tanaka, Y., et al. (1984), 'Effect of vitamin D3 on the pancreatic secretion of insulin and somatostatin', *Acta Endocrinol (Copenh),* 105 (4), 528-33.

Tyan, Y. C., et al. (2005a), 'Proteomic analysis of human pleural effusion', *Proteomics,* 5 (4), 1062-74. (2005b), 'Proteomic profiling of human pleural effusion using two-dimensional nano liquid chromatography tandem mass spectrometry', *J Proteome Res,* 4 (4), 1274-86.

van der Kamp, H. J., et al. (1999), 'Influence of peritoneal loss of GHBP, IGF-I and IGFBP-3 on serum levels in children with ESRD', *Nephrol Dial Transplant,* 14 (1), 257-8.

Wang, H. Y., et al. (2010), 'Differential proteomic characterization between normal peritoneal fluid and diabetic peritoneal dialysate', *Nephrol Dial Transplant,* 25 (6), 1955-63.

Wieslander, A. P., et al. (1991), 'Toxicity of peritoneal dialysis fluids on cultured fibroblasts, L-929', *Kidney Int,* 40 (1), 77-9.

Williams, J. D., et al. (2002), 'Morphologic changes in the peritoneal membrane of patients with renal disease', *J Am Soc Nephrol,* 13 (2), 470-9.

Witowski, J. and Jorres, A. (2000), 'Glucose degradation products: relationship with cell damage', *Perit Dial Int,* 20 Suppl 2, S31-6.

Witowski, J., et al. (2003), 'Mesothelial toxicity of peritoneal dialysis fluids is related primarily to glucose degradation products, not to glucose per se', *Perit Dial Int,* 23 (4), 381-90.

Young, G. A., Kendall, S., and Brownjohn, A. M. (1993), 'Complement activation during CAPD', *Nephrol Dial Transplant,* 8 (12), 1372-5.

7

Peritoneal Dialysate Effluent During Peritonitis Induces Human Cardiomyocyte Apoptosis and Express Matrix Metalloproteinases-9

Ching-Yuang Lin and Chia-Ying Lee
College of Medicine, China Medical University,
China Medical University Hospital, Taichung
Taiwan

1. Introduction

Cardiovascular event and infection are the first and second leading causes of death in the peritoneal dialysis (PD) populations (Parfrey and Foley, 1999; Go et al., 2004; Schiffrin et al., 2007; USRDS, 2008); both events are closely related. PD-related peritonitis is the crucial infection in PD patients (Aslam et al., 2006; Bender et al., 2006). Peritoneal toxin should be absorbed to the systemic circulation and might induce cardiotoxicity. After an episode of severe infection in dialysis patients, risk of death from cardiovascular events is increased sevenfold for 6 months and continues to rise for up to 48 months (Ishani et al., 2005; Bender et al., 2006). It has been considered to play a significant role in up to one sixth of patient deaths occurring during the course of PD therapy (Fried et al., 1996). In 41.5% of patients with peritonitis-related mortality, immediate cause of death was a cardiovascular event (Pe´ rez Fontan et al., 2005). Clinical findings indicate that a peritonitis episode may culminate in cardiovascular event (Fried et al., 1996; Bender et al., 2006): high incidence of peritonitis is accompanied by greater risk of death (Maiorca et al., 1993; Fried et al., 1996; Piraino, 1998), and cardiovascular events contribute to risk of peritonitis-related death in patients undergoing PD (Digenis et al., 1990; Firanek et al., 1991; Lupo et al., 1994). However, the possible mechanisms connecting PD-related peritonitis and cardiac mortality have not been addressed.

Growing evidence implicates cardiomyocyte apoptosis as a mechanism contributing to various types of heart disease (Olivetti et al., 1997; Haunstetter and Izumo, 1998; Narula et al., 1999). Cardiomyocyte apoptosis could result in a loss of contractile tissue, compensatory hypertrophy of myocardial cells, reparative fibrosis, and heart failure. In animal models, endotoxin (Natanson et al., 1989; Ramana et al., 2006), exotoxin (Natanson et al., 1989; Sibelius et al., 2000), and inflammatory mediator (Mann, 1999) play important roles in cardiomyocyte apoptosis. In PD patients with infectious peritonitis, expression of inflammatory mediators and cytokines increase in PD effluent (PDE) and correlate with treatment outcome (Lai et al., 2000; Wang and Lin, 2005). Yet there are no data on effects of peritonitis PD effluent (PPDE) on cardiomyocytes viability and apoptosis.

Bcl-2 protein family members are the best characterized proteins that are directly involved in the regulation of apoptosis (Cory and Adams, 2002). Bcl-2 and its closest homologues,

Bcl-x_L and Bcl-w, potently inhibit apoptosis in response to many cytotoxic insults. Bax and Bak are well known proapoptotic members of the Bcl-2 protein family. Regulation of apoptosis is highly dependent on the ratio of anti-apoptotic to pro- apoptotic proteins. Conditions that induce myocardial stress cause complex alterations in levels of Bcl-2 family proteins (Bishopric et al., 2001).

Cardiac Bcl-2 gene expression has been shown to be regulated by GATA-4 both in vitro and in vivo (Kobayashi et al., 2006). GATA-4 is a transcription factor enriched in cardiac tissue that is essential for various cardiomyocyte physiological and adaptive responses. An early event in the cardiotoxicity induced by the antitumor drug doxorubicin is GATA-4 depletion, which in turn causes cardiomyocyte apoptosis (Aries et al., 2004; Suzuki and Evans, 2004). GATA-4 has also been shown to upregulate transcription of the anti-apoptotic genes Bcl-2 (Kobayashi et al., 2006) and Bcl-x_L (Aries et al., 2004; Suzuki and Evans, 2004) in cardiomyocytes, and to play a central role in regulating the survival or apoptosis of cardiomyocytes. Although previous studies have suggested the importance of apoptosis regulation and GATA-4 expression in various heart diseases, their role in PD peritonitis-related cardiotoxicity has not been elucidated.

Cardiac extracellular matrix (ECM) lends structural support and integrity to the myocardium and facilitates conversion of cardiomyocyte contraction into pump function (Caulfield JB et al., 1979; Sato S et al., 1983; Thompson MM et al., 2002). Integrity of original ECM is thought to play a key role in determining extent of remolding after myocardial infarction and matrix metalloproteinases (MMPs) play crucial roles in regulation of ECM. Inflammatory response and cardiac pro-matrix metalloproteinase (MMP)-9 are critical to heart failure (Jugdutt BI, 2003; Shah AP et al., 2009). Increasing MMP-9 level and activity may develop in a special group of patients with exposure to peritonitis toxin in their cardiomyocytes.

To clarify the relationship between PD-related peritonitis and high cardiac mortality, we postulated that during PD-related peritonitis, proapoptotic pathways are activated and MMP-9 protein is also expressed in cardiomyocytes.

To test this hypothesis, human cardiomyocytes were cultured and treated with PPDE. The possible underlying signaling pathways of cardiotoxicity and enhancing MMP-9 expression in cultured human cardiomyocytes after stimulated by PPDE were examined.

2. Human cardiomyocytes culture

This research was approved by the China Medical Hospital Institutional Review Board. Written informed consent was obtained from each individual. Human cardiomyocytes obtained from the myocardial ventricular resection specimens of patients undergoing cardiac surgery were isolated as previously described (Hsin-Hui Wang et al., 2010).

3. Characterization of human cardiomyocytes in primary culture

To characterize cardiomyocytes, muscle markers desmin and myocyte-specific protein a-sarcomeric actinin were detected (Fig. 1). CAPON, recently documented as endogenous protein expressed in guinea pig cardiomyocytes, interacts with nitric oxide synthase to accelerate cardiac repolarization by inhibition of L-type calcium channels. Expression of endogenous CAPON protein in cultured cardiomyocytes was detected by immunofluorescent staining and confocal microscopy (Fig. 1). Both action potential duration

(APD) and peak L-Type calcium current (IcaL) were APD_{10}, APD_{50}, APD_{75} and APD_{90}: 95.4 ± 10.6, 289.2 ± 15.6, 308.2 ± 15.4, and 318.4 ± 16.4 msec, respectively, with peak IcaL density of −10.2 ± 0.9 pA/pE at ± 10 mV (n=6).

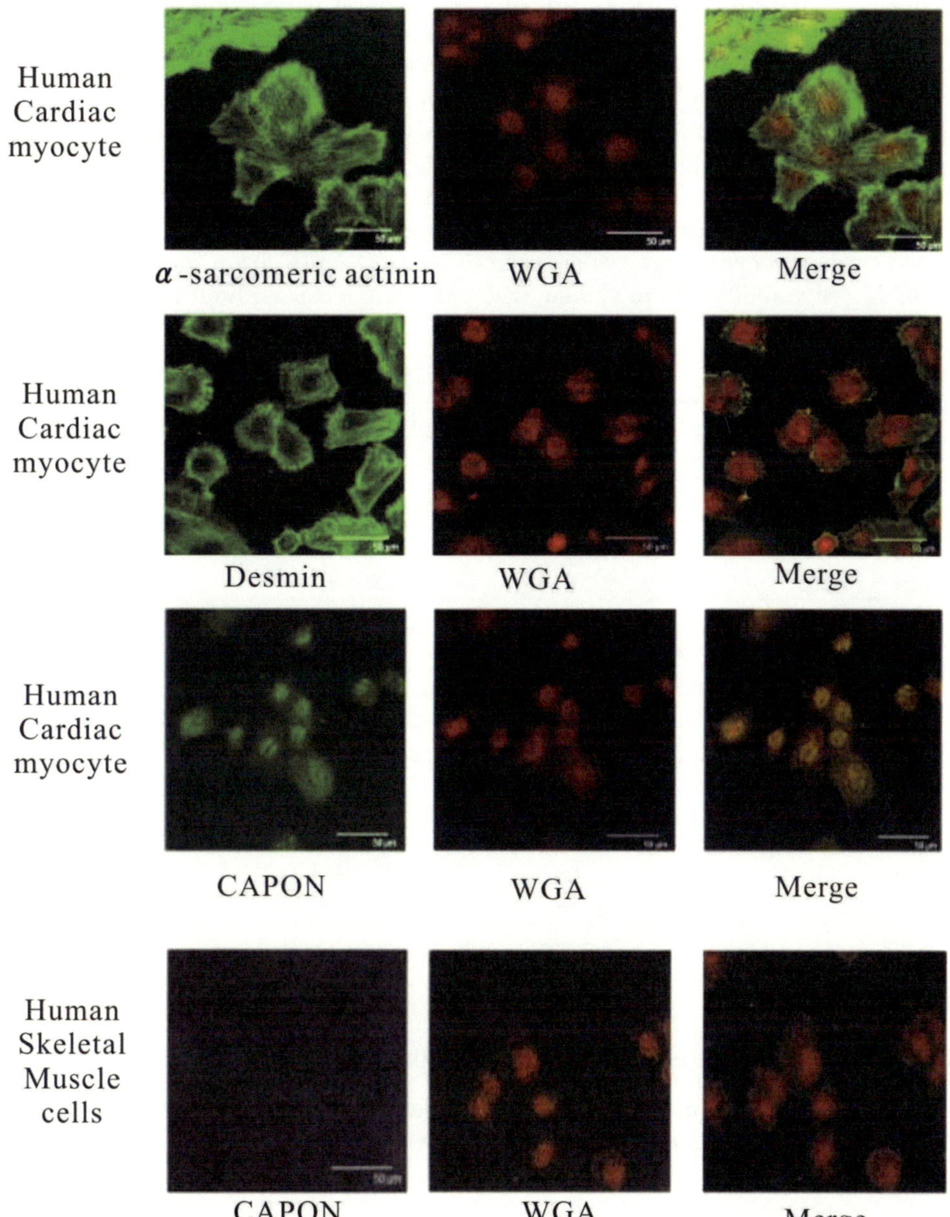

Fig. 1. Characterization of human cardiomyocytes by immunostaining of cardiomyocyte markers. Double labeling of cardiomyocytes with WGA (red) and α-sarcomeric actinin (green) (first line)or desmin (green) (second line) or CAPON (green) (third line). Negative control using cultured human skeletal muscle cells was stained with CAPON (last line).

4. PPDE induces cell death in human cardiomyocytes

Cardiac cell death is believed to play a major contributory role in development and progression of myocardial dysfunction (Haunstetter and Izumo, 1998). To assess whether PPDE treatment induced cardiac cell death, cell viability were evaluated by MTT assay. Doxorubicin-induced cardiotoxicity, which has been well described (Shan et al., 1996), was used as a positive control. MTT assay showed PDE during peritonitis- and doxorubicin-induced human cardiomyocyte cell death as both dose- (Fig. 2A and Table 1) and time-dependent (Fig. 2B and Table 2). When cardiomyocytes were pre-exposed to 12.5, 18, or 25 mg/ml PDE during peritonitis for 24h, cell viabilities were 70.6 ± 5.7%, 58.7 ± 9.7%, and 41.6 ± 7.8%, respectively, all significantly lower than in cardiomyocytes without pre-treatment ($P < 0.05$) (Fig. 2A). This change was even more profound in the 48 h treatment group (Fig. 2B). When cardiomyocytes were pre-exposed to 25 mg/ml PDE from stable PD patients for 24 and 48 h, cell viabilities were similar with cardiomyocytes without pre-treatment (data not shown).

	% of apoptosis		
Treatment	0	12.5 mg/ml	25 mg/ml
Medium only	1.0 ± 2.7	10.4 ± 2.8	11.8 ± 3.2
PBS only	2.2 ± 3.1	10.2 ± 3.2	10.8 ± 3.6
Medium + DOXO	9.7 ± 2.4	28.5 ± 4.1[a]	41.2 ± 4.5[a]
Medium + SPDE	0.7 ± 2.5	10.2 ± 2.7	12.4 ± 3.5
Medium + PPDE	9.7 ± 2.6	32.4 ± 3.8[a]	48.6 ± 4.8[a]

Table 1. Dose dependent manner of PPDE induced cell apoptosis in cultured human cardiomyocytes

	% of apoptosis		
Treatment	0	24 h	48 h
Medium only	1.0 ± 2.7	11.5 + 2.7	12.1 + 3.2
PBS only	2.2 ± 3.1	10.4 + 2.6	11.5 + 3.4
Medium + DOXO	9.7 ± 2.4	34.8 + 3.6[a]	42.2 + 4.2[a]
Medium + SPDE	0.7 ± 2.5	12.2 + 3.2	13.6 + 3.2
Medium + PPDE	9.7 ± 2.6	48.2 + 4.7[a]	57.6 + 4.4[a]

Table 2. Time dependent manner of PPDE induced cell apoptosis in cultured human cardiomyocytes

5. PPDE induces apoptosis in human cardiomyocytes

The above lend substantial evidence of apoptosis playing a critical role in cardiomyocyte cell death associated with several cardiac diseases (Olivetti et al., 1997; Haunstetter and Izumo, 1998). To explore whether PPDE during peritonitis challenge induces human cardiomyocyte apoptosis, we assessed apoptotic cell death by flow cytometry. Comet assays were also performed for determination of DNA damage. Doxorubicin, which can induce cardiomyocytes apopotosis (Kim et al., 2003), was used as a positive control. After cell incubation with 25 mg/ml PPDE peritonitis for 24 h, apoptosis was detected by flow cytometry (Tables 1 and 2). Analyses indicated little cardiomyocyte apoptosis with non-exposed condition (control group) and exposure with 25 mg/ml SPDE from stable PD

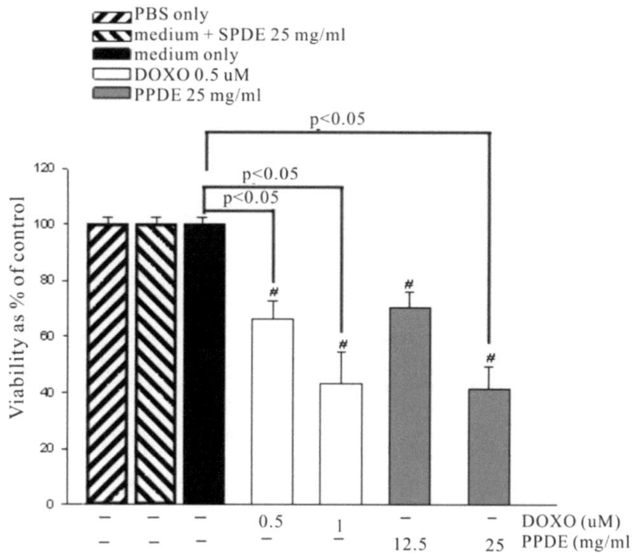

(a)

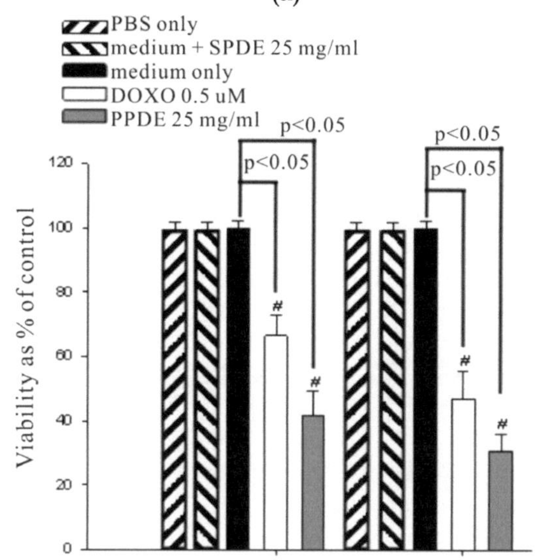

(b)

Fig. 2. Cell viability reduced after treatment with PPDE. Human cardiomyocytes were treated with PPDE during peritonitis. Cell viability was determined by MTT assay. (A) Cells were incubated with various concentration of peritoneal dialysate effluent during peritonitis (PPDE) (12, 5, 18, 25 mg/ml) (n=8) or doxorubicin (0.5, 1 μM; Doxo) as a positive control for 24 hr. (■) treated with medium only (□) or Doxo pretreatment; (B) cell were treated with PPDE (25 ng/ml) for 24 or 48 hrs. (n=8) and controls Data are expressed as mean ± SD of 8 different PPDE. # P<0.01 versus medium only control, * P<0.05, ** P<0.01. (: treated with PBS only) (: treated with medium and stable peritoneal dialysate effluent (SPDE) without peritonitis) (treated with medium and peritonitis peritoneal dialysate effluent (PPDE))

patients (Tables 1 and 2). By contrast, doxorubicin and PPDE induced apoptosis in 34.8–48.6% of human cardiomyocytes after treated for 24 h. Finally, PPDE induced DNA damage was determined by Comet assay (Fig. 3): higher concentrations of PPDE resulted in greater numbers of damaged cells.

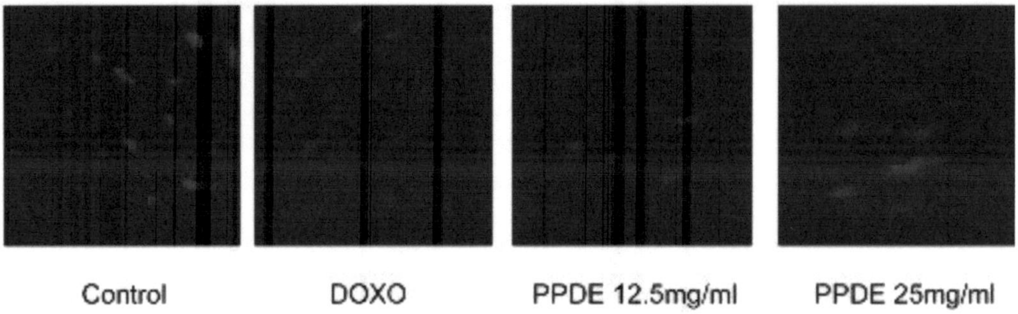

Fig. 3. PPDE treatment induces apoptosis in cultured human cardiomyocytes. Cardiomyocyte DNA damage was determined by the Comet assay. Cardiomyocytes were treated with PPDE (12.5 or 25 mg/ml) or Doxo (0.5 μM) as a positive control for 24 h, and then the Comet assay was performed.

6. PPDE induced Bax increase and suppression of GATA-4 expression in human cardiomyocytes

The Bcl-2 family of proteins are key regulators of the stress- induced apoptotic pathway (Bishopric et al., 2001); to determine their role in regulation of PPDE induced cardiomyocyte apoptosis, mRNA concentrations of prosurvival proteins Bcl-2 and Bcl-xL and proapoptotic protein Bax were measured in human cardiomyocytes by quantitative real-time RT-PCR (Fig. 4A). Compared to the no-exposure control group, Bcl-2/Bax and Bcl-xL/Bax ratios dropped significantly following 4 h of PPDE treatment (Fig. 4B; $P < 0.05$ vs. control). Western blotting analysis for Bcl-2, Bcl-xl, and Bax protein expression in the same experimental conditions obtained similar results (Fig. 6A). These data indicated that PPDE treatment decreased Bcl-2/Bax and Bcl-xL/Bax ratios, resulting in increase Bax expression in human cardiomyocytes.

Transcription factor GATA-4 has been identified as a specific myocardial survival factor which induces transcription and expression of Bcl-2 and which is associated with cell survival (Ancey et al., 2002; Kitta et al., 2003; Aries et al., 2004; Suzuki and Evans, 2004). To characterize mechanisms underlying PPDE activity in human cardiomyocytes, mRNA and protein expression of GATA-4 were measured. For cardiomyocytes exposed to PPDE, GATA-4 mRNA expression decreased fivefold relative to no-exposure control cells by quantitative real-time RT-PCR ($P < 0.05$) (Fig. 5A). Western blots of nuclear GATA-4 protein expression in PPDE exposed human cardiomyocytes also showed lower levels than the control group (Fig. 5B,C), suggesting that PDE during peritonitis treatment decreases levels of GATA-4 gene expression in human cardiomyocytes.

7. PPDE does not contain inflammatory mediators

To evaluate whether PPDE was enriched in pro-apoptotic mediators, TRAEL, FasL, TNFa, IL-6, and IL-1 were measured by enzyme-linked immunoassay by commercial ELISA kit.

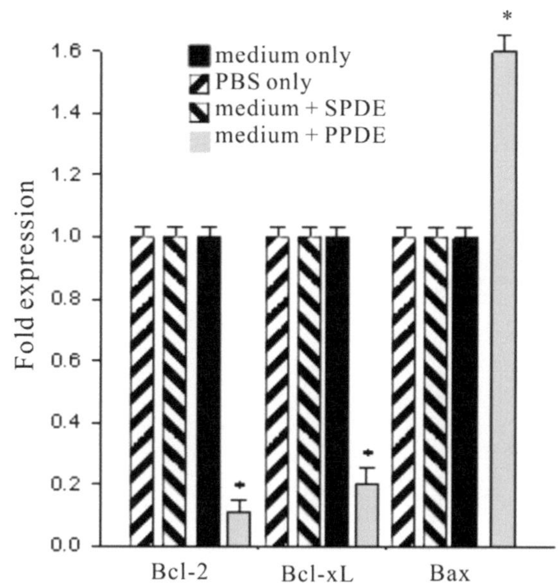

(a)

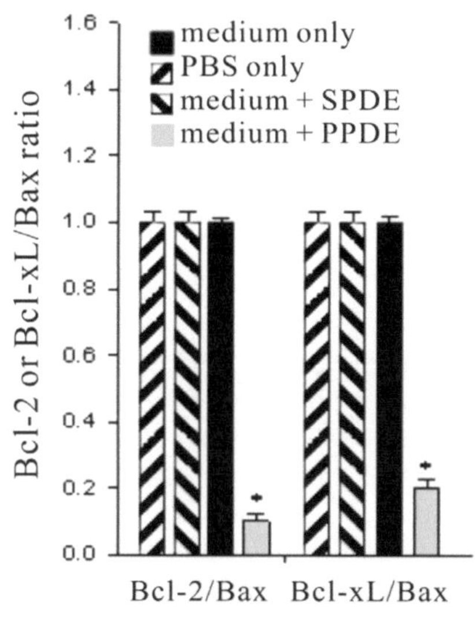

(b)

Fig. 4. (A) PPDE treatment upregulates Bax gene expression in cultured human cardiomyocytes. Human cardiomyocytes were treated with or without PPDE (25 mg/ml), and then total RNA was prepared following 4 h of treatment. Bcl-2, Bcl-xL, and Bax mRNA expression levels in cardiomyocytes were determined by quantitative real-time RT-PCR. (n=8) Data are expressed as the mean ± SD of 8 different PPDE.* P<0.01 versus control. (B)Bcl-2/Bax and Bcl-xL/Bax ratio of experiment (A). Data are expressed as mean ± SD of 8 different PPDE. * P<0.01 versus control. ■: no treatment, medium only ; ▨: no treatment PBS only ; ▧: medium + stable PDE without peritonitis(SPDE) (treated with medium and peritonitis peritoneal dialysate effluent (PPDE).

Cultured supernatant from peripheral blood mononuclear cells stimulated with lippolysaccharide was used as positive control; TRAEL, FasL, TNFa, and IL-1 were undetectable in 25 mg/ml PPDE (data not shown). The lower limit of sensitivity was 0.70 pg/ml.

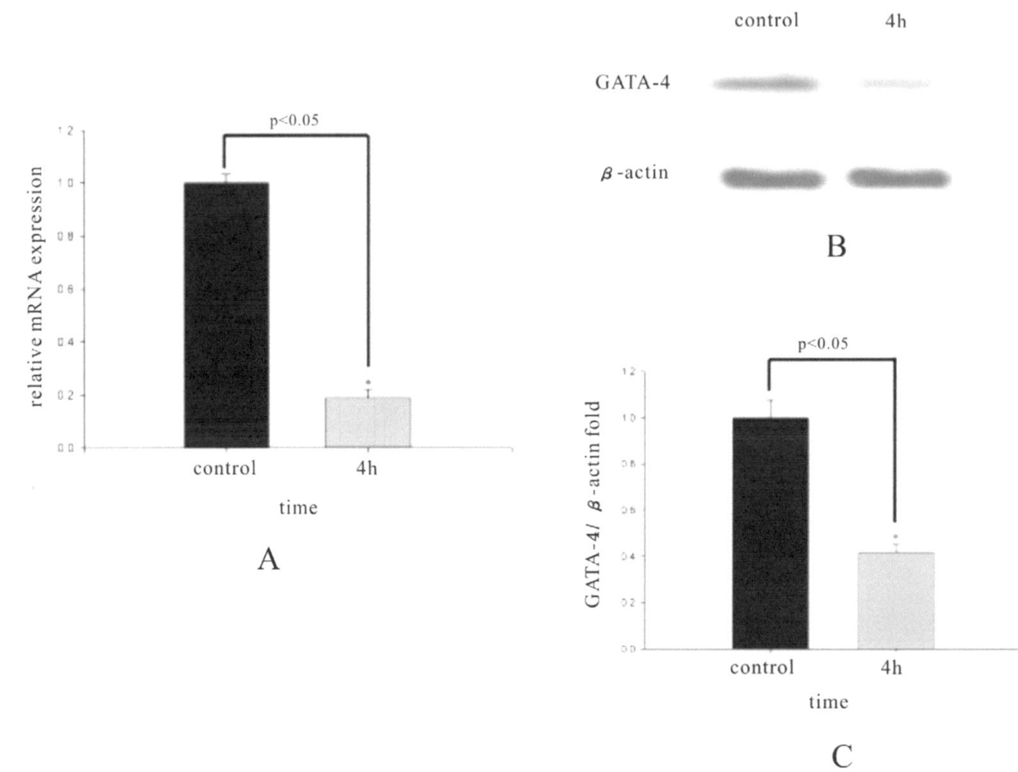

Fig. 5. Effects of PPDE on expression of cardiac GATA-4 mRNA and protein. Cultured human cardiomyocytes were treated with or without PPDE (25 mg/ml), and then protein extracts and total RNA were prepared following 4 h of treatment. A: GATA-4 mRNA expression levels in cultured human cardiomyocytes as determined by quantitative real-time RT-PCR. B: Western blot showing GATA-4 protein levels. C: GATA-4 protein levels in cultured human cardiomyocytes, ascertained by densitometry. Data are expressed as mean ± SD of 8 different PPDE. * P<0.01 versus control.

8. Role of ERK pathway in PPDE induced cardiotoxicity

We next examined possible signaling mechanisms regulating PPDE-induced cardiomyocyte apoptosis. The GATA-4 molecule contains putative ERK phosphorylation sites, and recent studies have shown that some survival factors (Morimoto et al., 2000; Kitta et al., 2001, 2003) induce activity of GATA-4 via MEK/ERK-dependent phosphorylation. Therefore, we explored activity of MEK/ERK signaling pathways in PPDE treated cardiomyocytes. Figure 6 shows ERK phosphorylation significantly reduced in cells exposed to PPDE peritonitis, suggesting that PPDE inhibits the ERK signaling pathway, consistent with the idea that the ERK pathway is crucial for GATA-4 activity and cardiomyocyte survival.

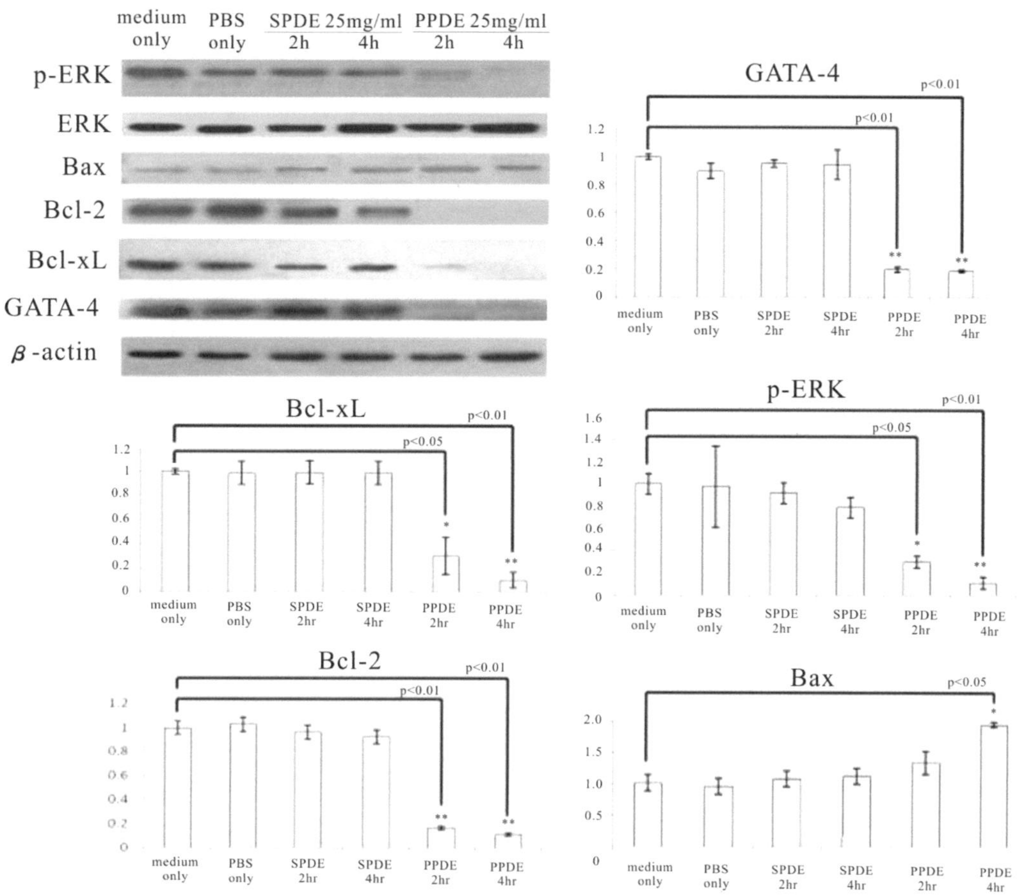

Fig. 6. PPDE treatment reduces ERK phosyhorylation, GATA4, Bcl-2, Bcl-xL expression and enhances Bax expression in cultured human cardiomyocytes. Cardiomyocytes were treated with medium only, PBS only, SPDE (25 mg/ml) for 2 and 4 hours and PPDE (25 mg/ml) for 2 and 4 hours. Cell lysates were separated by SDS-PAGE and specific monoclonal antibodies were used to detect phosphorylated and total ERK, and Bax, Bcl-2, Bcl-xL, GATA4 expression. Representative blots from 8 separate experiments were shown. Quantitative densitometry expressed as phosphorylated protein relative to total protein. Data are expressed as the mean ± SD of 8 different PPDE .* P<0.01 versus control. Medium only, PBS only and SPDE (25 mg/ml) in medium were used as negative controls.

9. PPDE induces MMP-9 expression in cultured human cardiomyocytes

Expression of MMP-9 protein was noted, accompanied by enhanced MyD88, IRAK1 and NF-kB phosphorylation in cultured human cardiomyocytes treated by PPDE.(Fig. 7). We also found MMP-9 co-localized with macrophages and myofibroblasts in autopy specimens of cardiac tissue from patients with end-stage renal disease by immunostaining using confocal microscopic imaging. (Fig. 8)

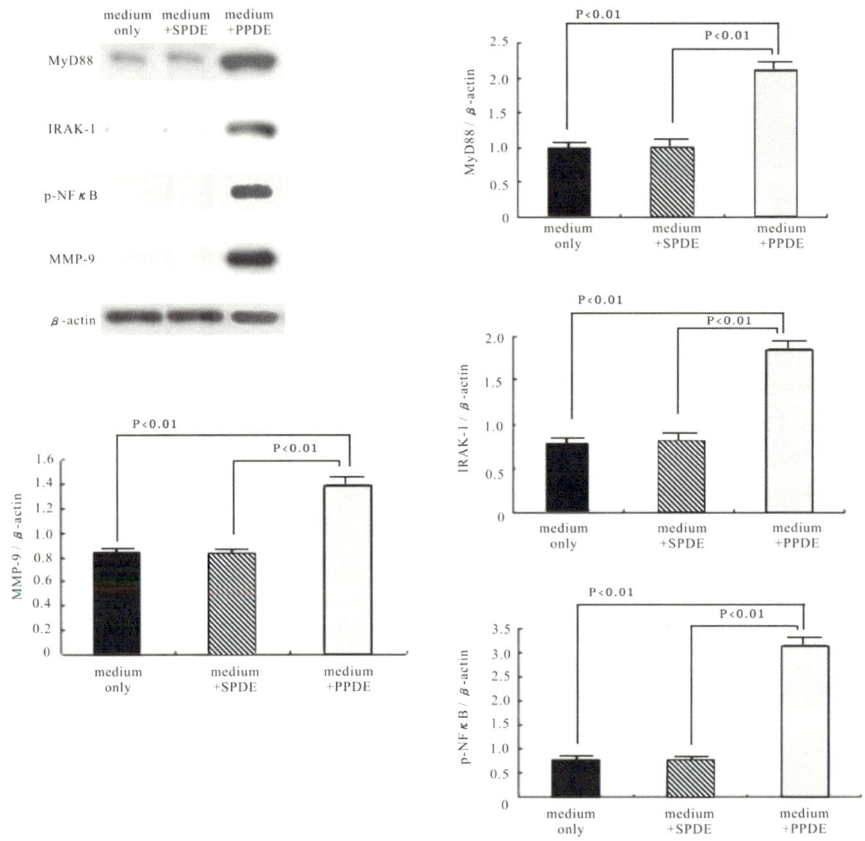

Fig. 7. Effects of PPDE (25 mg/ml) on the expression of MyD88, IRAK-1, MMP-9 protein and NFκB phosphorylation. Cultured human cardiomyocytes were treated with medium only, medium + SPDE (25 mg/ml) and medium + PPDE (25 mg/ml), and then protein extracted for western blot analysis. Data are expressed as the mean±SD of 8 different PPDE. *P<0.01 versus control.

10. PPDE induces MMP-9 expression via MyD88/IRAK1/p65 signal pathway

To determine whether MyD88-dependent signaling pathway in cultured human cardiomyocytes will be modulate by PPDE, we studied MyD88 protein expression in cultured human cardiomyocytes after treated with PPDE. The result showed cultured human cardiomyocytes express MyD88 after PPDE treatment (Fig. 9). To further study MyD88-dependent signaling pathway in cultured human cardiomyocytes after treated with PPDE, we compared the difference of cytoplasm IRAK1-1 expression with and without PPDE treatment in cultured human cardiomyocytes. PPDE enhanced cytoplasmic IRAK1 expression when compared to the SPDE and medium only (Fig. 10).

NF-κB is an important transcription factor to induce chronic inflammation in myocarditis; and contains a transactivation domain which is involved in the MyD88-dependent pathway that produces many pro-inflammatory cytokines. Increased nuclear NF-κB/p65 expression with PPDE treatment in cultured human cardiomyocytes was observed (Fig. 11).

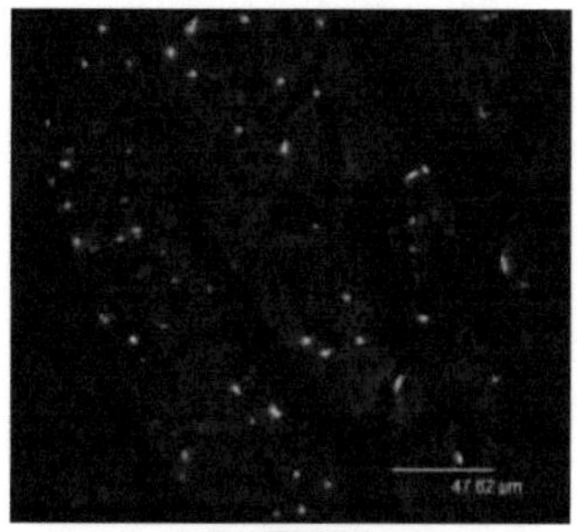

CAPON

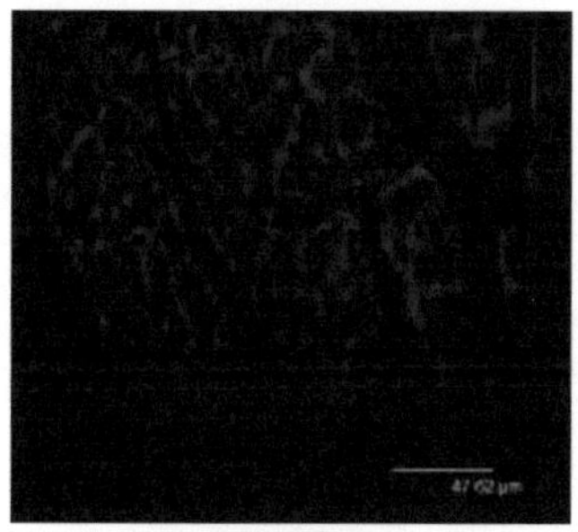

MMP-9

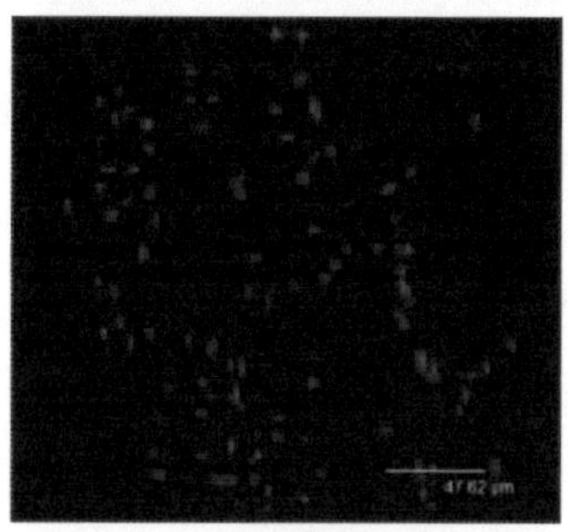

nuclei

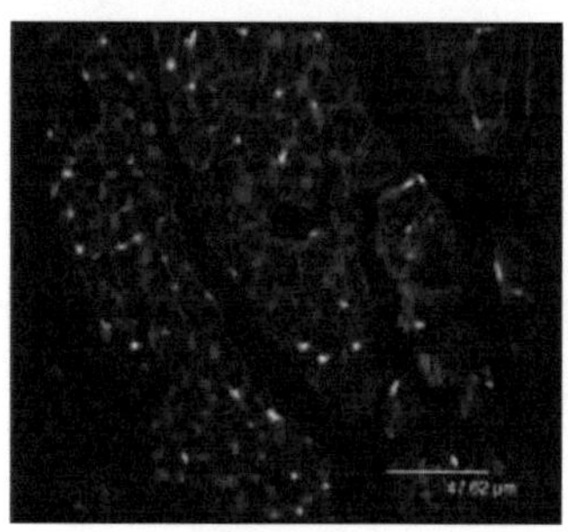

Merge

Fig. 8. MMP-9 co-localized with cardiomyocytes in cardiac tissue of patient with uremic cardiomyopathy. Double labeling of cardiomyocytes with CAPON(green), MMP-9(red) and nuclei(blue).

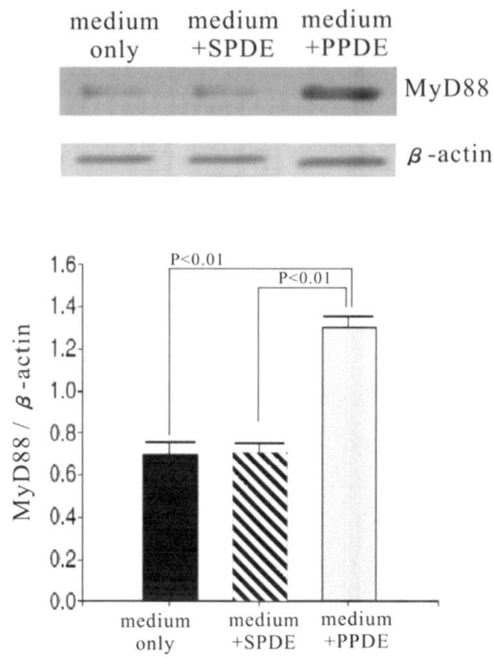

Fig. 9. Cultured human cardiomyocytes express MyD88 after PPDE (25 mg/ml) stimulation. Representative western blot results of 8 different PPDE were shown.

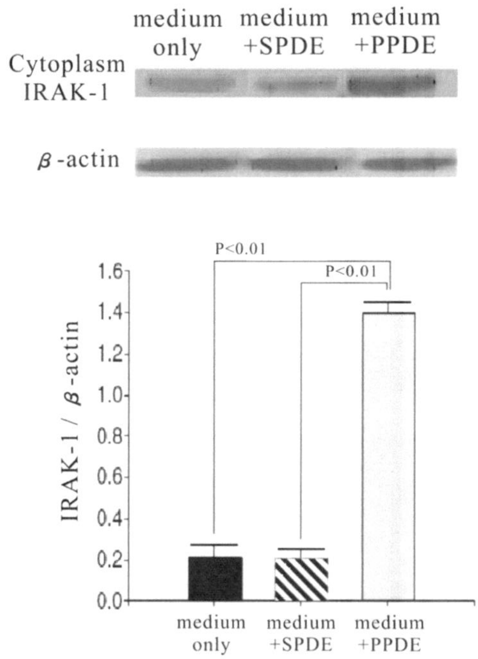

Fig. 10. Increased cytoplasm interleukin receptor-associated kinase-1 (IRAK-1) expression in cultured human cardiomyocytes after PPDE (25 mg/ml) stimulation. Representative western blot results of 8 different PPDE were shown.

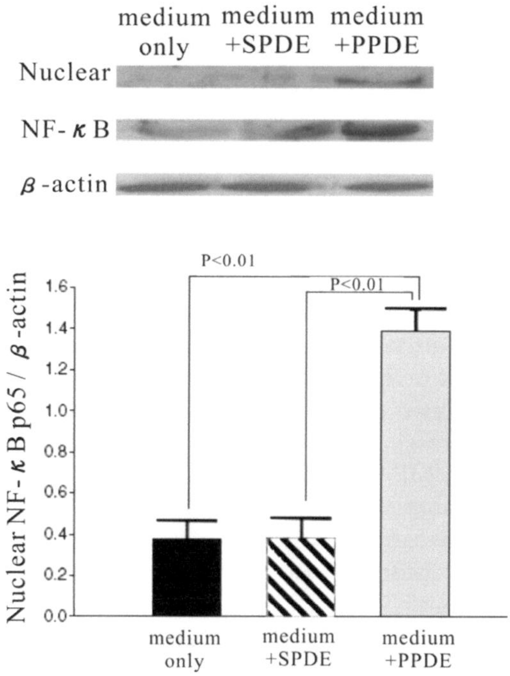

Fig. 11. Cultured human cardiomyocytes were stimulated with PPDE (25 mg/ml) for shown and expression of nuclear NF-κB/p65 was detected by western blot. Increased expression of nuclear NF-κB/p65 was noted. Representative western blot results of 8 different PPDE were shown.

11. Conclusion

Our study demonstrated that PPDE contains potent pro-apoptotic factors and causes an imbalance between proapoptotic and prosurvival pathways, inducing apoptosis in human cardiomyocytes. This study revealed a possible mechanism of PD-related, peritonitis-induced cardiotoxicity. These novel findings constitute the first direct evidence linking PD peritonitis and cardiomyocyte apoptosis. Cardiovascular events are the major cause of death in PD patients with peritonitis. Our findings demonstrated the central role of apoptosis in PD peritonitis-associated cardiovascular events, and provided an explanation for the high incidents of cardiovascular events in PD-related peritonitis.

Cardiomyocyte death is important in the pathogenesis of cardiac disease in end-stage renal disease (Parfrey and Foley, 1999). Cardiomyocyte death induces LV compensatory LV hypertrophy, and eventually leading to dilatation with systolic dysfunction. LV hypertrophy appears to be an important, independent, determinant of survival in patients with end stage renal diseases (Silberberg et al., 1989). Our study yields direct cellular evidence of PPDE from PD patients as cardiotoxic. In end-stage renal disease, cardiomyocyte death may be caused by continual LV overload, decreased large and small coronary vessel perfusion, hyperparathyroidism, and malnutrition (Parfrey and Foley, 1999). Our data provide another possible cause of cardiac cell death in patients undergoing PD.

Previous studies suggested that the elevated plasma concentration of MMP-9 were likely due to an enhanced release from the infarcted myocardium (Inokubo, Y., et al., 2001; Rosemberg, G.A. et al., 1996). Furthermore, it is well documented that both neutrophil and MMP-9 have a synergistic effect in inflammatory injury (Steinberg, J. et al., 2001). In our previous studies, we also found MMP-9 co-localized with macrophages and myofibroblasts in human myocardial infarcted tissue. In the present study we demonstrated MMP-9 co-localized in human uremic myocardium. These results suggest both macrophage from post myocardial infarction to heart failure and activated cardiomyocytes can express MMP-9 protein. The increase of MMP-9 activity and levels not only can be used as the marker of post myocardial infarction, but also involved the pathogenesis of cardiac remodeling. Our results provided some new information in terms of diagnostic and therapeutic implications in a special group of patients with uremic cardiomyopathy in PD patients.

In conclusion, we demonstrated for the first time that PPDE contains potent pro-apoptotic factors that regulate expression of GATA-4 and Bcl-2 families, inducing cultured cardiomyocyte apoptosis. MMP-9 expression provided some new information of cardiac remodeling. Findings illustrate a pivotal role of apoptosis and cardiac remodeling in PD peritonitis-associated cardiovascular events, explain high cardiac mortality in PD-related peritonitis, and pinpoint apoptotic events as a marker and potential therapeutic target for PD peritonitis-induced cardiotoxicity.

12. References

Ancey C, Corbi P, Froger J, Delwail A, Wijdenes J, Gascan H, Potreau D, Lecron JC. (2002). "Secretion of IL-6, IL-II and LIF by human cardiomyocytes in primary culture." Cytokine 18:199–205.

Aries A, Paradis P, Lefebvre C, Schwartz RJ, Nemer M. (2004). "Essential role of GATA-4 in cell survival and drug-induced cardiotoxicity." Proc Natl Acad Sci USA 101:6975–6980.

Aslam N, Bernardini J, Fried L, Burr R, Piraino B. (2006). "Comparison of infectious complications between incident hemodialysis and peritoneal dialysis patients." Clin J Am Soc Nephrol 1:1226–1233.

Bender FH, Bernardini J, Piraino B. (2006). "Prevention of infectious complications in peritoneal dialysis: Best demonstrated practices." Kidney Int 103(Suppl): S44–S54.

Bishopric NH, Andreka P, Slepak T, Webster KA. (2001). "Molecular mechanisms of apoptosis in the cardiac myocyte." Curr Opin Pharmacol 1:141–150.

Caulfield JB, Borg TK. (1979). "The collagen network of the heart." Lab Invest 40: 364-72.

Cory S, Adams JM. (2002). "The Bcl2 family: Regulators of the cellular life-or-death switch." Nat Rev Cancer 2:647–656.

Firanek CA, Vonesh EF, Korbet SM. (1991). "Patient and technique survival among an urban population of peritoneal dialysis patients: An 8-year experience." Am J Kidney Dis 18:91–96.

Fried LF, Bernardini J, Johnston JR, Piraino B. (1996). "Peritonitis influences mortality in peritoneal dialysis patients." J Am Soc Nephrol 7:2176–2182.

Go AS, Chertow GM, Fan D, McCulloch CE, Hsu CY. (2004). "Chronic kidney disease and the risks of death, cardiovascular events, and hospitalization." N Engl J Med 351:1296–1305.

Haunstetter A, Izumo S. (1998). "Apoptosis: Basic mechanisms and implications for cardiovascular disease. Circ Res 82:1111–1129.

Inokubo, Y., Hanada, H. and Ishizaka, H. (2001). "Plasma levels of Matrix metalloproteinase-9 and tissue inhibitor of metalloproteinase-1 are increased in the coronary circulation in patients with acute coronary syndrome." Am. Heart J. 141:211-217.

Ishani A, Collins AJ, Herzog CA, Foley RN. (2005). "Septicemia, access and cardiovascular disease in dialysis patients: The USRDS Wave 2 study." Kidney Int 68:311–318.

Jugdutt BI. (2003). "Ventricular remodeling after infarction and the extracellular collagen Matrix: when is enough enough?" Circulation 108: 1395-403.

Kim Y, Ma AG, Kitta K, Fitch SN, Ikeda T, Ihara Y, Simon AR, Evans T, Suzuki YJ. (2003). "Anthracycline-induced suppression of GATA-4 transcription factor: Implication in the regulation of cardiac myocyte apoptosis." Mol Pharmacol 63:368–377.

Kitta K, Clement SA, Remeika J, Blumberg JB, Suzuki YJ. (2001). "Endothelin-I induces phosphorylation of GATA-4 transcription factor in the HL-I atrial-muscle cell line." Biochem J 359:375–380.

Kitta K, Day RM, Kim Y, Torregroza I, Evans T, Suzuki YJ. (2003). "Hepatocyte growth factor induces GATA-4 phosphorylation and cell survival in cardiac muscle cells." J Biol Chem 278:4705–4712.

Kobayashi S, Lackey T, Huang Y, Bisping E, Pu WT, Boxer LM, Liang Q. (2006). "Transcription factor gata4 regulates cardiac BCL2 gene expression in vitro and in vivo." FASEB J 20:800- 802.

Lai KN, Lai KB, Lam CW, Chan TM, Li FK, Leung JC. (2000). "Changes of cytokine profiles during peritonitis in patients on continuous ambulatory peritoneal dialysis." Am J Kidney Dis 35:644–652.

Lupo A, Tarchini R, Carcarini G, Catizone L, Cocchi R, De Vecchi A, Viglino G, Salomone M, Segoloni G, Giangrande A. (1994). "Long-term outcome in continuous ambulatory peritoneal dialysis: A I0-year-survey by the Italian Cooperative Peritoneal Dialysis Study Group." Am J Kidney Dis 24:826–837.

Mann DL. (1999). "Inflammatory mediators in heart failure: Homogeneity through heterogeneity." Lancet 353:1812–1813.

Morimoto T, Hasegawa K, Kaburagi S, Kakita T, Wada H, Yanazume T, Sasayama S. (2000). "Phosphorylation of GATA-4 is involved in alpha I-adrenergic agonist-responsive transcription of the endothelin-I gene in cardiac myocytes." J Biol Chem 275:13721–13726.

Narula J, Pandey P, Arbustini E, Haider N, Narula N, Kolodgie FD, Dal Bello B, Semigran MJ, Bielsa-Masdeu A, Dec GW, Israels S, Ballester M, Virmani R, Saxena S, Kharbanda S. (1999). "Apoptosis in heart failure: Release of cytochrome c from mitochondria and activation of caspase-3 in human cardiomyopathy." Proc Natl Acad Sci USA 96:8144–8149.

Natanson C, Danner RL, Elin RJ, Hosseini JM, Peart KW, Banks SM, MacVittie TJ, Walker RI, Parrillo JE. (1989). "Role of endotoxemia in cardiovascular dysfunction and mortality. Escherichia coli and Staphylococcus aureus challenges in a canine model of human septic shock." J Clin Invest 83:243–251.

Olivetti G, Abbi R, Quaini F, Kajstura J, Cheng W, Nitahara JA, Quaini E, Di Loreto C, Beltrami CA, Krajewski S, Reed JC, Anversa P. (1997). "Apoptosis in the failing human heart." N Engl J Med 336:1131–1141.

Parfrey PS, Foley RN. (1999). "The clinical epidemiology of cardiac disease in chronic renal failure." J Am Soc Nephrol 10:1606–1615.

Pe´ rez Fontan M, Rodr´ıguez-Carmona A, Garc´ıa-Naveiro R, Rosales M, Villaverde P, Valde´ s F. (2005). "Peritonitis-related mortality in patients undergoing chronic peritoneal dialysis." Perit Dial Int 25: 274–284.

Ramana KV, Willis MS, White MD, Horton JW, DiMaio JM, Srivastava D, Bhatnagar A, Srivastava SK. (2006). "Endotoxin-induced cardiomyopathy and systemic inflammation in mice is prevented by aldose reductase inhibition." Circulation 114:1838–1846.

Rosemberg, G.A., Navratil, M., Barone, F. and Feuerstein, G. (1996). "Proteolytic cascade enzymes increase in focal cerebral ischemia in rat." J. Cereb. Blood Flow Metab. 16: 360-366.

Sato S, Ashraf M, Millard RW. (1983). "Connective tissue changes in early ischemia of porcine myocardium: an ultrastructural study." J Mol Cell Cardiol 15: 261-75.

Schiffrin EL, Lipman ML, Mann JF. (2007). "Chronic kidney disease: Effects on the cardiovascular system." Circulation 116:85–97.

Shah AP, Niemann JT, Youngquist S, Heyming T, Rosborough JP. (2009). "Plasma endothelin-1 level at the onset of ischemic ventricular fibrillation predicts resuscitation outcome." Resuscitation 80: 580-3.

Shan K, Lincoff AM, Young JB. (1996). "Anthracycline-induced cardiotoxicity." Ann Intern Med 125:47–58.

Sibelius U, Grandel U, Buerke M, Mueller D, Kiss L, Kraemer HJ, Braun-Dullaeus R, Haberbosch W, Seeger W, Grimminger F. (2000). "Staphylococcal alpha-toxin provokes coronary vasoconstriction and loss in myocardial contractility in perfused rat hearts: Role of thromboxane generation." Circulation 101:78–85.

Silberberg JS, Barre PE, Prichard SS, Sniderman AD. (1989). "Impact of left ventricular hypertrophy on survival in end-stage renal disease." Kidney Int 36:286–290.

Steinberg, J., Fink, G., Picone, A ., Searles, B., Schiller, H,. Lee, H.M. and Nieman, G. (2001). "Evidence of increased matrix metalloproteinase-9 concentration in patients following cardiopulmonary bypass." J. Extra.Corpor. Technol. 33: 218-222.

Suzuki YJ, Evans T. (2004). "Regulation of cardiac myocyte apoptosis by the GATA-4 transcription factor." Life Sci 74:1829–1838.

Thompson MM, Squire IB. (2002). "Matrix metalloproteinase-9 expression after myocardial infarction: physiological or pathological?" Cardiovasc Res 54: 495-8.

U.S. Renal Data System. (2008). USRDS 2008 Annual Data Report: Atlas of Chronic Kidney Disease and End-Stage Renal Disease in the United States, National Institutes of Health, National Institute of Diabetes and Digestive and Kidney Diseases, Bethesda, MD.

Wang HH, Lin CY. (2005). "Interleukin-I2 and -I8 levels in peritoneal dialysate effluent correlate with the outcome of peritonitis in patients undergoing peritoneal dialysis: Implications for the Type I/Type II T-cell immune response." Am J Kidney Dis 46:328- 338.

Wang HH, Li PC, Huang HJ, Lee TY, Lin CY. (2011). "Peritoneal Dialysate Effluent During Peritonitis Induces Human Cardiomyocytes Apoptosis by Regulating the Expression of GATA-4 and Bcl-2 Families" J.cell. Physiol. 226(1):94-102.

8

A Renal Policy and Financing Framework to Understand Which Factors Favour Home Treatments Such as Peritoneal Dialysis

Suzanne Laplante and Peter Vanovertveld
[1]Baxter Healthcare Corporation, EMEA Health Outcomes, Brussels,
[2]Baxter Healthcare Corporation,
Western Europe Government Affairs & Public Policy, Zurich,
[1]Belgium
[2]Switzerland

1. Introduction

Dialysis services are expensive. Typically, a country spends 1 to 2% of its healthcare budget treating less than 0.1% of its population that requires dialysis (De Vecchi et al, 1999). In western countries, 90% of the patients are treated with haemodialysis in a dialysis centre attached or affiliated to a hospital.

The literature shows that when given the choice, up to 50% of dialysis patients will prefer to perform the procedure at home (Jager et al, 2004, Goovaerts et al, 2005) . Performing dialysis at home can generate significant cost savings to high income country healthcare systems and societies while improving survival, reducing morbidity (i.e., dialysis-related complications, hospital acquired infection, etc.) and increasing patient's quality of life. Furthermore, patients' satisfaction with care is higher with home modalities (Fadem SZ, 2011). Home dialysis therefore represents an opportunity for healthcare systems to improve health gains in their population while reducing the cost per case of a dialysis patient.

In a survey of 6595 nephrology healthcare professionals, 56% mentioned home/self-care modalities as the preferred long-term dialysis modalities (Ledebo & Ronco, 2008). Yet, in western countries only 10% of the patients are treated at home with either peritoneal dialysis or home haemodialysis. Canada, the Netherlands, the UK and the Scandinavian countries have a much higher (20-30%) usage of home modalities.

Reimbursement and organization of renal care have often been cited as being responsible for the differences observed between countries. This chapter will review the organization and financing of dialysis in 14 countries and suggests a 4-pillar framework to explain the differences observed between countries. Correcting or addressing each of these 4 pillars will be essential for home modalities such as peritoneal dialysis to benefit a significant number of patients in a country. This chapter will propose a few avenues for this.

2. The framework

A 4-pillar framework (Figure 1) was postulated as an explanation of the extent to which home dialysis modalities are used. The 4 pillars can be described as follows:

Pillar 1 - Home target: the presence of a peritoneal dialysis or home dialysis target, i.e., a specific proportion of dialysis patients that should be treated at home, ideally within a specified time frame.
Pillar 2 - Organization of renal services: with a particular focus on the absence of undesired financial imbalance favouring one modality over the other (i.e., provider-driven demand rather than based on patient's needs), the availability of a well-structured pre-dialysis education program for stage 4 patients, the availability of home assistance for elderly patients, and the presence of a renal replacement therapy career or "home first" guideline/policy.
Pillar 3 - Incentives: either financially or quality-based for home dialysis.
Pillar 4 - Tracking: a renal registry or some other form of tracking system to monitor dialysis quality and/or clinical outcomes such as survival, hospitalizations, complications, etc. and to plan future dialysis needs.

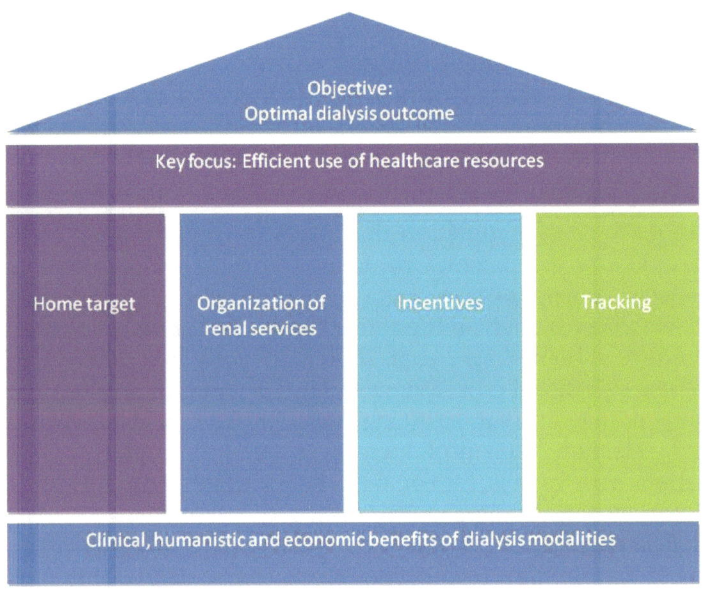

Fig. 1. Framework for renal policy and reimbursement

3. The analysis

Publicly available information on the organization of dialysis care in 14 target countries was reviewed and scored using a semi-quantitative scoring algorithm based on the 4-pillar framework (Table 1). The relationship between the score and the percent of patients performing dialysis at home (as per the latest information available, i.e., 2008 data from the European Renal Association-European Dialysis and Transplant Association renal registry, the United States Renal Data System, the Canadian Organ Replacement Register, the MNC Medical Netcare report for Germany and a publication by Gloor, 2010 for Switzerland) was explored with a regression analysis. An analysis of variance was performed to identify which factors of the 4-pillar framework were more associated with a higher usage of home modalities. The evolution of home dialysis usage during the a 5-year period (2004 to 2008) in countries where the data was available was plotted on a graph to identify trends and try to relate them to changes in the respective local healthcare system.

Pillar	Score	Description
1 Home target	+1	per 15% target
2 Organization of renal services		
Provider-driven demand	-2	Provider "profit" largely favouring in-centre modalities
	-1	Important in-centre haemodialysis over capacity or tariffs too low to cover all costs
	0	No significant provider profit imbalance between modalities
Pre-dialysis education	-1	Presence of information bias due to prescriber being also provider of dialysis services
	0	No well organized pre-dialysis education
	+1	Pre-dialysis education in usage in most of the centres. Could be secured in a guideline or other official document.
Assisted dialysis	-1	Significant hurdles to supply and/or finance
	0	Per case basis
	+1	Official tariff
Payment flow	-1	Payment for home modalities via a different channel than in-centre modalities
	+1	Payment for all modalities going through hospital
RRT career/home guideline/policy	0	Absence of guideline/policy recommending home modalities
	+1	Presence of a guideline or other official recommendation/document favouring home modalities
3 Incentive	0	No incentive for home modalities
	+1	Presence of an incentive (e.g., key performance indicator, bonus scheme) favouring home
4 Tracking	0	No registry or other means of tracking the epidemiology and survival of dialysis patients
	+1	Existence of a registry recording/reporting incidence and prevalence with or without survival
	+2	Existence of a registry recording/reporting in addition some intermediate quality indicators with or without recommendations for changes
	+3	Existence of a registry recording/reporting final quality indicators such as evolution of survival with time, infections and hospitalizations rates

Table 1. Scoring criteria

4. Results

4.1 Pillar 1 - Home target

Some countries (Figure 2) have set a target for dialysis patients to be treated at home. This target is either for peritoneal dialysis as in Norway (30%), for home haemodialysis as in the UK (10-15%) or for home dialysis (i.e., peritoneal dialysis and home haemodialysis) as in Denmark (45%). The issuing body could be a government body or a government-appointed committee like in the UK or Denmark or an independent group of experts like Sweden or the nephrologist association like in Finland. In only a few instances (Austria, Denmark, Stockholm County) was this target accompanied by a timeline. Evidence of an implementation plan could not be found in any of the countries surveyed, except maybe in Ontario, one of the Canadian provinces (Provincial Peritoneal Dialysis Coordinating Committee, 2006).

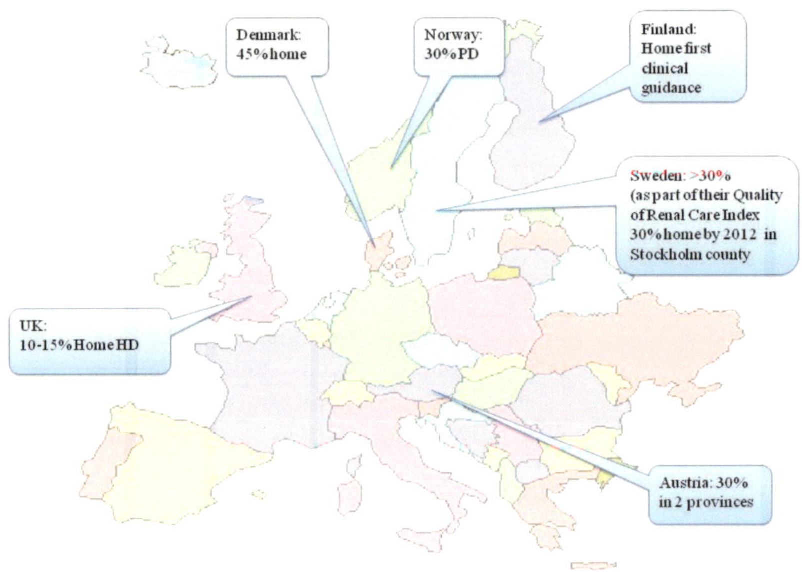

Fig. 2. Home targets

4.2 Pillar 2 – organization of renal services

Except for the USA, all countries have a public healthcare system. However, even in the USA, most dialysis patients are covered under the public system, Medicare (Mendelssohn DC, 2009). Dialysis providers are financed through either an overall department budget (e.g., Finland, some parts of Austria) or via a retrospective fee-for-service or prospective payment system like disease related groups. Transport costs and expensive medications such as erythropoietin stimulating agents or phosphate binders are paid through a different channel, increasing the difficulty for an exact comparison of costs between in-centre and home modalities. Medical monitoring is most of the time included within the tariff. In-centre haemodialysis has often the highest tariff and chronic ambulatory peritoneal dialysis the lowest. In some countries like Italy, the tariffs are more than 10 years old. In others like in the UK, France and the Nordic countries, a good tracking system of costs is in place and tariffs are updated on a yearly basis. In France, Austria, Denmark and Switzerland the payment for home modalities is made via a different channel than in-centre modalities, therefore not contributing to the revenues of the dialysis centre where the prescriber of dialysis sits.

Healthcare tariffs are commonly set as closely as possible to the real costs. This is done in order to avoid creating an imbalance in "profitability" between services that would lead to an increased usage of one service over the others based on the "profits" it generates to the provider rather than based on the benefits it can bring to patients. In healthcare financing, this is called provider-driven demand. Most healthcare system would track healthcare costs (i.e., using paid tariffs) per type of provider, but provider costs are not publicly available. Therefore, the real costs of dialysis were not available for most countries and we could not estimate if there was a major difference in provider's "profit" between home and in-centre modalities. However, based on the most recent analysis performed in Belgium (Cleemput et al, 2010) where automated peritoneal dialysis with more biocompatible and/or non glucose-based solutions is used in about 60% of the peritoneal dialysis patients, it can be seen that peritoneal dialysis costs to a dialysis provider (i.e., excluding transport and medications in the case of Belgium) are slightly lower than in-centre haemodialysis and in the same range as limited-care haemodialysis (Figure 3).

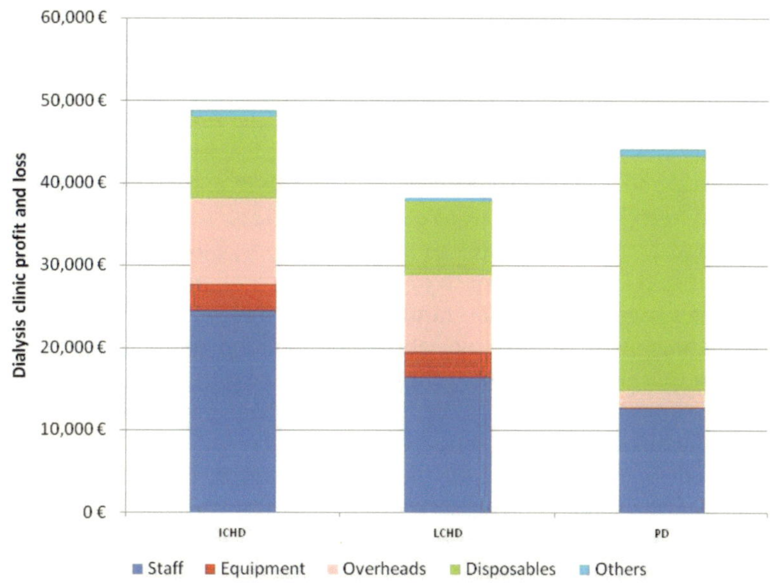

Fig. 3. 2006 costs of PD and HD to Belgium dialysis providers (Cleemput et al, 2010)

Therefore, the peritoneal dialysis and in-centre haemodialysis tariffs should not be too wide apart, otherwise it is likely to create a disproportionate "profit" in favour of in-centre haemodialysis. A large difference in tariffs in favour of in-centre modalities was found in most countries. In the USA, however, the recent changes in the tariffs are creating the reverse effect, i.e., disproportionate profit in favour of peritoneal dialysis. This was done on purpose, recognizing the overall lower healthcare costs associated with peritoneal dialysis (Berger et al, 2009; Cleemput et al, 2010; Figure 4) and changing the tariff setting method from cost-based to value-based.

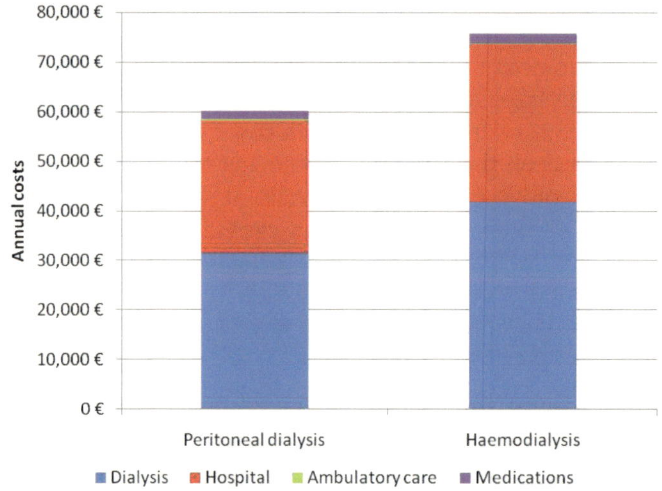

Fig. 4. 2006 Belgian total healthcare costs for dialysis patients (excluding transport; n=7230; Cleemput et al, 2010)

Well structured pre-dialysis education programs (where chronic kidney disease stage 4 patients are walked through the complications of the disease, the various renal replacement therapy modalities and the prevention measures to be taken to delay further decline in their renal function) exist mainly in Nordic countries. The USA has just implemented its new chronic kidney disease education program in 2010 and they are the only country so far with a payment attached to it (Medicare, 2010; Young et al, 2011).

Nursing assistance at home is available in some countries, but sometimes the financing is obscure and it is left to the nephrologist to organize.

Although most countries have some kind of guidelines on haemodialysis, peritoneal dialysis, or the management of anaemia, etc., none of them have a holistic guideline that sees end stage renal disease patients as cycling between various renal replacement therapies, therefore requiring focusing on the "big picture" rather than on each decision point separately (Braun Curtin et al, 2003). Finland, however, has a "home first" approach. It was originally developed by the Helsinki hospital (Honkanen & Rauta, 2008) but is followed throughout the country and is further supported by the nephrologist and patient associations' quality of renal care criteria (Kidney and Transplant Patients Association, 2006). The British National Institute for Health and Clinical Excellence is currently preparing a clinical guideline for peritoneal dialysis. The draft that has been circulated for consultation (National Institute for Health and Clinical Excellence, 2011) mentioned the need to have patient-centred care where the patients' needs and preferences are taken into account and where patients are enabled to make informed decisions on their options. The draft guidance also refers to the renal replacement therapy career concept. How this guideline will be implemented remains unclear at this moment.

4.3 Pillar 3 – incentives

In 2001, Belgium implemented a bonus scheme to favour the treatment of patients outside of the hospital premises (Royal Decree, 2006), and although PD benefited from it at the beginning, limited care HD was the great winner of this bonus scheme. The USA is currently starting its Quality Incentive Program focusing on indicators such as anaemia and urea reduction ratio (Medicare, 2011). This is in fact a penalty scheme where payment is reduced by up to 2% if the dialysis provider fails to reach the quality standards. The UK has also recently published its quality standards for chronic kidney disease, but no intention to link them to payment has been announced yet (National Institute for Health and Clinical Excellence, 2010). In the Netherlands, the Hans Mak Institute is qualifying dialysis centres (including an on-site inspection and a patients' survey every 3 years); the standards as well as the results of the qualification are publicly available for patients to consult on their website (Hans Mak Institute, 2011).

4.4 Pillar 4 – tracking

Renal registries exist in many countries. The data recorded are often only limited to the number of incident and prevalent patients as well as mortality. Morbidity indicators such as infections or hospitalizations are rarely recorded. Registries are not often used for planning purposes.

4.5 Scores

Scores varied from -2 in Germany to +5 in Denmark, Sweden, Canada and Netherlands. All Nordic countries scored 4 or 5. The total score of each country is displayed in Figure 5 and a detailed description of the scoring results is given in Table 2.

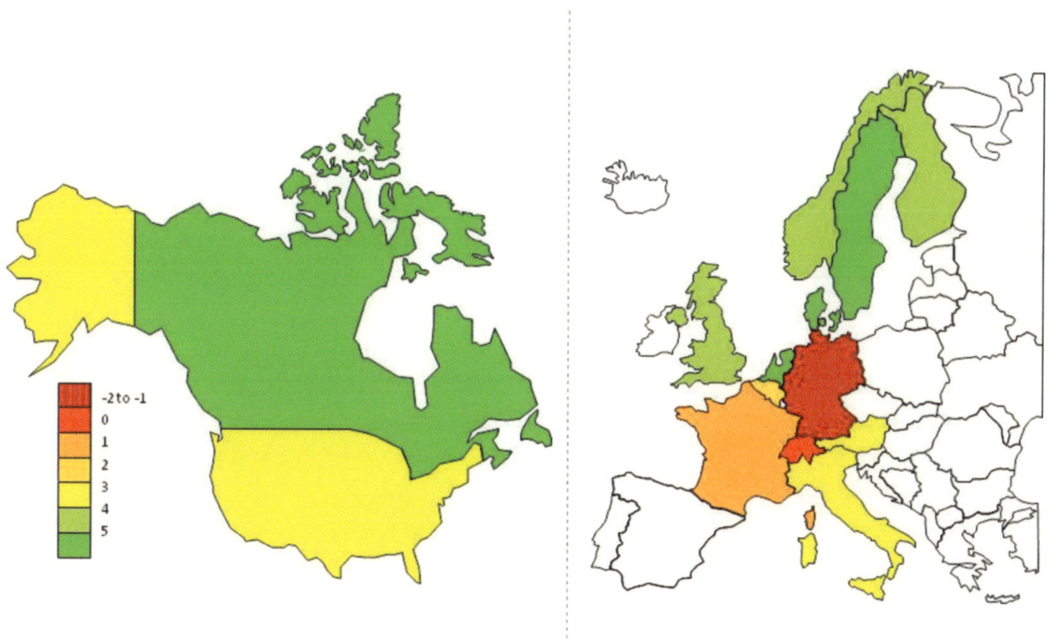

Fig. 5. 4-pillar framework total score

Country	Target	Provider-driven demand	Pre-dialysis education	Assisted dialysis	Payment flow	Clinical guidelines favouring RRT career/home modalities	Incentive	Tracking	Over-all rating	Home dialysis usage (2008)
Denmark	+3 45% home dialysis in 10 years (National Board of Health, 2006)	See under payment flow	+1 Implemented in most centres with some state of the art, but no mandatory requirement or tariff	-1 Financing is to be organized by nephrologist with municipa-lities	-1 No DRG earned by hospital for home modaliti-es (corrected in 2011)	+1 Health technology assessment report supporting home modalities		+2 Tracking quality indicators. Link possible with national healthcare database to track hospitaliza-tions	5	27.9%
Sweden	30% home by 2012 in largest county >20% PD (Renal Care Index, 2007)		+1 Documented in 2007 renal guidelines	Possible on a per case basis	+1	+1 Quality of renal care index Renal guidelines 2007	Quality of renal care index	+2 Tracking quality indicators and practice (cross-sectional report)	5	26.5%
Finland			+1 Secured in good renal patient management criteria from the kidney and liver patient association	On a per case basis	+1 Financing via hospital budget (i.e., based on real costs)	+1 Home first guidance followed throughout the country and secured in local policies and good renal patient management criteria from the neprhologist and patient associations		+1	4	25.5%

Table 2. Continued

Country	Target	Provider-driven demand	Pre-dialysis education	Assisted dialysis	Payment flow	Clinical guidelines favouring RRT career/home modalities	Incentive	Tracking	Over-all rating	Home dialysis usage (2008)
Netherlands		-1 Important in-centre HD over capacity	+1 Necosad guidance on pre-dialysis information	+1 Tariff for home HD and PD with nursing assistance	+1	+1 HansMak Institute guidelines		+2 HansMak Institute quality standards	5	22.4%
Canada	30% PD by 2010 in the largest province (Ontario)		+1	+1	+1	+1 Canadian Society of Nephrology favouring home dialysis		+1	5	21.7%
UK	+1 2002/2005 NICE guidance recommending 10-15% HHD	HHD tariff only indicative in 2011/2012 and requires negotiation between provider and NHS trust	+1	-1 No specific tariff, costs have to be assumed by dialysis centre or additional payment needs to be negotiated with NHS trust	+1	2011 NICE guidance on PD 2011 NICE chronic kidney disease quality standards recommending home dialysis	2011/2012 incentive for arterio-venous permanent access will increase the "profit" gap between HD and PD	+2	4	19.1%
Norway	+2 30% PD	-1 The use of HHD is slowed by several administrative hurdles to secure payment	+1	-1 Service available but no formal tariff, i.e., costs assumed by service provider	+1			+2 2009 report foresee lack of capacity in the future and the need to increase usage of home modalities	4	16.6%
Italy	General intent to treat more patients at home	-1 All tariffs not completely covering provider costs. Over in-centre HD capacity.		See incentive	+1	+1 Home first (in certain provinces)	+1 Some incentives to patients in Piemonte and Puglia	+1	3	11.4%

Table 2. Continued

Country	Target	Provider-driven demand	Pre-dialysis education	Assisted dialysis	Payment flow	Clinical guidelines favouring RRT career/home modalities	Incentive	Tracking	Over-all rating	Home dialysis usage (2008)
Belgium	See Incentive	-2 Large provider profit imbalance favouring ICHD	Recognized as an area that needs improvement in 2010 health technology agency report	+1 Tariff for PD and HHD	+1		+1 Bonus scheme favouring "out-of-hospital" modalities	+1	2	9.8%
Austria	+1 30% PD or home (in 2 provinces)	-1 No tariff for HHD. Only PD solutions reimbursed in some provinces.		+1 In some provinces as of 2009	-1 Home treatments funded via sickness funds (i.e., outside hospital budget). No tariff for HHD.		+1 Important lack of dialysis capacity in centres	+2 Tracking of dialysis quality indicators and patients' quality of life	3	8.8%
Switzerland	+1 Swiss dialysis contract with providers overall supports home modalities first	-1 In-centre HD overcapacity. Smaller provider profit with PD, no provider profit with HHD.	-1 Conflict of interest (prescriber is also the provider)	+1 Small payment to helping relative	+1			-1	0	8.6%
France	General intent to use the modality which is most appropriate to the patient	-1 MD honorarium penalizing home therapies Some regional authorities have recently set home dialysis targets		+1	-1 Payment flow penalizing home therapies			+2 Started in 2002 and covering most of the country now	1	8.4%

Table 2. Continued

Country	Target	Provider-driven demand	Pre-dialysis education	Assisted dialysis	Payment flow	Clinical guidelines favouring RRT career/home modalities	Incentive	Tracking	Over-all rating	Home dialysis usage (2008)
USA (Medicare)		Provider profit favouring in-centre modalities. New payment favouring home therapies as of 2010	New pre-dialysis education tariff as of 2010	-1	+1		New quality incentive performance scheme to be in place in 2010/2011	+3	3	8.0%
Germany	Promotion of HHD by 2 large providers (KfH and PHV)	-2 Large in-centre HD over capacity. Low tariff overall forcing high efficiency of provider and therefore favouring in-centre modalities despite better margins for PD and limitations in number of HD patients per nephrologist	-1 Conflict of interest (prescriber is also the provider)	-1 Nursing assistance has to be assumed by providers	+1			+1 Via Quality Assurance in Dialysis program of Medical Netcare GmbH (commissioned by G-BA) since 2007	-2	4.5%

Table 2. Scoring

5. Analysis

5.1 Regression analysis

The regression analysis reveals a significant ($p<0.001$) correlation between the total score and the use of home dialysis. In countries like Denmark or Sweden where the score was 5, 26-27 % of their dialysis patients are treated at home. At the opposite end of the spectrum, Germany, which obtained a score of -2 is using home dialysis in only 4.2% of its dialysis population (Figure 5).

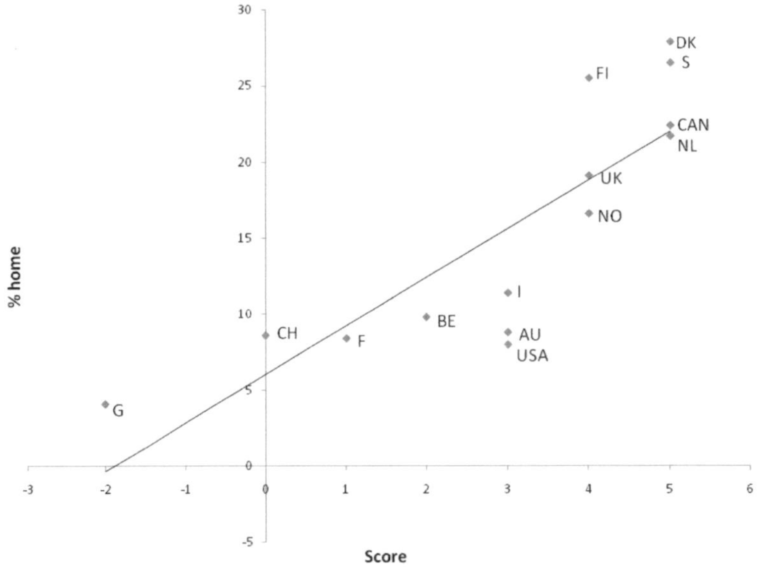

$r^2=0.694$; $p<0.001$. AU: Austria; BE: Belgium; CAN: Canada; CH: Switzerland; DK: Denmark; F: France; FI: Finland; G: Germany; I: Italy; NL: the Netherlands; NO: Norway; S: Sweden; UK: United Kingdom; USA: United States of America

Fig. 6. Correlation between framework score and percent use of home dialysis

5.2 Analysis of variance

The analysis of variance showed that 3 factors were significantly predictive of home usage. These were pre-dialysis education ($p<0.001$), clinical guidelines/policies favouring home modalities ($p=0.002$) and (the absence of) provider-driven demand ($p=0.035$).

5.3 Time trends

The usage of home modalities over the 2004-2008 period was plotted on a graph to identify trends (Figure 6). Three different trends were observed. Small (3-5%) upward trends were observed in Denmark, Finland, Sweden and Canada, countries that already have a large proportion of their dialysis patients at home. A larger upward trend was observed in Austria (14%), but as the home usage was small to start with, this increase does not result in a significant absolute increase in home usage. The second trend was observed in countries like Belgium the USA, and Germany. These countries have a low usage of home modalities and there is no indication that this is changing. The third trend is seen in the Netherlands and in the UK, where home dialysis usage has markedly dropped over the 2004-2008 period, from 27.7% to 22.4% in the Netherlands and from 25.9% to 19.1% in the UK, a 19% drop in the Netherlands and a 26% drop in the UK. It is interesting to note that these two countries implemented healthcare reforms during that time that had an overall objective of increasing competition among providers (that led to the opening of private dialysis centres) in the hope of decreasing healthcare costs.

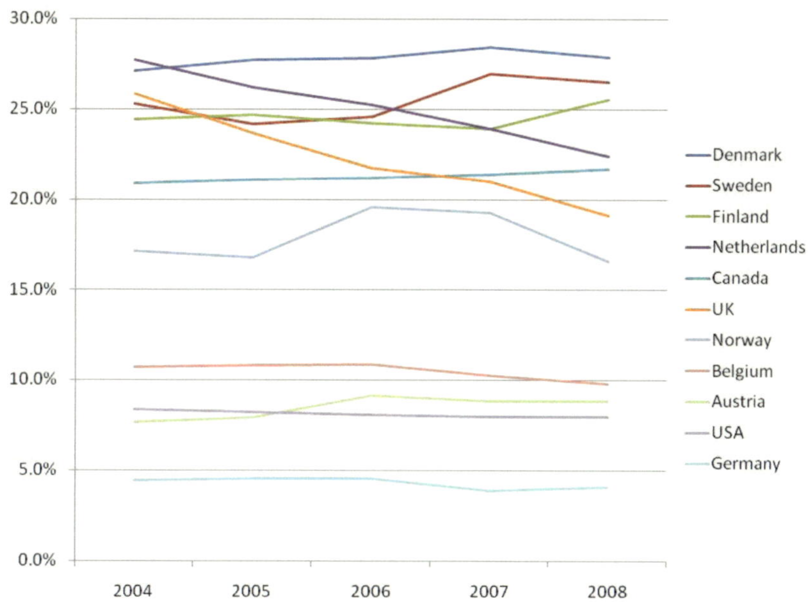

Fig. 7. Evolution of home dialysis usage over the 2004-2008 period

6. The recommendations

The 14 systems analyzed provide a series of possible avenues for change in local renal policy and reimbursement in order to create an environment that promotes home therapies such as peritoneal dialysis.

6.1 Pillar 1 – home target

Considering that 70% of patients are eligible for peritoneal dialysis and that when offered, 50% of them would choose peritoneal dialysis (Jager et al, 2004), a 35% target for peritoneal dialysis appears reasonable. For home haemodialysis, the literature cites approximately 10-15%. Therefore, ultimately, the goal should be to have around 45-50% of patients treated at home (35% peritoneal dialysis, 10-15% home haemodialysis). This target should be accompanied with an implementation plan to ensure better results. This implementation plan has been lacking in most countries that have such a target so far.

Recommendation 1: Set a reasonable proportion of patients (e.g., 10 to 15% over the current level up to 35% for peritoneal dialysis and 15% home haemodialysis) that should be treated at home within a set time frame (e.g., 5 years).

6.2 Pillar 2 – organization of renal services

The financing of dialysis in most countries with a high usage of home modalities is characterized by limited financial imbalance between modalities so that provider-driven demand (i.e., when the demand for a service is based on the benefits to the provider rather than the benefits to the patient) is avoided. This was a significant factor in the analysis of variance. Furthermore, in these countries, all payments are made via the same entity, i.e., the dialysis clinic.

Recommendation 2: Correct provider-driven demand by adjusting reimbursement levels to real costs or healthcare system value and use similar payment flow for in-centre and home modalities. Make healthcare costs more transparent by tracking provider costs and making them available to public.

Pre-dialysis education is well structured and organized in most countries with a high usage of home modalities. As mentioned earlier, when patients are informed of the various modalities, 50% of them will choose a home based therapy. The proportion is only slightly lower (35%) in the case of unplanned urgent start (Rioux et al, 2011). Pre-dialysis education, if performed in an unbiased way, should lead to a large increase in the use of home modalities. This factor was also significant in the analysis of variance.

Recommendation 3: Drive the development of high quality, unbiased, and ideally independent pre-dialysis education programs by providing adequate reimbursement for this activity.

Assisted dialysis is seldom available but is seen as a means to support home treatment. Assistance is not recommended for all patients but should be available for patients in some situations. For example, it can be useful while being trained for peritoneal dialysis or home haemodialysis; for patients who have had an urgent and unplanned start on dialysis to enable them to be discharged home before training starts; for patients or carers approaching burnout; for frail elderly patients who may not be able to manage all of their dialysis themselves; or for patients with particular mobility or dexterity problems who require assistance to enable dialysis at home.

Recommendation 4: Facilitate and actively encourage the adoption of home dialysis through the provision and reimbursement of assisted home dialysis.

Guidelines/policies on home dialysis were found in all countries with a high usage of home modalities. This was a significant factor in the analysis of variance.

Recommendation 5: Establish a holistic approach of dialysis care in an overall dialysis care guideline/policy integrating the patient "renal replacement therapy career" or "home first" concepts.

6.3 Pillar 3 - incentive

The Belgian financial incentive was effective in moving patients from in-centre haemodialysis to modalities where patients take more responsibility for their own therapy. This is the only example of a financial incentive available at the country level in the 14-country sample. The Italian incentive is only available in two provinces, while in Austria the incentive is the lack of resources rather than a financial incentive. These may not be sufficient to counteract the payment flow issue in Austria and the provider-driven demand in both countries. However, limited care haemodialysis performed in a hospital environment should be excluded of such a financial incentive as it defeats the purpose of home, i.e., no impact on hospital acquired infections, lower impact on patient's schedule and quality of life.

Penalties or incentives on outcomes have only been recently implemented in dialysis and their impact is yet to be measured. However, there are examples in other fields of medicine, e.g., the Centers for Medicare and Medicaid Services and Premier Hospitals Quality Incentive Demonstration program on 34 key performance indicators for 5 target diseases where a bonus or penalty is given to hospital lying outside of the norm (top and last 2 deciles); UK Quality Outcomes Framework to increase delivery of chronic care; Centers for Medicare and Medicaid Services non-payment for iatrogenic conditions, nosocomial infections and other similar complications; UK fine program on methicilin-resistant *Staphylococcus aureus* and *Clostridium difficile* infections. In their recent paper, Finkelstein et al, 2011, suggested a series of 12 quality improvement domains adapted from the Kidney Disease Outcomes Quality Initiative recommendations that could represent good targets for a dialysis related quality incentive.

Recommendation 6: Implement a financial incentive (that could be temporary until the target is reached) that will reward centres achieving a certain proportion of patients treated at home.

Recommendation 7: Implement a penalty for poor outcomes such as survival or hospitalizations/complications and/or for failing to meet set centre home dialysis targets.

6.4 Pillar 4 – tracking

With the exception of the US (great quality registry but low usage of home) and Canada (low quality of registry but high usage of home), countries with a high usage of home modalities have good renal registries that track not only incidence, prevalence and mortality, but also quality indicators, morbidities (such as complications or hospitalizations) and changes in survival over time.

Recommendation 8: Establish a renal registry that will track morbidity (e.g., hospitalizations, days in hospitals, infections, complications, etc.) and changes in survival over time and use the data to assess impact of renal care policies and to plan future needs for renal services and healthcare professional training.

The recommendations are summarized in Table 4.

Framework pillar	Recommendation number	Recommendation
Home target	1	Set a reasonable proportion of patients (e.g., 10 to 15% over the current level up to 35% for PD and 15% home HD) that should be treated at home within a set time frame (e.g., 5 years).
Organization of renal services	2	Correct provider-driven demand by adjusting reimbursement levels to real costs or healthcare system value and use similar payment flow for in-centre and home modalities. Make healthcare costs more transparent by tracking provider costs and making them available to public.

Framework pillar	Recommendation number	Recommendation
	3	Drive the development of high quality, unbiased, and ideally independent pre-dialysis education programs by providing adequate reimbursement for this activity.
	4	Facilitate and actively encourage the adoption of home dialysis through the provision and reimbursement of assisted home dialysis
	5	Establish a holistic approach of dialysis care in an overall dialysis care guideline/policy integrating the patient "RRT career" concept.
Incentives	6	Implement a financial incentive (that could be temporary until the target is reached) that will reward centres achieving a certain proportion of patients treated at home.
	7	Implement a penalty for poor outcomes such as survival or hospitalizations/complications and/or for failing to meet set centre home dialysis targets.
Tracking	8	Establish a renal registry that will track morbidity (e.g., hospitalizations, days in hospitals, infections, complications, etc.) and changes in survival over time and use the data to plan future needs for renal services and healthcare professional training.

Table 4. Recommendation for change in renal services

7. Discussion

The cross-sectional nature of the analysis prevents the identification of a causal relationship between the score on the 4-pillar framework and the use of home modalities. The recent changes in the US and in the UK will be kept on the radar screen for their impact on home modalities. Small (3-5%) upward trends in the usage of home modalities were observed in most Nordic countries and Canada from 2004 to 2008, all countries that scored highly on the framework. The common themes between these 4 countries are the lack of provider-driven demand, well structured pre-dialysis education programs, and clinical guidelines/policies favouring home modalities, i.e., the 3 factors identified as significant in the analysis of variance. On the other hand, the remarkable decrease in usage of home modalities observed in the UK and the Netherlands while these countries are trying to let the market forces play a more active role seems to be detrimental to therapies such as home dialysis that generate savings outside of the budget scope of the dialysis providers. Provider efficiency may not always be compatible with overall healthcare system efficiency.

With lower income countries such as Hong-Kong, Mexico and Latin America having a high usage of peritoneal dialysis and higher income countries having a high usage of haemodialysis, it is tempting to conclude that peritoneal dialysis might be an inferior good, i.e., one for which the usage is decreasing as income increases (like cheap cars or inter-city bus transport). However, our analysis showed that countries such as the Nordics, that have an elevated gross domestic product, also have a high usage of home modalities. This is not supporting an inferior good status for peritoneal dialysis.

It is likely that no single factor is the secret weapon and that any change in the usage of home modalities will be the result of the inter-relation of the various factors described by the 4-pillar framework and maybe other factors not taken into consideration in this analysis (Chaudhary et al, 2011, Finkelstein FO et al, 2011). Nevertheless, it is reasonable to think that improving the score on the 4-pillar framework, and especially on the 3 factors identified by the analysis of variance (i.e., absence of provider-driven demand, well structured pre-dialysis education programs, clinical guidelines favouring home) would impact on the usage of home modalities.

8. Conclusions

The analysis of the organization of dialysis services in 14 countries allowed the identification of several factors organized in a 4-pillar framework that favour the use of home modalities. Furthermore, several avenues for improvement were identified in the course of the analysis and have been used to suggest a series of 8 recommendations for change in renal policy and reimbursement. Some of these recommendations are in the process of being implemented (although secondary to a process totally independent from this analysis) in some countries. It will be interesting to assess the impact of the USA quality incentive program, the pre-dialysis education program and the new reimbursement tariffs on the usage of home dialysis in the years to come.

9. References

Berger A, Edelsberg J, Inglese GW et al. Cost comparison of peritoneal dialysis versus hemodialysis in end-stage renal disease. Am J Managed Care 2009; 15(8): 509-518.

Braun Curtin R, Becker B, Kimmel PL et al. An integrated approach to care for patients with chronic kidney disease. Sem Dialysis 2003 ; 16(5) : 399-402.

Chaudhary K, Sangha H, Khanna R. Peritoneal dialysis first: rationale. Clin J Am Soc Nephrol 2011; 6:447-456.

Cleemput I, Beguin C, de la Kethule Y et al. Organisation et financement de la dialyse chronique en Belgique. Health Technology Assessment (HTA). Bruxelles Centre federal d'expertise des soins de sante (KCE) 2010. KCE Reports 124B. Accessed on November 30, 2010, Available from:
http://www.kce.fgov.be/index_fr.aspx?SGREF=14844&CREF=14962

De Vecchi AF, Dratwa M, Wiedemann ME. Healthcare systems and end-stage renal disease (ESRD) therapies - an international review : costs and reimbursement/funding of ESRD therapies. Nephrol Dial Transplant 1999; 14(Suppl 6): 31-41.

Fadem SZ, Walker DR, Abbott G et al. Satisfaction with renal replacement therapy and education: the American Association of Kidney Patients survey. Clin J Am Soc Nephrol 2011; 6 epub.

Finkelstein FO, Ezekiel OO, Raduc R. Development of a peritoneal dialysis program. Blood Purif 2011;31:121-124.

Gloor HJ, Eine Lanze fuer peritonealdialyse. Bull Medecins Suisses 2010; 91(40): 1582-1584.

Goovaerts T, Jadoul M, Goffin E. Influence of pre-dialysis education programme (PDEP) on the mode of renal replacement therapy. Nephrol Dial Transplant 2005; 20: 1842-1847.

Hans Mak Institute quality system. Accessed on 08 March 2011, Available from: http://www.hansmakinstituut.nl/xcms/text/pid/131106/mid/116295

Honkanen EO, Rauta VM. What happened in Finland to increase home hemodialysis? Hemodial Int 2008; 12:S11-S15.

Jager KJ, Korevaar JC, Dekker FW et al. The effect of contraindications and patient preference on dialysis modality selection in ESRD patients in The Netherlands. Am J Kidney Dis 2004; 43: 891-899.

Kidney and Transplant Patients Association. Kidney patient's criteria for good management in Finland. 2006, Accessed on 08 March 2011, Available from: http://www.musili.fi/fin/julkaisut_ja_tuotteet/esitteet/

Lebedo I, Ronco C. The best dialysis therapy? Results from an international survey among nephrology professionals. Nephrol Dial Transplant Plus 2008; 6: 403-408.

Medicare. Medicare program; End-Stage Renal Disease Quality Incentive Program. Federal Register 2011; 76(3): 628-646.

Medicare learning Network. Coverage of Kidney Disease Patient Education Services - JA6557. Accessed on 08 March 2011, Available from: https://www.cms.gov/ContractorLearningResources/downloads/JA6557.pdf.

Mendelssohn DC, Wish JB. Dialysis delivery in Canada and the United States: a view from the trenches. Am J Kidney Dis 2009; 54(5): 954-964.

National Board of Health, Danish Center for Evaluation and Health Technology Assessment. Dialysis in chronic renal failure. A health technology assessment. Copenhagen: HTA 2006; 8(3)

National Institute for Health and Clinical Excellence. Draft 2011 Kidney disease: peritoneal dialysis in the treatment of chronic kidney disease stage 5. London: National Institute for Health and Clinical Excellence. Accessed on 08 March 2011, Available from: http://guidance.nice.org.uk/CG/Wave23/9/Consultation/Latest

National Institute for Health and Clinical Excellence. Draft quality standards for chronic kidney disease in adults. 2010. Accessed on 08 March 2011, Available from: http://www.nice.org.uk/media/5CD/DB/ChronicKidneyDiseaseQualityStandard.pdf

Provincial Peritoneal Dialysis Coordinating Committee. Provincial peritoneal dialysis joint initiative: Strategy on the delivery of PD in Ontario. November 2006. Accessed on 14 April 2011, Available from: http://www.improvementpractices.com/UploadFiles/Resource%20Manual%20-%20Section%201.pdf

Renal Care Index 2007. A comparison of renal care in the Swedish counties. Health Consumer Powerhouse. Stockholm and Brussels. 2007. Accessed on 18 March 2011. Available from: http://www.healthpowerhouse.se/index.php?option=com_content&view=category&layout=blog&id=49&Itemid=70

Rioux JP, Cheema H, Bargman JM et al. Effect of an in-hospital chronic kidney disease education program among patients with unplanned urgent-start dialysis. Clin J Am Soc Nephrol 2011;6(4): 799-804.

Royal Decree of Belgium of March 24, 2006. Accessed on 08 March 2011, Available from http://www.inami.fgov.be/care/fr/hospitals/pdf/hospitals018.pdf

Young HN, Chan MR, Yevzlin AS, Becker BN. The rationale, implementation and effect of Medicare CKD education benefit. Am J Kidney Dis 2011; 57(3): 381-386.

9

Nutritional Considerations in Indian Patients on PD

Aditi Nayak, Akash Nayak, Mayoor Prabhu and K S Nayak
Nephrology [Clinical Nephrology] Hyderabad, Andhra Pradesh, India

1. Introduction

Malnutrition inevitably accompanies Chronic Kidney Disease (CKD) and dialysis. Markers of malnutrition like low serum albumin have been shown to correlate independently with higher mortality in dialysis patients (1).Malnutrition is seen in both Hemodiaysis (HD) and Peritoneal Dialysis (PD) patients. The incidence has been described at 10-70% in HD and 18-51% in PD patients (2,3). The causes of malnutrition in dialysis patients can be manifold-dialysis factors, biochemical factors, gastrointestinal factors, miscellaneous factors, and low socio-economic status (4). Miscellaneous factors include depression, multiple medications, recurrent hospitalizations, and underlying illness. Modality of dialysis also affects nutritional status. There are factors unique to each both PD and HD that may contribute to the overall malnutrition. In PD, loss of albumin in PD fluid may range from 5.5-11.8 gms per day (5).In comparison, low flux dialysers account for amino acid losses of 5.6-7.1 gm/day in HD patients(6).Thus PD patients maintain lower serum albumin than age and weight controlled HD patients. Other causes responsible for hypoalbuminemia in PD patients include older age, etiology of renal failure, transport status, and chronic inflammation. Anorexia can result from distention due to fluid in the abdomen. Episodes of peritonitis can cause protein losses of upto 15 gm per day (7). Overhydration, and early satiety due to absorption of glucose from PD fluid can also be a cause of malnutrition in PD (8).Hospitalisation of dialysis patients is estimated to lead to them missing upto 20% of their lunches and dinners, with calorie deficits of upto 3000kcal/week (9).Other factors may ultimately impinge upon a dialysis patients nutritional well being. Blindness, amputations, dementia, depression and stroke are some factors adding to the nutritional challenges. Disabilities are more in HD patients than in PD, and is also more common in diabetics than non diabetics (10).As the number of diabetics on PD increased exponentially, malnutrition is also expected to increase with the same rate. Even though malnutrition is very common and strongly predicts outcome, malnutrition is not thought to directly cause death. Rather, a combination of malnutrition, inflammation and cardiovascular disease may be interrelated in dialysis (11,12). Serum levels of CRP and interleukin-6 (IL-6, which is a pivotal proinflammatory cytokine involved in systemic inflammation) were found to be significantly elevated in malnourished HD and PD patients. As a marker of systemic inflammatory reaction, serum CRP is now regarded as the best predictor for development of cardiovascular disease in the general population as well as in dialysis patients .These factors led to the proposal that malnutrition be characterised as Type1 and Type 2 (12).Type 1 malnutrition is related to the uremic syndrome per se and can be corrected by adequate dialysis. It is characterised by a normal/low serum albumin, absence of inflammation and comorbidity, low food intake and decreased protein catabolism. Type 2 malnutrition is thought to be 'cytokine driven' and is clinically more severe, characterised by hypoalbuminemia, inflammation, comorbidity and increased protein catabolism. Thus, it is clear that malnutrition and co morbidities play a major role in determining outcomes in patients on PD. Assessment and treatment of nutritional problems in PD may lead to overall better performance on PD, better quality of life, and increased longevity. Methods of assessment of nutritional status, the interpretation and limitations of the same, approaches towards the optimum treatment strategies, and future directions in the management of nutritional status in PD patients is dealt with at length in this chapter in the following pages.

2. Global perspective

The prevalence of malnutrition in PD patients varies based upon the method of assessment used(13).For unclear reasons, longitudinal studies have shown that after initiation on PD, following an initial improvement, nutritional status gradually declines (14,15,16). There is clear association between malnutrition and poor outcome in PD patients, but the relevant studies including the much quoted CANUSA study (17) were based on Caucasian populations. It is not yet known whether the relationship is also applicable for Asian populations and whether Asian PD patients have distinct and unique nutritional issues compared to their Western counterparts. Also, it is not clear whether the reported superior survival of Asian patients can be related to better preservation of nutritional status (18,19).There is a general feeling that the incidence of malnutrition is essentially similar in Western and Asian populations, but the incidence of severe malnutrition is lower in Asian populations (20,21,22,23). Lesser activation of a systemic inflammatory reaction in Asian PD patients is suggested, and that circumstance may partially explain their lower incidence of malnutrition as compared with Western PD patients(24)Lesser incidence of metabolic acidosis in Asian patients has also been reported (25). It appears that correction of metabolic acidosis improves the nutritional status of Asian PD patients, which is consistent with the results from earlier reports in Western PD patients. Reported data indicate that dietary protein and energy intakes are not much different, although actual dietary intake of nutrients is independently influenced by the delivered dialysis dose and RRF in Asian PD patients(26). The effect of peritoneal membrane transport characteristics on long-term nutritional status remains controversial (27).Establishing a relationship between dialysis adequacy and nutritional status (and clinical outcome) would give nutrition a central role and thus have important therapeutic implications. Important nutritional issues that need further investigation in Asian PD patients include determining daily diet requirements for maintenance of a positive nitrogen balance, establishing an optimum method to assess nutritional status, and developing preventive and therapeutic strategies to manage malnutrition.

3. Indian scenario

The lack of a Renal Registry system in India prevents an exact estimation of the incidence of renal failure and ESRD in India. Estimates suggest that an average of 160,000 new patients require dialysis every year in India (28).Several problems mar the optimum use of PD in our patients. An initial prescription is usually limited to 3 exchanges of 2-L bags (29).Most patients are unable to afford 4 exchanges, or the use of newer/biocompatible solutions. Currently about 6000 patients are receiving PD in the country. Malnutrition in Indian patients is often severe and multifactorial. Reasons include late initiation of PD, protein restriction in the pre dialysis period, intercurrent infections, comorbidity, and dietary factors. Patients almost invariably fall short of recommended dietary intakes (30). The mean age of our CAPD patients is lower than that of PD patients in Western countries (31), and most of our PD patients are malnourished at PD initiation (20). Comorbidities may also be different in Indian PD patients. Vegetarianism is very common in India which means that patients do not get animal source protein in their diet. Dietary habits in India are complex with many patients being pure vegetarians, some who occasionally partake of meat in the diet and some who are regular non vegetarians. This makes nutritional assessment and management difficult. Data on Indian patients nutritional status is scant. A recent trial showed that malnutrition at initiation of PD was predictive of higher incidence of peritonitis. Patients were categorized into malnourished or well-nourished groups on the basis of Subjective Global Assessment (SGA) scores. Malnourished patients experienced significantly more peritonitis episodes (1 vs. 0.2 annually) than did patients with a normal nutritional status. On univariate analysis, SGA, nutritional risk index, serum albumin, and daily calorie intake were significantly associated with peritonitis. On multivariate regression analysis, only SGA was a significant predictor of peritonitis. Peritonitis-free survival was better in patients showing normal nutrition than showing malnutrition (32).Indian PD patients are thought to consistently fail to achieve NKF-KDOQI recommended calorie and protein intake, which was confirmed in some Indian studies (31).There is an overall paucity of good data from India. Assessment of nutritional status, and the management of malnutrition, all remain suboptimal at present.

4. Assessment of nutritional status in PD patients

An ideal assessment of nutritional status of a patient draws from a detailed history, clinical examination including anthropometry and biochemical tests. There is no ideal and 100% effective method available at present. Current strategies of evaluating nutritional status vary from centre to centre and depend on many factors including economic considerations. In a country like India it is impossible to perform too frequent and cumbersome investigations especially when they are expensive. The different available tools for nutritional assessment are discussed here

5. Subjective Global Assessment (SGA)

This is probably the most widely used method of nutritional assessment. It is simple and inexpensive. It is based on the clinicians ability to make an assessment of the overall nutritional status based on a medical history and clinical examination, to derive a final score. In general, 60% of the clinician's rating of the patient is based on the results of the medical history, and 40% on the physical examination. The clinician rates each medical history and physical examination parameter as either an A, B, or C. Although originally used to categorize surgical patients, this nutritional classification system has been shown to be a reliable nutritional assessment tool for dialysis patients(14,33). SGA is limited by the very fact that it is subjective and may not be entirely reproducible due to observer variability. In addition, its ability to detect small variations in nutritional status is limited. One parameter, the degree of anorexia, has been reported to be a strong predictor of mortality in haemodialysis patients [34].

6. Serum Albumin and Prealbumin

Serum albumin has been, by far, the most commonly used marker of nutrition status in CKD patients, and it is a powerful predictor of mortality in PD patients (17).However Serum albumin as a marker of malnutrition has several caveats. The low serum albumin level observed in PD patients may reflect mostly the acute-phase response and resulting albumin losses in dialysate and urine, and only to a lesser extent poor nutrition status. The patient's clinical status must be examined when evaluating changes in the serum albumin concentration, which is weakly and inversely correlated with serum acute phase proteins (35). Prealbumin is thought to be a better marker than serum albumin due to its shorter half life, and better correlation to the nutritional status. However Prealbumin is also a negative acute phase reactant (36).Also the prealbumin levels are related to the residual renal function (36,37).Hence both these markers may not be the ideal reflection of nutritional status.

7. Serum Transferrin

Serum Transferrin, though initially thought to reflect nutritional status, is now not widely used. It is almost universally low in dialysis patients and reflects iron status predominantly.

8. Protein equivalent of total nitrogen appearance (nPNA)

The use of nPNA as an estimate of protein intake is simple to use in the clinical setting. nPNA approximates DPI only when the patient is in nitrogen equilibrium or steady state. It will change inanabolic or catabolic situations and needs to be interpreted accordingly.

9. Anthropometry and hand grip strength

The anthropometric parameters that are generally assessed include body weight, height, skeletal frame size, skin-fold thickness, midarm muscle circumference, percentage of the body mass that is fat, the percentage of usual body weight, the percentage of standard body weight and the body mass index (BMI) [38,39,40]. These various measures provide different information concerning body composition, and it is therefore advantageous to measure more than one of these parameters. Moreover these tests are cheap and easy to perform. There is focus on hand grip strength as a nutritional assessment tool as it has been demonstrated to predict mortality on PD patients (41).It is recommended to use some of these tests singly or in combination, for diagnosis of malnutrition and also for follow up of patients.

10. Body composition measurements

A-dual energy xray absorptiometry

This is considered superior to other currently available techniques. With DEXA, bone mineral, fat mass (FM), and LBM distribution are estimated directly, without making assumptions about the two-compartment model. However, the assessment of LBM by DEXA is subject to flaws, because it assumes that 72% of the LBM compartment is water. Given that PD patients can exhibit abnormal hydration status, DEXA might not be a very precise method for assessing LBM in dialyzed patients. Therefore, measurement of LBM by DEXA should be combined with estimation of the extracellular fluid volume by the tracer dilution technique. Provides accurate data on body composition which are superior to anthropometry, creatinine kinetics and bioelectrical impedance [42,43].

B-Bioimpedance Analysis (BIA)

Bioimpedance analysis is based on the measurement of resistance and reactance when a constant alternating electrical current is applied to a patient, by empirical equations. However BIA is highly influenced by the hydration status .It is recommended that BIA be attempted only when the patient is at his oedema free weight. Our own experience with the use of BIA in CAPD patients showed good results (44).

C-creatinine kinetics

Creatinine kinetics is based on creatinine excretion in urine and dialysate. LBM estimated from creatinine kinetics depends on the creatinine content in the diet and the metabolic degradation of creatinine. Variations observed during repeated measures of LBM estimated using creatinine kinetics is unacceptably high (45).
From the available tests we recommend relying on a panel of nutritional markers rather than any one particular test. We recommend assessment of nutritional status at least every 6 months. Ideally, body weight, serum albumin, SGA, protein intake as assessed from dietary recall or nPNA, and an assessment of protein stores and iron stores (serum transferrin) would be necessary. A prospective decline in nutritional status would prompt a detailed evaluation. A cost effective but complete strategy for Indian patients would be a 6 monthly battery of tests that includes

- Serum albumin
- Serum Transferrin Saturation
- SGA
- Anthropometrics/Hand Grip Strength.

While inexpensive, these tests would enable assessment of all necessary parameters.

11. Nutritional intervention strategies

It is important to individualise strategies for each patient rather than slavishly adhere to guidelines or formulae. Considerations towards cost, palatability, culture, and comorbidity should be considered. We recommend using the services of a renal dietician in addition to the expertise of the treating Physician. In consultation with the patient, a unique and exclusive plan is drawn up for each patient.

12. Daily Protein Intake

While a Daily Protein Intake(DPI) of 1.3g/kg/day is recommended, there is no conclusive evidence to show that lower protein intakes impact upon nutritional status in PD. Some studies have shown that a DPI of 1.0-1.2g/kg/day is adequate to maintain positive nitrogen balance (46,47). We would recommend a daily protein intake of > 1.0g/kg/day as sufficient if the patient has no declining trend in nutritional parameters. At a DPI of < 0.9g/kg/day, we would reassess the patients nutritional status. Our own experience with the use of 0.8

g/kg/day of protein, supplemented with keto analogues 0.4g/kg/day, when compared with a traditional protein diet of 1.2g/kg/day showed that the keto-group had improvement on parameters like appetite, anthropometry, serum albumin and a decrease in serum cholesterol and fasting blood sugar (48).

MANAGEMENT OF MALNUTRITION IN PD PATIENTS-

NON DIALYTIC MEASURES

Preserve residual renal function
Prevent catabolic factors
  Correct acidosis
  Treat comorbidity and inflammation
Maintain optimal nutrition
  Nutritional counseling
  Nutritional supplementation (oral, enteral, or parenteral)
Correct anemia
Encourage exercise
Emotional and social support

DIALYSIS RELATED MEASURES

Optimize dialysis dose
Avoid potential sources of inflammation
  during the PD procedure
  Peritonitis
  Bioincompatible PD solutions
Attention to fluid, electrolyte and acid base balance.
Encourage anti-inflammatory diets

NOVEL APPROACHES

Use PD fluids with nutritional supplements
Appetite stimulants
Anti inflammatory diets
  Dietary fibre, Phytoestrogens,Omega-3 fatty acids
  Glycation End Product Inhibitor, PPAR-agonist, Antioxidants

Table. 1.

13. Dietary energy intake

A dietary energy intake of > 35kcal/kg/day is essential for PD patients. In elderly patients 30 kcal/kg/day may suffice. It is important to consider glucose absorption from the PD fluid. This can account for upto 100-200 g/24 hours.

LIPIDS

A diet with no more than 30% of total calories from fat should be encouraged. No more than 10% should derive from saturated fat.

CARBOHYDRATES

Complex carbohydrates are encouraged over refined carbohydrates.

SODIUM AND WATER

This is individualised based upon urine output, fluid status and blood pressure. We recommend 3-4 grams of salt intake / day in patients where ultrafiltration is easily achieved.

POTASSIUM

With residual renal function, we allow upto 100 meq/ day of K unless the patient is on ACE inhibitors or ARBs. As dialysate contains no potassium, even in anuric PD patients we allow upto 100 meq/ day.

CALCIUM

We attempt to achieve calcium balance with supplementation of calcium/ Vit D as needed.

PHOSPHORUS

Phosphorus restricted diets are often impractical to achieve as they lead to malnutrition. Ideally phosphorus intake should be limited to 0.6-1.2g/ day. Most PD patients need the use of Phosphate binders. We target a serum phosphorus of 4.5-5.5 mg/ dL. The choice of phosphate binders is individualised.

IRON

We target a serum transferring saturation of 20% or higher. We prefer the intravenous route of iron supplementation, for reasons of ease, compliance and effectiveness.

14. Correction of metabolic acidosis

Metabolic acidosis is an important stimulus for net protein catabolism and elicits the transcription of genes for proteolytic enzymes in muscle including the ubiquitin–proteasome pathway. The correction of metabolic acidosis decreases protein degradation and improves nitrogen balance. This has been proven for PD patients (49).Oral sodium bicarbonate can be used to achieve this goal.

15. Dose of dialysis

The relationship between delivered dose of dialysis and nutrition is controversial. Overall, prospective studies of adequacy and nPNA or DPI have not shown any correlation.

16. Additional nutritional support

PD patients who may need additional support include patients with peritonitis, hospitalisation or gastroparesis. We recommend support with oral supplements of fortified energy and protein, intraperitoneal amino acids, nasogastric feeding or parenteral nutrition.

17. Amino acid based PD fluids

In a prospective, randomized, open-label study that evaluated the role of amino-acid dialysate on the nutrition status of malnourished PD patients, patients who replaced 1 daily exchange of traditional dialysate with amino-acid dialysate showed better evolution in markers of nutrition than did patients who continued to use dextrose dialysate only(50).

18. Appetite stimulants

The use of appetite stimulants such as megestrol acetate, cannabinoids, and cyproheptadine may be a tempting part of a new strategy for malnourished PD patients. Megestrol acetate has been suggested for use as an appetite stimulant in HD and PD patients (51,52); however, it is associated with several side effects, including hypogonadism, impotence, and increased risk of thromboembolism.

ANTI INFLAMMATORY DIET

A recent study with HD patients suggested a trend toward a reduction in the serum concentration of C-reactive protein (CRP) after 8 weeks' ingestion of an isoflavone soy-based supplement(phytoestrogen based diet) (53).High fiber consumption in non-renal subjects was shown to lower the risk of elevated CRP (54). The anti-inflammatory effects of the omega-3 fatty acids, mainly eicosapentaenoic acid, found in fish oil are also well recognized.

ANTI INFLAMMATORY PHARMACOTHERAPY

This includes statins, ACEIs, PPAR agonists, and anti-oxidative agents, such as a- and g-tocopherol.

ANTICYTOKINE THERAPY

These are still experimental.Interleukin-1 receptor antagonists are in trial. Recombinant insulin-like growth factor (rhIGF-1) may induce an anabolic response in patients in whom the primary cause of malnutrition is a low protein intake (55).

19. Conclusions

Nutritional management of PD patients is challenging, and vital to the patients long term survival and well being. A multi disciplinary approach, with a patient centric plan is necessary to achieve long term compliance and success. Consideration to cultural, economic and medical issues is paramount to develop a workable plan, especially in a country as large and diverse as India.

20. References

[1] Joki N, Hase H, Tanaka Y, *et al.* Relationship between serum albumin level before initiating haemodialysis and angiographic severity of coronary atherosclerosis in end-stage renal disease patients. Nephrol DialTransplant 2006;21:1633–9.

[2] Bergström J, Lindholm B. Nutrition and adequacy of dialysis: how do hemodialysis and CAPD compare? Kidney Int 1993;43(suppl 40):39–50.

[3] Kopple J. McCollum Award Lecture, 1996: protein– energy malnutrition in maintenance dialysis patients. Am J Clin Nutr 1997;65:1544–57.

[4] Hakim R, Levin N. Malnutrition in hemodialysis patients. Am J Kidney Dis 1993;21:125–37.

[5] Blumenkrantz MJ, Kopple JD, Moran JK, Coburn JW. Metabolic balance studies and dietary protein requirements in patients undergoing continuous ambulatory peritoneal dialysis. Kidney Int 1982;21:849–61

[6] Ikizler TA, Flakoll PJ, Parker RA, Hakim RM. Amino acid and albumin losses during hemodialysis. Kidney Int 1994;46:830–7

[7] Bannister DK, Acchiardo SR, Moore LW, Kraus AP Jr. Nutritional effects of peritonitis in continuous ambulatory peritoneal dialysis (CAPD) patients. J Am Diet Assoc 1987;87:53–6.
[8] Sezer S, Tutal E, Arat Z, *et al.* Peritoneal transport status influence on atherosclerosis/inflammation in CAPD patients. J Ren Nutr 2005;15:427–34.
[9] Laville M, Fouque D. Nutritional aspects in hemodialysis. Kidney Int Suppl 2000;(76):S133–9.
[10] United States Department of Health and Human Services, Public Health Service, National Institutes of Health, National Institute of Diabetes and Digestive and Kidney Diseases, Division of Kidney, Urologic, and Hematologic Diseases. USRDS 2007 annual data report. Atlas of end-stage renal disease in the United States. Bethesda: United States Renal Data System; 2007.
[11] Bergström J, Lindholm B. Malnutrition, cardiac disease and mortality—an integrated point of view. *Am J Kidney Dis* 1998; 32:1–10.
[12] Stenvinkel P, Heimbürger O, Lindholm B, Kaysen GA, Bergström J. Are there two types of malnutrition in chronic renal failure? Evidence for relationships between malnutrition, inflammation and atherosclerosis (MIA syndrome). *Nephrol Dial Transplant* 2000; 15: 953–60.
[13] Wang T, Heimbürger O, Bergström J, Lindholm B. Nutritional problems in peritoneal dialysis: an overview. *Perit Dial Int* 1999; 19(Suppl 2):S297–303
[14] Young GA, Kopple JD, Lindholm B, Vonesh EF, DeVecchi A, Scalamogna A, et al. Nutritional assessment of continuous ambulatory peritoneal dialysis patients: an international study. Am J Kidney Dis 1991; 17:462–71.
[15] Davies SJ, Phillips L, Griffiths AM, Russel LH, Naish PF, Russel GI. What really happens to people on longterm peritoneal dialysis? Kidney Int 1998; 54:2207–17.
[16] Johansson A, Samuelsson O, Haraldsson B, Bosaeus J, Attman P-O. Body composition in patients treated with peritoneal dialysis. Nephrol Dial Transplant 1998; 13:1511–17.
[17] Churchill DN, Taylor DW, Keshaviah PR, and the CANUSA Peritoneal Dialysis Study Group. Adequacy of dialysis and nutrition in continuous peritoneal dialysis: association with clinical outcomes. *J Am Soc Nephrol* 1996; 7:198–207
[18] Wong JS, Port FK, Hulbert-Shearon TE, Carroll CE, Wolfe RA, Agodoa LY, *et al.* Survival advantage in Asian American end-stage renal disease patients. *Kidney Int* 1999; 55:2515–23.
[19] Held PJ, Brunner F, Odaka M, Garcia JR, Port FK, Gaylin DS. Five-year survival for end-stage renal disease patients in the United States, Europe, and Japan, 1982 to 1987. *Am J Kidney Dis* 1990; 15:451–7.
[20] Chung SH, Na MH, Lee SH, Park SJ, Chu WS, Lee HB. Nutritional status of Korean peritoneal dialysis patients. *Perit Dial Int* 1999; 19(Suppl 2):S517–22.
[21] Kumano K, Kawaguchi Y. Multicenter cross-sectional study for dialysis dose and physician's subjective judgment in Japanese peritoneal dialysis patients. Group for the Water and Electrolyte Balance Study in CAPD. *Am J Kidney Dis* 2000; 35:515–25.
[22] Wang AY, Sea MM, Ip R, Law MC, Chow KM, Lui SF, *et al.* Independent effects of residual renal function and dialysis adequacy on actual dietary protein, calorie, and other nutrient intake in patients on continuous ambulatory peritoneal dialysis. *J Am Soc Nephrol* 2001; 12: 2450–7.

[23] Kang EW, Goo YS, Lee SC, Han SH, Yoon SY, Choi SR, *et al.* Factors affecting malnutrition in continuous ambulatory peritoneal dialysis patients: a cross-sectional study. *Korean J Nephrol* 2002; 21:943–55.
[24] Noh H, Lee SW, Kang SW, Shin SK, Choi KH, Lee HY, *et al.* Serum C-reactive protein: a predictor of mortality in continuous ambulatory peritoneal dialysis patients. *Perit Dial Int* 1998; 18:387–94.
[25] Kang DH, Lee R, Lee HY, Han DS, Cho EY, Lee CH, *et al.* Metabolic acidosis and composite nutritional index (CNI) in CAPD patients. *Clin Nephrol* 2000; 53: 124–31.
[26] Mak SK, Wong PN, Lo KY, Tong GM, Fung LH, Wong AK. Randomized prospective study of the effect of increased dialytic dose on nutritional and clinical outcome in continuous ambulatory peritoneal dialysis patients. *Am J Kidney Dis* 2000; 36:105–14.
[27] Oreopoulos DG. The optimization of continuous ambulatory peritoneal dialysis. *Kidney Int* 1999; 55: 1131–49
[28] Modi GK, Jha V. The incidence of end-stage renal disease in India: a population-based study. *Kidney Int* 2006; 70:2131–3.
[29] Abraham G, Mathew M, Gopalakrishnan P, Sankarasubbaiyan S, Shroff S. Are three exchanges suitable for Asian patients on peritoneal dialysis? *Perit Dial Int* 2003; 23(Suppl 2):S45–7.
[30] Prasad N, Gupta A, Sinha A, Singh A, Sharma RK, Kumar A, et al. A comparison of outcomes between diabetic and nondiabetic CAPD patients in India. Perit Dial Int 2008; 28:468–76.
[31] Prasad N, Gupta A, Sinha A, Sharma RK, Kumar A, Kumar R. Changes in nutritional status on follow-up of an incident cohort of continuous ambulatory peritoneal dialysis patients. J Ren Nutr 2008; 18:195–201.
[32] Prasad N, Gupta A, Sharma RK, Sinha A, Kumar R. Impact of nutritional status on peritonitis in CAPD patients. *Perit Dial Int* 2007; 27:42–7.
[33] Enia G, Sicuso C, Alati G, Zoccali C: Subjective global assessment nutrition in dialysis patients. J Am Soc Nephrol 1:323, 1991
[34] Kalantar-Zadeh, Block G, McAllister CJ, Humphreys MH, Kopple JD. Appetite and inflammation, nutrition, anemia and clinical outcome in hemodialysis patients. Am J Clin Nutr 2004; 80: 299–307 (B)
[35] Gabay C, Kushner I. Acute-phase proteins and other systemic responses to inflammation. N Engl J Med 1999; 340: 448–454 (C)
[36] Heimbürger O, Qureshi AR, Blaner WS, Berglund L, Stenvinkel P. Hand-grip muscle strength, lean body mass, and plasma proteins as markers of nutritional status in patients with chronic renal failure close to start of dialysis therapy. Am J Kidney Dis 2000; 36:1213–25.
[37] Jacob V, Marchant PR, Wild G et al. Nutritional profile of CAPD patients. Nephron 1995; 71: 16–22 (B)
[38] Woodrow G, Oldroyd B, Smith MA et al. Measurement of body composition in chronic renal failure: comparison of skinfold anthropometry and bioelectrical impedance with dualenergy X-ray absorptiometry. Eur J Clin Nutr 1996; 50: 295–301
[39] Jones CH, Newstead C, Will EJ et al. Assessment of nutritional status in CAPD patients: serum albumin is not a useful measure. Nephrol Dial Transplant 1997; 12: 1406–1413

[40] Szeto CC, Kong J, Wu AKL et al. The role of lean body mass as a nutritional index in Chinese peritoneal dialysis patients— comparison of creatinine kinetics method and anthropometric method. Perit Dial Int 2000; 20: 708–714
[41] Wang AYM, Sea MMM, Ho ZSY, Lui SF, Li PKT, Woo J. Evaluation of handgrip strength as a nutritional marker and prognostic indicator in peritoneal dialysis patients. Am J Clin Nutr 2005; 81: 79–86
[42] Borovnicar DJ, Wong KC, Kerr PG et al. Total body protein status assessed by different estimates of fat-free mass in adult peritoneal dialysis patients. Eur J Clin Nutr 1996; 50: 607–616
[43] Stenver DI, Godfredsen A, Hilsted J, Nielsen B. Body composition in hemodialysis patients measured by dual-energy X-ray absorptiometry. Am J Nephrol 1995; 15: 105–110
[44] Brundavani V, Nayak K.S, Vinny J, Fatima P, Subhramanyam S.V, Sinoj K.A Bioelectric impedance vector analysis (BIVA) for nutritional health assessment in CAPD patients-an Indian study. Perit Dial Int 2005: Vol 25(2) (Abstract)
[45] Bhatla B, Moore H, Emerson P, Keshaviah P, Prowant B, Nolph KD, et al. Lean body mass estimation by creatinine kinetics, bioimpedance, and dual energy X-ray absorptiometry in patients on continuous ambulatory peritoneal dialysis. ASAIO J 1995; 41:M442–6.
[46] Blumenkrantz MJ, Kopple JD, Moran JK, Coburn JW. Metabolic balance studies and dietary protein requirements in patients undergoing CAPD. Kidney Int 1982; 21: 849–861
[47] Giordano C, De SG, Pluvio M et al. Protein requirement of patients on CAPD: a study on nitrogen balance. Int J Artif Organs 1980; 3: 11–14
[48] Brundavani V, Nayak K.S, Vinny J, Fatima P, Kanchana D, Subhramanyam S.V. Dietary protein quality evaluation: ammonia acid score and relative protein digestibility of Indian renal diets. Perit Dial Int 2005:Vol 25(2).(Abstract)
[49] Szeto CC, Wong TYH, Chow KM, Leung CB, Li PKT. Oral sodium bicarbonate for the treatment of metabolic acidosis in peritoneal dialysis patients: a randomized placebo-control trial. J Am Soc Nephrol 2003; 14: 2119–2126
[50] Li FK, Chan LY, Woo JC, Ho SK, Lo WK, Lai KN, et al. A 3-year, prospective, randomized, controlled study on amino acid dialysate in patients on CAPD. Am J Kidney Dis 2003; 42: 173–83
[51] Costero O, Bajo MA, del Peso G, Gil F, Aguilera A, Ros S, et al. Treatment of anorexia and malnutrition in peritoneal dialysis patients with megestrol acetate. Adv Perit Dial 2004; 20:209–12.
[52] 52-. Rammohan M, Kalantar-Zadeh K, Liang A, Ghossein C.Megestrol acetate in a moderate dose for the treatment of malnutrition-inflammation complex in maintenance dialysis patients. J Ren Nutr 2005; 15:345–55.
[53] 53- Fanti P, Asmis R, Stephenson TJ, Sawaya BP, Franke AA. Positive effect of dietary soy in ESRD patients with systemic inflammation—correlation between blood levels of the soy isoflavones and the acute-phase reactants. Nephrol Dial Transplant 2006; 21:2239–46.
[54] King DE, Egan BM, Geesey ME. Relation of dietary fat and fiber to elevation of C-reactive protein. Am J Cardiol 2003; 92:1335–9.

[55] Fouque D, Peng SC, Shamir E, Kopple JD. Recombinant human insulin-like growth factor-1 induces an anabolic response in malnourished CAPD patients. Kidney Int 2000; 57:646–54

10

Hyponatremia and Hypokalemia in Peritoneal Dialysis Patients

Sejoong Kim
Department of Internal Medicine, Gachon University of Medicine and Science
Korea

1. Introduction

Imbalance of sodium and potassium in patients on peritoneal dialysis (PD) is not uncommon. Sodium is the major extracellular cation; however, its concentrations are mainly affected by water balance, as well as sodium balance. Potassium is the major intracellular cation, and serum potassium concentrations are very low, compared with its intracellular components. Hyponatremia and hypokalemia are associated with severe consequences, respectively. I will review development of hyponatremia and hypokalemia in incident PD patients, and describe recently emerging evidence related to hyponatremia and hypokalemia in PD patients.

2. Hyponatremia in PD patients

2.1 Hyponatremia in hospitalized patients

Hyponatremia is one of the most common electrolyte disorders in hospitalized patients (Anderson et al., 1985; Zevallos et al., 2001). Daily incidence and prevalence of hyponatremia are approximately 1% and 2.5%, respectively. Two thirds of all hyponatremia was hospital-acquired. Normovolemic state (so-called syndrome of inappropriate secretion of antidiuretic hormone) is the most commonly seen clinical setting of hyponatremia. Hyponatremia, defined as a serum sodium level less than 135 mEq/L, was increased by 20% in inpatients with congestive heart failure (Gheorghiade et al., 2007). The fatality rate for hyponatremic patients was 60-fold that for patients without documented hyponatremia (Anderson et al., 1985). Hyponatremia is an independent predictor of death and myocardial infarction in middle-aged and elderly community subjects, respectively (Sajadieh et al., 2009). Hyponatremic patients with congestive heart failure are associated with a 75% increase in 60- to 90-day mortality, compared with normonatremic patients (Gheorghiade et al., 2007). Therefore, even mild hyponatremia has a poor prognosis.

2.2 Pathophysiology of hyponatremia in PD patients

The prevalence of hyponatremia is approximately 10% in PD patients (Zevallos et al., 2001). Because fluid and electrolyte balance in these patients is dependent on nonrenal routes, PD-related hyponatremia has been suggested to differ pathophysiologically from non-PD-related hyponatremia. Regulation of a normal serum sodium concentration is dependent on the content of sodium and potassium, as well as total body water. Despite a low rate of glomerular filtration, the normal kidney can regulate serum sodium concentrations independent of solute and water balance. Whereas, in PD patients without residual renal function, solute and water balance through peritoneal membrane plays an important role in development of hyponatremia (Nolph et al., 1980). Sodium removal by convective transport predominates over diffusive transport in patients on PD, thereby requiring augmentation of ultrafiltration volume in order to increase sodium removal (Nolph et al., 1980). Due to the Gibbs–Donnan effect created by negatively charged proteins in the plasma space, and sodium sieving by aquaporins, the typical dialysate sodium concentration is substantially lower than the plasma sodium concentration (Rippe & Venturoli, 2008). As a result of this sieving, the early part of a PD dwell removes mostly water, and sodium removal occurs later in the dwell as the dialysate Na^+ concentration decreases, creating a higher gradient for diffusive transport of sodium. As a result of its longer dwell times, continuous ambulatory PD removes more sodium per ultrafiltration volume than automated PD (Rippe & Venturoli, 2008).

The serum sodium concentration accounts for the balance of three components: mainly sodium, potassium, and body water. The basis for hyponatremia is a negative balance for sodium plus potassium and/or a positive balance for water. Vasopressin can control water permeability in the normally functioning nephron, which leads to electrolyte-free water retention. In dialysis patients without residual renal function, the role of vasopressin is limited; therefore, solute balance may play a more important role in development of hyponatremia (Zanger, 2010). Hypotonic hyponatremia may occur in PD patients, either from free water retention or loss of electrolyte, such as sodium or potassium. If hyponatremia is accompanied by a quantitatively appropriate gain in weight, a gain of electrolyte-free water is the basis for hyponatremia (Cherney et al., 2001). In the absence of this weight gain, loss of sodium from the extracellular fluid (ECF) space will lead to movement of water into the intracellular fluid (ICF), to restore the equilibrium between intra- and extracellular osmolality. Loss of potassium, along with an ECF anion, such as chloride or bicarbonate, results in potassium efflux from ICF into ECF, with a shift of sodium into the cell for maintenance of electroneutrality (Nguyen & Kurtz, 2004). The net effect is loss of sodium from the ECF, with development of hyponatremia (Cherney et al., 2001). In patients without weight gain, loss of intracellular potassium, with an intracellular anion, such as phosphate, will contribute to development of hyponatremia, due to movement of water from the ICF into the ECF.

2.3 De novo hyponatremia in incident PD patients

In order to control bias on pre-existing hyponatremic conditions, we observed development of hyponatremia in incident PD patients, and evaluated factors contributing to its development. We conducted a 1-year observational study at a single PD center at Gachon University Gil Hospital, South Korea (Lee et al., 2010). Fifty-one incident PD patients were enrolled. All patients were ethnic Koreans and older than 18 years. The same protocol used in our previous report was used in performance of the peritoneal equilibration test (PET) and measurement of dialysis adequacy at 1 and 13 months after the start of PD (Kim et al., 2009). Patients with hyponatremia ($Na^+ < 135$ mEq/L) at month 1 were excluded. At month 13, patients were divided according to their serum sodium levels into hyponatremic ($Na^+ <$ 135 mEq/L) and normonatremic ($Na^+ \geq 135$ mEq/L) groups.

Between the two groups, there were no significant differences in baseline demographics of patients beginning PD, including age, sex, height, cause of end-stage renal disease, co-morbidity, biocompatible fluid, and CAPD versus automated PD. Sixteen percent of enrolled patients had de novo hyponatremia 13 months after initiation of PD. Initial serum albumin levels of the hyponatremia group were significantly lower than those of the normonatremic group (p = 0.022; Table 1). Median levels of initial serum sodium in the hyponatremia group were also slightly lower than those in the normonatremic group; however, the difference was not significant. At month 13, the hyponatremia group showed no significant difference in serum albumin levels, compared to the normonatremic group.

Parameters	Month 1		Month 13	
	HN	NN	HN	NN
Serologic parameters				
C-reative protein (mg/dL)	0.15	0.13	0.26	0.13
Glucose (mg/dL)	173	130	160	120*
Creatinine (mg/dL)	7.6	7.4	10	7.9
Albumin (mg/dL)	3.1*	3.7	3.4	3.6
Cholesterol (mg/dL)	179	171	200	189
Sodium (mEq/L)	136	140	134*	139
Potassium (mEq/L)	3.7	4.2	3.8	4.3
Chloride (mEq/L)	99	101	95*	101
Total CO_2 (mEq/L)	23.4	23.0	22.3	25.9
Peritoneal function and adequacy tests				
D/P Cr	0.64	0.67	0.75*	0.66
Maximum dip in DPNa	0.071	0.070	0.091	0.071
Ultrafiltration capacity (mL)	800	875	700	900
Weight (kg)	66.5	65.8	66.5	65.5
nPNA (g/kg/day)	0.81	0.88	0.79	0.88
Total Kt/Vurea	2.05	2.28	2.19	2.12
GFR (L/week/1.73m^2)	44.8	45.1	53.1*	43.8

Table 1. Serum levels of the parameters at months 1 and 13 (Lee et al., 2010). Values are presented as the median. HN, hyponatremia; NN, normonatremia. D/P Cr, dialysate-to-plasma creatinine ratio at 4 hours; Maximum dip in DPNa, the difference between the initial D/P sodium and the lowest D/P sodium; nPNA, protein equivalent of total nitrogen appearance normalized to desirable body weight (generating rate of urea); GFR, Glomerular Filtration Rate (average of creatinine clearance and urea clearance). * *P*-value < 0.05, hyponatremia group vs. normonatremic group.

No significant differences were observed in serum C-reactive protein, creatinine, cholesterol, potassium, or total CO_2 between the two groups after 13 months. Several parameters changed from month 1 to 13 in PD patients with de novo hyponatremia. Serum albumin levels in the hyponatremia group showed a moderate, but not significant increase ($p = 0.058$), from 3.10 to 3.45 mg/dL. During the 12-month period, no statistical difference was observed in serum glucose, creatinine, cholesterol, potassium, chloride, and total CO_2 levels.

At month 1, the two groups showed no significant differences in peritoneal function and adequacy tests. In contrast, at month 13, the D/P Cr was increased to 0.748 in the hyponatremia group, compared with 0.662 in the normonatremic group ($p = 0.007$). The glomerular filtration rate measured at month 13 was slightly higher in the hyponatremia group ($p = 0.021$). No other measure of peritoneal function and adequacy differed between the two groups. Changes in peritoneal function and adequacy tests in PD patients with de novo hyponatremia were observed after 12-month treatments. The D/P Cr showed a significant increase ($p = 0.036$) from 0.644 to 0.748. The glomerular filtration rate tended to be higher at 12 months (44.8 vs. 53.1 L/week/1.73m^2, $p = 0.063$). A trend toward a decrease in nPNA was seen in the hyponatremia group at month 13; however, the difference was not significant.

We found that the increase in D/P Cr at month 13 was significantly higher in the hyponatremia group. The lower fluid removal during a single PD exchange in high transporters was not only due to a decrease in the ultrafiltration rate, but also an increase in the peritoneal fluid absorption rate (Wang et al., 1998). The decrease in the ultrafiltration rate in high transporters is likely due to a rapid decrease in the osmotic gradient resulting from increased absorption of glucose from the dialysate. The increased fluid absorption rate may be the result of increased peritoneal interstitial hydraulic conductivity, as the peritoneal hydrostatic pressure gradient is unlikely to be higher in high transporters. Therefore, subjects in the hyponatremia group, who were high transporters, showed lower fluid removal, which might lead to free water gain.

Of particular interest, in this study, despite reduced ultrafiltration capacity, there were no changes of body weight in the hyponatremic groups. This finding suggests that hyponatremia in incident PD patients can occur due not only to free water gain, but also additional causes, including catabolic states or malnutrition. Patients with de novo hyponatremia had low levels of initial serum albumin and low levels of nPNA at month 13. Serum albumin and nPNA are markers for nutrition and a well-known predictor of mortality in PD patients; therefore, these conditions may also contribute to de novo hyponatremia (Perez-Flores et al., 2007). Diuretics, which were prescribed to maintain urine output, may also affect development of hyponatremia (Sonnenblick et al., 1993). However, there was no significant difference between the two groups, although approximately half of patients were prescribed diuretics in the current data.

The majority of the patients still had residual renal function since all the enrolled patients were incident cases of peritoneal dialysis. The residual renal function tended to be higher at 12 months in hyponatremic group. Excessive peritoneal ultrafiltration may, by provoking intravascular volume depletion, play a causative role in the decline in residual renal function (Konings et al., 2005; Konings et al., 2003). In the present study, it is possible that increased D/P Cr and, consequently, lower peritoneal ultrafiltration volume in the hyponatremic group might provide a lower risk of intravascular volume depletion and higher probability of relative increase of residual renal function.

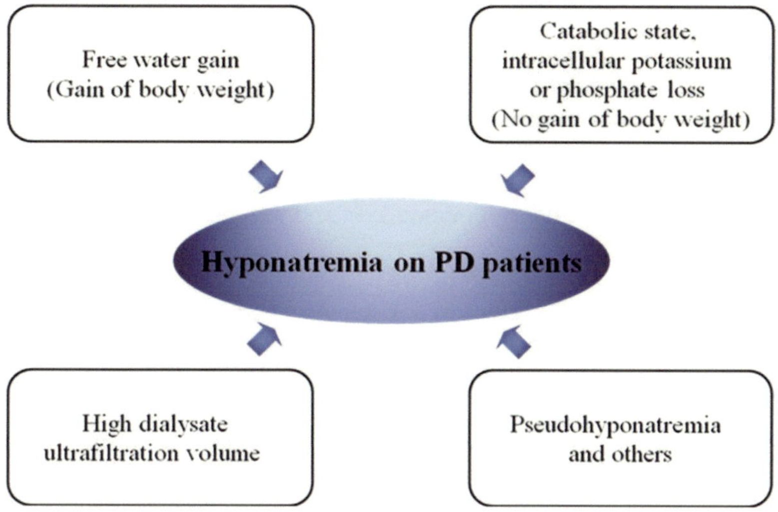

Fig. 1. Pathophysiology of hyponatremia in PD patients

Our findings showed that the maximum dip in D/PNa did not differ between the two groups, while D/P Cr was significantly higher in the hyponatremia group. The sieving coefficient for sodium is higher in high transport patients compared, with low transport patients (Wang et al., 1997). However, no significant differences were found in our study. Discrepancies between studies may be explained by small differences in D/P Cr. The average D/P Cr in the hyponatremia and normonatremic groups classified both as high-average transporters. We observed higher serum glucose levels at month 13 in the hyponatremia group, while no change in glucose or uric acid was observed in the hyponatremia group from month 1 to 13. Hyperglycemia is associated with a decrease in the serum sodium concentration (Roscoe et al., 1975). The expected decrease in the serum sodium concentration is 1.35 mEq/L for every 100 mg/dL increase in the blood glucose concentration (Roscoe et al., 1975). Therefore, higher serum glucose levels in the hyponatremia group were related to the decrease in serum sodium levels.

2.4 Summary of hyponatremia in PD patients

The primary cause of hyponatremia is free water gain by the ECF, which is often paralleled by an increase in body weight. Intracellular potassium or phosphate loss, pseudohyponatremia, and catabolic states are less common causes of hyponatremia (Cherney et al., 2001)(Fig. 1). Some studies have demonstrated a relationship between the incidence of PD-associated hyponatremia and the catabolic state (Zevallos et al., 2001). They reported that tissue catabolism combined with intracellular potassium and phosphate loss may lead to hyponatremia in PD patients. Other studies have shown that the main determinant of PD sodium loss is the net dialysate ultrafiltration volume (Uribarri et al., 2004). Treatment with icodextrin-based dialysis solution regimes has also been implicated as a risk factor for hyponatremia (Gradden et al., 2001). Increased serum NT-Pro-BNP, a predictor of mortality in PD and hemodialysis patients, was found to play a role in development of hyponatremia, water balance disturbance, anemia status, and hypoalbuminemia in the PD patient group (Adachi & Nishio, 2008).

3. Hypokalemia in PD patients

3.1 Pathophysiology of hypokalemia in PD patients

A third of PD patients, in whom potassium removal by PD does not explain the occurrence of hypokalemia, are frequently hypokalemic (Oreopoulos et al., 1982; Rostand, 1983). Some studies have noted that 36% of PD patients have a serum potassium level less than 3.5 mEq/L at some time during their course and that 20% require potassium supplementation (Spital & Sterns, 1985). In addition, hypokalemia is an independent predictor of mortality in PD patients (Szeto et al., 2005).

Potassium homeostasis is maintained by two different balances: the internal balance, representing potassium redistribution between intracellular and extracellular compartments, and the external balance, representing potassium interchange between the organism and the environment (Adrogue & Wesson, 1992). Since fluid and electrolyte balance in these patients is dependent on nonrenal routes, PD-related hypokalemia also differs pathophysiologically from non-PD-related hypokalemia. Daily consumption of potassium exceeds daily elimination with PD; therefore, PD fluid has never contained potassium. Enhanced large intestine secretion of potassium in direct proportion to dietary potassium intake, which is an additional route of potassium removal, plays an important role in maintenance of potassium balance in patients with renal insufficiency (Bastl et al., 1977; Mathialahan et al., 2005).

Figure 2 shows the pathophysiology of hypokalemia in PD patients. Serum potassium levels in PD patients are associated with nutritional status and severity of coexisting comorbid conditions. Hypokalemia in PD patients is due to a shift of potassium into the intracellular space, probably due to insulin release during the continuous dwell of the dialysis solution containing glucose (Tziviskou et al., 2003). Thus, cellular uptake may play an important role in the pathogenesis of hypokalemia. Muscle biopsy studies have shown higher intracellular potassium content in PD patients, compared with hemodialysis patients (Lindholm et al., 1986). Ongoing loss of potassium in dialysate may be another important factor contributing to hypokalemia (Szeto et al., 2005). The main driving force for elimination of potassium is the diffusive gradient between blood and PD fluid (Brown et al., 1973; Nolph et al., 1980).

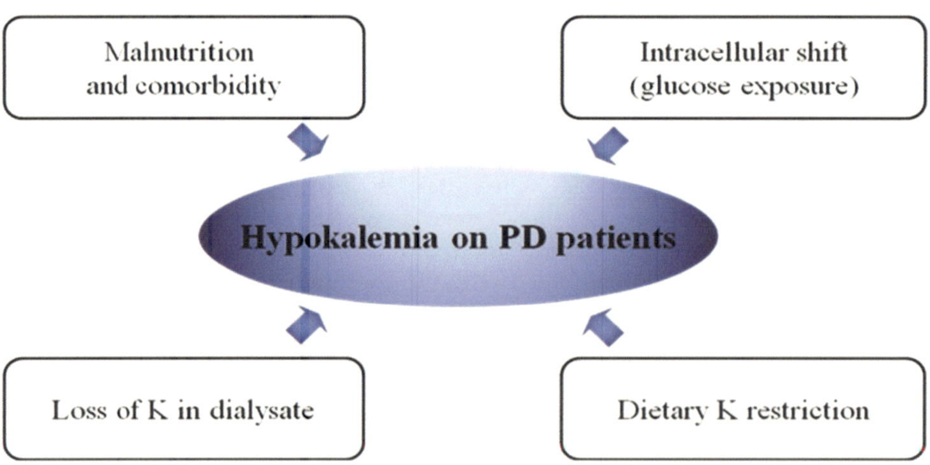

Fig. 2. Pathophysiology of hypokalemia in PD patients

Due to the low concentration of serum potassium, removal of convective fluid, under most circumstances, contributes little to potassium removal (Brown et al., 1973; Nolph et al., 1980). In addition, end stage renal disease patients are instructed to restrict potassium-rich foods, such as fruits and vegetables.

3.2 De novo hypokalemia in incident PD patients

This study (Jung et al., 2009) was undertaken in order to investigate clinical features and factors related to de novo hypokalemia in incident PD patients over the 1-year observational period using the same protocol (Lee et al., 2010), which is designed for control of bias on pre-existing hypokalemic conditions.

Eighty-two incident PD patients who were normokalemic at month 1 of PD were enrolled in the study. According to the plasma potassium levels at month 13, patients were divided into hypokalemic ($K^+ < 3.5$ mEq/L) and normokalemic (3.5 mEq/L $\leq K^+ < 5.5$ mEq/L) groups. Eight patients who showed hyperkalemia at month 13 were excluded. Blood, peritoneal function tests, and dialysis adequacy and nutritional status data were taken at months 1 and 13. The two groups, those with and those without hypokalemia, did not differ significantly in age, sex, height, and causes of end-stage renal disease. Medication history of ACE inhibitors or angiotensin II receptor blockades and diuretics were not significantly different between the two groups. No statistical differences were found between the two groups with respect to the Davies comorbidity index, biocompatible fluid, and continuous ambulatory PD versus automated PD.

The incidence of hypokalemia in patients starting PD was 7.3% over the 1-year observation period. Whereas the initial serum potassium and albumin levels at month 1 did not differ between the two groups, serum albumin level in the hypokalemia group showed a significant decrease from 3.1 to 2.9 mg/dL at month 13 ($p = 0.014$)(Table 2). In contrast, no significant differences were observed in serum C-reactive protein, glucose, cholesterol, and total CO_2 between the two groups at month 13. At month 1, the hypokalemia group showed higher serum phosphorus levels and lower cholesterol levels.

At month 1, the two groups showed no significant differences. nPNA at month 1 was also similar between the hypokalemic and normokalemic groups. However, at month 13, the nPNA was significantly lower in the hypokalemia group, compared with that in the normokalemic group. Other measurements determined for peritoneal function, including D/P Cr and daily glucose exposure, did not differ between the two groups.

In the current study, the incidence of hypokalemia in our PD patients, 7.3% in one year, appears relatively low, compared with that of previous reports (Kim et al., 2007; Oreopoulos et al., 1982; Rostand, 1983). This is probably because our result was from newly starting PD patients. We demonstrated an association between development of hypokalemia in incident PD patients and decreases in serum albumin and nPNA. This poor nutritional status can lead to de novo hypokalemia. In PD patients, insulin hormone, stimulated by the continuous glucose peritoneal dwell, can generate an increase of potassium redistribution into the intracellular compartment (Tziviskou et al., 2003). In the present study, the presence of diabetes and daily glucose load did not differ between the two groups, suggesting that intracellular potassium redistribution may not be the main mechanism of hypokalemia in our PD patients. In a cross-sectional study, the serum potassium level of PD patients was correlated with ultrafiltration volume (Kim et al., 2007). However, in our longitudinal study, no difference in ultrafiltration volume was observed between the two groups at month 13.

This finding is consistent with the previous study showing that convective fluid removal contributes little to potassium elimination (Brown et al., 1973; Nolph et al., 1980).

	Month 1		Month 13	
	HK	NK	HK	NK
Serologic parameters				
C-reative protein (mg/dL)	0.53	0.15	0.36	0.18
Glucose (mg/dL)	158	138	137	127
Creatinine (mg/dL)	7.6	7.6	8.6	9.4
Albumin (mg/dL)	3.1	3.7	2.9*	3.7
Cholesterol (mg/dL)	125*	163	163	174
Sodium (mEq/L)	136	139	136	139
Potassium (mEq/L)	4.1	4.2	3.4*	4.5
Chloride (mEq/L)	101.5	102.0	98.0	101.0
Total CO_2 (mEq/L)	19.5	23.0	23.5	22.1
Calcium (mg/dL)	8.5	8.5	8.6	8.9
Phosphorus (mg/dL)	5.6 *	4.2	3.7	4.6
Peritoneal function and adequacy tests				
D/P Cr	0.68	0.67	0.69	0.67
Ultrafiltration capacity (mL)	675	850	800	800
Weight (kg)	63.8	66.0	66.0	63.6
nPNA (g/kg/day)	0.89	0.91	0.66*	0.91
Total Kt/Vurea	2.37	2.05	1.94	1.98
GFR (L/week/1.73m^2)	47.0	41.1	48.5	42.6
Glucose exposure (g/day)	130	120	163	120

Table 2. Serum parameters at months 1 and 13 (Jung et al., 2009). Values are presented as median values. HK, hypokalemia; NK, normokalemia. D/P Cr, dialysate-to-plasma creatinine ratio at 4 hours; nPNA, protein equivalent of total nitrogen appearance normalized to desirable body weight (generating rate of urea); GFR, Glomerular Filtration Rate (calculated as the mean of the values for creatinine and urea clearances) * P-value < 0.05, hypokalemia group vs. normokalemic group.

3.3 Summary of hypokalemia in PD patients

Ten to 58% of patients on PD are known to develop hypokalemia (K^+ < 3.5 mEq/L)(Khan et al., 1996; Rostand, 1983; Spital & Sterns, 1985). The wide range of prevalence of hypokalemia may depend on dietary consumption of potassium according to the study population or ethnicity. Compared with Caucasians, Asians and African Americans tend to have lower daily potassium intake (Gao et al., 2009; Kant et al., 2007; Szeto et al., 2005). In a group of 266 Chinese PD patients, prevalence was reported as 20.3%, and hypokalemia was found to be an independent predictor of mortality, although causes of death in the hypokalemic group did not differ from those in the normokalemic group (Szeto et al., 2005). In other Asian PD patients, hypokalemia can be considered a nutrition marker, such as serum albumin or normalized protein nitrogen appearance (nPNA) (Chuang et al., 2009; Szeto et al., 2005). Therefore, hypokalemia is associated with poor clinical outcomes, including malnutrition and death. New evidence points to a link between hypokalemia and the risk of peritonitis. Hypokalemia and malnutrition may increase the incidence of Enterobacteriaceae peritonitis, which is caused by impairment of gut mobility, small bowel overgrowth with colonic flora, and bacterial translocation across the bowel wall (Berg, 1992; Casafont et al., 1997; Chuang et al., 2009). Particularly in diabetic patients, hypokalemia may be associated with impaired bowel motility and bacterial overgrowth (Shu et al., 2009). A study of 140 Asian PD patients found a higher incidence of peritonitis in hypokalemic patients, compared with normokalemic patients, and the incidence of peritonitis due to Enterobacteriacea was found to be higher in the hypokalemic group, compared with the normokalemic group (Chuang et al., 2009). Both hypokalemia and markers of malnutrition may be independent risk factors for development of peritonitis. Further studies are warranted for determination of whether correction of hypokalamia can result in reduced risk of peritonitis.

4. Conclusion

Hyponatremia occurs frequently in patients undergoing PD. Therefore, one must understand its pathophysiology, since the therapeutic strategy differs from that of non-PD-related hyponatremia. Incidence of PD-associated hyponatremia is mainly related to fluid overload. Tissue catabolism combined with intracellular potassium and phosphate loss may also lead to hyponatremia. Sodium loss through peritoneal membrane is associated with the dialysate ultrafiltration volume, although that may be of little effect. Hypokalemia also develops commonly in PD patients. Serum potassium levels in PD patients may be influenced by nutritional status and severity of coexisting comorbid conditions. Development of hypokalemia can be due to a shift of potassium into the intracellular space, which is related to insulin release during the continuous dwell of the dialysis solution containing glucose. Ongoing loss of potassium in dialysate may be another important factor contributing to hypokalemia; however, potassium loss may not be related to ultrafiltration volume. Recently, hypokalemia has been considered as a risk factor for peritonitis in PD patients. This common electrolyte imbalance in PD patients is associated with severe consequences, morbidity, and mortality. Therefore, hyponatremia and hypokalemia should be monitored more carefully in these patients.

5. References

Adachi, Y., & Nishio, A. (2008). N-terminal pro-brain natriuretic peptide in prevalent peritoneal dialysis patients, *Adv Perit Dial* 24:75-78.

Adrogue, H., & Wesson, D. 1992. Potassium. Houston: Libra and Gemini Publications. 48 p.

Anderson, R. J., Chung, H. M., Kluge, R., & Schrier, R. W. (1985). Hyponatremia: a prospective analysis of its epidemiology and the pathogenetic role of vasopressin, *Ann Intern Med* 102(2):164-168.

Bastl, C., Hayslett, J. P., & Binder, H. J. (1977). Increased large intestinal secretion of potassium in renal insufficiency, *Kidney Int* 12(1):9-16.

Berg, R. D. (1992). Bacterial translocation from the gastrointestinal tract, *J Med* 23(3-4):217-244.

Brown, S. T., Ahearn, D. J., & Nolph, K. D. (1973). Potassium removal with peritoneal dialysis, *Kidney Int* 4(1):67-69.

Casafont, F., Sanchez, E., Martin, L., Aguero, J., & Romero, F. P. (1997). Influence of malnutrition on the prevalence of bacterial translocation and spontaneous bacterial peritonitis in experimental cirrhosis in rats, *Hepatology* 25(6):1334-1337.

Cherney, D. Z., Zevallos, G., Oreopoulos, D., & Halperin, M. L. (2001). A physiological analysis of hyponatremia: implications for patients on peritoneal dialysis, *Perit Dial Int* 21(1):7-13.

Chuang, Y. W., Shu, K. H., Yu, T. M., Cheng, C. H., & Chen, C. H. (2009). Hypokalaemia: an independent risk factor of Enterobacteriaceae peritonitis in CAPD patients, *Nephrol Dial Transplant* 24(5):1603-1608.

Gao, S. K., Fitzpatrick, A. L., Psaty, B., Jiang, R., Post, W., Cutler, J., & Maciejewski, M. L. (2009). Suboptimal nutritional intake for hypertension control in 4 ethnic groups, *Arch Intern Med* 169(7):702-707.

Gheorghiade, M., Abraham, W. T., Albert, N. M., Gattis Stough, W., Greenberg, B. H., O'Connor, C. M., She, L., Yancy, C. W., Young, J., & Fonarow, G. C. (2007). Relationship between admission serum sodium concentration and clinical outcomes in patients hospitalized for heart failure: an analysis from the OPTIMIZE-HF registry, *Eur Heart J* 28(8):980-988.

Gradden, C. W., Ahmad, R., & Bell, G. M. (2001). Peritoneal dialysis: new developments and new problems, *Diabet Med* 18(5):360-363.

Jung, J. Y., Chang, J. H., Lee, H. H., Chung, W., & Kim, S. (2009). De novo hypokalemia in incident peritoneal dialysis patients: a 1-year observational study, *Electrolyte Blood Press* 7(2):73-78.

Kant, A. K., Graubard, B. I., & Kumanyika, S. K. (2007). Trends in black-white differentials in dietary intakes of U.S. adults, 1971-2002, *Am J Prev Med* 32(4):264-272.

Khan, A. N., Bernardini, J., Johnston, J. R., & Piraino, B. (1996). Hypokalemia in peritoneal dialysis patients, *Perit Dial Int* 16(6):652.

Kim, H.-W., Chang, J. H., Park, S. Y., Moon, S. J., Kim, D. K., Lee, J. E., Han, S. H., Kim, B. S., Kang, S.-W., Choi, K. H., Lee, H. Y., & Han, D.-S. (2007). Factors associated with hypokalemia in continuous ambulatory peritoneal dialysis patients, *Electrolyte Blood Press* 5:102-110.

Kim, S., Oh, J., Chung, W., Ahn, C., Kim, S. G., & Oh, K. H. (2009). Benefits of biocompatible PD fluid for preservation of residual renal function in incident CAPD patients: a 1-year study, *Nephrol Dial Transplant* 24(9):2899-2908.

Konings, C. J., Kooman, J. P., Gladziwa, U., van der Sande, F. M., & Leunissen, K. M. (2005). A decline in residual glomerular filtration during the use of icodextrin may be due to underhydration, *Kidney Int* 67(3):1190-1191.

Konings, C. J., Kooman, J. P., Schonck, M., Gladziwa, U., Wirtz, J., van den Wall Bake, A. W., Gerlag, P. G., Hoorntje, S. J., Wolters, J., van der Sande, F. M., & Leunissen, K. M. (2003). Effect of icodextrin on volume status, blood pressure and echocardiographic parameters: a randomized study, *Kidney Int* 63(4):1556-1563.

Lee, H. H., Choi, S. J., Lee, H. N., Na, S. Y., Chang, J. H., Chung, W., & Kim, S. (2010). De novo hyponatremia in patients undergoing peritoneal dialysis: a 12-month observational study, *Korean J Nephrol* 29:31-37.

Lindholm, B., Alvestrand, A., Hultman, E., & Bergstrom, J. (1986). Muscle water and electrolytes in patients undergoing continuous ambulatory peritoneal dialysis, *Acta Med Scand* 219(3):323-330.

Mathialahan, T., Maclennan, K. A., Sandle, L. N., Verbeke, C., & Sandle, G. I. (2005). Enhanced large intestinal potassium permeability in end-stage renal disease, *J Pathol* 206(1):46-51.

Nguyen, M. K., & Kurtz, I. (2004). New insights into the pathophysiology of the dysnatremias: a quantitative analysis, *Am J Physiol Renal Physiol* 287(2):F172-180.

Nolph, K. D., Sorkin, M. I., & Moore, H. (1980). Autoregulation of sodium and potassium removal during continuous ambulatory peritoneal dialysis, *Trans Am Soc Artif Intern Organs* 26:334-338.

Oreopoulos, D. G., Khanna, R., Williams, P., & Vas, S. I. (1982). Continuous ambulatory peritoneal dialysis - 1981, *Nephron* 30(4):293-303.

Perez-Flores, I., Coronel, F., Cigarran, S., Herrero, J. A., & Calvo, N. (2007). Relationship between residual renal function, inflammation, and anemia in peritoneal dialysis, *Adv Perit Dial* 23:140-143.

Rippe, B., & Venturoli, D. (2008). Optimum electrolyte composition of a dialysis solution, *Perit Dial Int* 28 Suppl 3:S131-136.

Roscoe, J. M., Halperin, M. L., Rolleston, F. S., & Goldstein, M. B. (1975). Hyperglycemia-induced hyponatremia: metabolic considerations in calculation of serum sodium depression, *Can Med Assoc J* 112(4):452-453.

Rostand, S. G. (1983). Profound hypokalemia in continuous ambulatory peritoneal dialysis, *Arch Intern Med* 143(2):377-378.

Sajadieh, A., Binici, Z., Mouridsen, M. R., Nielsen, O. W., Hansen, J. F., & Haugaard, S. B. (2009). Mild hyponatremia carries a poor prognosis in community subjects, *Am J Med* 122(7):679-686.

Shu, K. H., Chang, C. S., Chuang, Y. W., Chen, C. H., Cheng, C. H., Wu, M. J., & Yu, T. M. (2009). Intestinal bacterial overgrowth in CAPD patients with hypokalaemia, *Nephrol Dial Transplant* 24(4):1289-1292.

Sonnenblick, M., Friedlander, Y., & Rosin, A. J. (1993). Diuretic-induced severe hyponatremia. Review and analysis of 129 reported patients, *Chest* 103(2):601-606.

Spital, A., & Sterns, R. H. (1985). Potassium supplementation via the dialysate in continuous ambulatory peritoneal dialysis, *Am J Kidney Dis* 6(3):173-176.

Szeto, C. C., Chow, K. M., Kwan, B. C., Leung, C. B., Chung, K. Y., Law, M. C., & Li, P. K. (2005). Hypokalemia in Chinese peritoneal dialysis patients: prevalence and prognostic implication, *Am J Kidney Dis* 46(1):128-135.

Tziviskou, E., Musso, C., Bellizzi, V., Khandelwal, M., Wang, T., Savaj, S., & Oreopoulos, D. G. (2003). Prevalence and pathogenesis of hypokalemia in patients on chronic peritoneal dialysis: one center's experience and review of the literature, *Int Urol Nephrol* 35(3):429-434.

Uribarri, J., Prabhakar, S., & Kahn, T. (2004). Hyponatremia in peritoneal dialysis patients, *Clin Nephrol* 61(1):54-58.

Wang, T., Heimburger, O., Waniewski, J., Bergstrom, J., & Lindholm, B. (1998). Increased peritoneal permeability is associated with decreased fluid and small-solute removal and higher mortality in CAPD patients, *Nephrol Dial Transplant* 13(5):1242-1249.

Wang, T., Waniewski, J., Heimburger, O., Werynski, A., & Lindholm, B. (1997). A quantitative analysis of sodium transport and removal during peritoneal dialysis, *Kidney Int* 52(6):1609-1616.

Zanger, R. (2010). Hyponatremia and hypokalemia in patients on peritoneal dialysis, *Semin Dial* 23(6):575-580.

Zevallos, G., Oreopoulos, D. G., & Halperin, M. L. (2001). Hyponatremia in patients undergoing CAPD: role of water gain and/or malnutrition, *Perit Dial Int* 21(1):72-76.

11

Encapsulating Peritoneal Sclerosis in Incident PD Patients in Scotland

Robert Mactier and Michaela Brown
Glasgow Renal Unit, Western Infirmary, Glasgow, Scotland UK

1. Introduction

1.1 Background

Encapsulating peritoneal sclerosis (EPS) is a devastating and potentially life threatening complication of peritoneal dialysis (PD). EPS was first described in 1980 and is characterised by progressive peritoneal fibrosis and thickening with encasement of bowel loops (Ghandi el al 1980). EPS results from chronic intra-abdominal inflammation and fibrosis but the trigger for this is unknown. The aetiology is thought to be multi-factorial. Early clinical studies identified acetate dialysate and chlorhexidine as causes (Slingeneyer 1987, Oules et al 1983). However, despite the removal of these causal factors from clinical practice, EPS continues to occur. The duration of exposure to PD therapy represents the most consistent "risk factor" identified in studies to date (Kawanishi et al 2001, Kawanishi et al 2004, Rigby et al 1998, Brown MC et al 2009).

1.2 Diagnosis of EPS

The clinical features of EPS have been described in previous clinical studies (Kawanishi et al 2001, Kawanishi et al 2004, Rigby et al 1998, Nomoto et al 1996, Summers et al 2005, Brown MC et al 2009). The progressive peritoneal fibrosis compromises bowel motility and absorption, ultimately causing bowel obstruction (often sub-acute) and severe malnutrition. Typically EPS is also associated with progressive loss of ultrafiltration, causing fluid accumulation. Ascites may also develop (Perks et al 2004).

The clinical, radiological and pathological criteria for the diagnosis of EPS have been defined by the International Society for Peritoneal Dialysis (ISPD) in 2000 (Kawaguchi et al 2000) and these criteria should be met by all patients included in clinical and epidemiological studies in the post millennium. EPS may be diagnosed while the patient is on PD but many cases become apparent after stopping PD including after renal transplantation (Fieren et al 2007, Korte et al 2007, de Freitas DG et al 2007) Brown MC et al 2009).

1.3 "Incidence" of EPS

EPS is an infrequent complication in patients after more prolonged exposure to PD but the exact incidence is unknown. Most previous studies are from Japan/Northeast Asia, where the duration of PD therapy tends to be longer. Multi-centre studies from Japan report "incidence" rates of 0.8-2.5% of PD patients (Kawanishi et al 2001, Kawanishi et al 2004, Nomoto et al). Whether the findings from these studies can be extrapolated to Western populations and practice is uncertain. A recent case series from the UK identified 27 cases of EPS, representing an "incidence" of 3.3% in their PD population over 7 years (Summers et al 2005). An earlier Australian case series identified 54 cases over 14 years, representing an "incidence" of 0.7% (Rigby et al 1998). The data from these studies is summarised in Table 1 below.

Study Country Year of publication	Nomoto *et al* Japan 1996	Rigby *et al* Australia 1998	Lee *et al* Korea 2003	Kawanishi *et al* Japan 2001	Kawanishi *et al* Japan 2004	Summers *et al.* UK 2005	Brown MC *et al.* UK 2009
Number of EPS Cases*	**62**	**54 (46)**	**31**	**17**	**48**	**27 (23)**	**46**
Dates of Study	1980 - 1994	1980 - 1994	1981 - 2002	1999 - 2001	1999 - 2003	1998 – 2003	2000-2007
Denominator Population (prevalent + incident patients)	6923	7374	3888	2216	1958	810	1638
Overall "Incidence"	**0.9%**	**0.7%**	**0.8%**	**0.8%**	**2.5%**	**3.3%**	**2.8%**
Mean PD Exposure (yrs)	5.1	4.3	5.8	10	4.3	6.1	5.4
Mortality (over study period)	43.5 %	56 %	25.8 %	35 %	37.5 %	29.6 %	56.5%

* The number of EPS cases who did not meet the ISPD 2000 criteria for EPS is shown in brackets in the second row of Table 1.

Table 1. "Incidence" of EPS reported from previous studies

1.4 Incidence of EPS

The true incidence of EPS has been difficult to establish because:

EPS is uncommon,

EPS is associated with poor survival rates,

misdiagnosis or delayed diagnosis of EPS may occur, especially if the patient develops symptoms after PD has been discontinued,

most epidemiological studies describing the "incidence" of EPS have been retrospective.

In addition most previous studies have included both incident and prevalent patients on PD on the start date of follow up which does not allow an accurate calculation of incidence (Kawanishi et al 2001, Kawanishi et al 2004, Rigby et al 1998, Nomoto et al 1996, Summers et al 2005). To calculate a true incidence of EPS a cohort of patients must be followed from the start of PD to identify all cases diagnosed thereafter. To address this we reported the incidence of EPS in all patients starting PD in Scotland in the time period 01 January 2000 - 31 December 2007 (Brown MC et al 2009). The rate of EPS in this study was 1.5% (19 EPS cases observed in 1238 incident PD patients) or an incidence of 4.9 per 1000 person years. This study showed that the incidence of EPS was 0% in first year of PD, rising progressively to 8.1% (CI 3.6-17.6) at >4-5 years; 8.8% (CI 3.2-23.1) at >5-6 years and 5.0% (CI 1.2-23.8) at >6 years PD exposure (Table 2). It is possible that greater awareness of EPS may have led to increased diagnosis of milder cases but the mortality rate was similar to rates reported in previous studies (Table 1) and was 42% at 1 year after diagnosis.

Cumulative PD Exposure	PD Cohort (n=1238)	EPS Cases (n=19)	Incidence (%)	95% Confidence Intervals
< 1 year	480	0	0	0
1-2 years	326	2	0.6	0.2 - 2.1
2-3 years	202	4	2.0	0.8 - 5.0
3-4 years	114	4	3.5	1.4 - 8.7
4-5 years	62	5	8.1	3.6 - 17.6
5-6years	34	3	8.8	3.2 - 23.1
> 6 years	20	1	5.0	1.2 - 23.8

Table 2. Incidence rates of EPS related to total duration of PD exposure (not necessarily continuous)

It is noticeable that there is a dramatic increase in the proportion of patients developing EPS after 4 years of PD (1 in 12 patients at risk). Thus analysis of this incident PD patient cohort up to December 2007 showed that the incidence of EPS increased significantly with PD duration but the confidence limits of the observed incidence of EPS were wide as the number of cases of EPS was low and the PD patient follow up was relatively short. However, 806 patients (66%) of the PD cohort had had less than 2 years PD exposure by the end of 2007 so the incidence of EPS in this patient cohort is likely to increase after longer follow up. This could be addressed by reporting the incidence of EPS in this same cohort of PD patients after a longer period of follow up.

1.5 Study aims

The primary aims of the current study were:

a. describe all of the cases of encapsulating peritoneal sclerosis (EPS) occurring between 01 January 2000 - 30 June 2009 in the above cohort of patients who had commenced peritoneal dialysis (PD) in Scotland between 01 January 2000 - 31 December 2007
b. calculate the true incidence of EPS in this PD cohort.

2. Methods

2.1 Patients

The cohort of patients aged over 18 years who started peritoneal dialysis (PD) between 01 January 2000 and 31 December 2007 in Scotland (n= 1238) was identified from the Scottish Renal Registry. We sent each of the 10 adult renal units in Scotland a list of their patients in this cohort and a note of the diagnostic features of EPS. We asked them to identify known or *potential* cases diagnosed after 01 January 2000. All units were originally approached in the summer of 2006 and at intervals thereafter.

2.2 Inclusion criteria for EPS diagnosis

Casenotes and electronic patient records for each possible case were examined by one data collector (MC Brown) to ensure all met the ISPD diagnostic criteria (Kawaguchi et al 2000). To confirm the diagnosis of EPS a patient had to have:
clinical features **and**
either typical radiological **and/or**
histopathological features.
Clinical features include abdominal pain, nausea, vomiting, abdominal distension, anorexia, weight loss, unexplained/resistant anaemia, unexplained fever, elevated inflammatory markers, loss of ultrafiltration, bowel obstruction and/or unexplained ascites. Typical radiological features include ascites, typically loculated with multiple strands or septations, peritoneal thickening, thickening of bowel wall, calcification, thickened mesentery and/or matted bowel in the central abdomen. Positive pathology included the typical macroscopic appearance at laparotomy or laparoscopy or biopsy consistent with EPS with gross interstitial thickening with loss of mesothelium.

2.3 Exclusion criteria for EPS diagnosis

Exclusion criteria for EPS were met if there was an alternative explanation for the above findings:
previous bowel perforation,
TB,
cirrhosis,
intraperitoneal (IP) malignancy/chemotherapy,
VP shunt or TIPSS,
IP lavage with disinfectant or talc contamination

2.4 Calculation of EPS incidence rates

We have assumed that the individual units had adequate systems locally to identify patients diagnosed with EPS since 2000. In addition we looked for EPS in the European Dialysis and Transplantation Association (EDTA) coded causes of death in the Scottish Renal Registry records to identify any additional cases. To calculate the incidence and rates per time on PD we have only included patients who developed EPS and who were first exposed to PD after 01 January 2000. The rates are given as the incidence with the 95% confidence intervals.
All cases have been used to describe the clinical presentation. Cases of EPS in this national cohort of incident patients on PD were used to calculate incidence rates between 01 January 2000 and 30 June 2009. Statistical analyses were performed using SPSS®. The incidence of

EPS was calculated as number of EPS cases divided by number of patients at risk, taking into account the person-time during which events were observed and time elapsed before EPS diagnosis.

2.5 PD- associated peritonitis

Peritonitis was defined as a PD effluent white cell count above 100 per mm^3. Peritonitis rates were calculated as the number of patient months on PD divided by number of infections and expressed as number of months between episodes.

3. Results

3.1 Patient demographics

31 of the 1238 patient cohort had developed EPS before 30 June 2009. The median duration of PD before the diagnosis of EPS was 4.0 years (interquartile range 2.9-5.2 years). The mean duration of exposure to PD of the patients who did not develop EPS was 1.8 years. The rate of peritonitis in the patients with EPS was 1 episode every 19.2 months which is very similar to the peritonitis rate in Scotland 2000-2009 (Scottish Renal Registry Report 2009).
The clinical details of the 31 patients who developed EPS have been compared with the patients who did not develop EPS in Table 3 below.

Patient demographics	EPS Cases (n=31)	PD Cohort (n=1207)
Median Age (IQR)	53.9 (43 - 64) years	55 (45 - 70) years
Proportion male	58%	55%
Proportion Caucasian	94.8%	>95%
Median number of peritonitis episodes (IQR)	2 (1-4)	1 (1-2)

Table 3. Summary of demographics of patients who did and did not develop EPS

The interquartile ranges (IQR) of median values are recorded in brackets.

3.2 Clinical presentation

Most patients had more than one clinical feature attributable to EPS. All patients had at least one of these three symptoms: abdominal pain, vomiting and/or abdominal distension (with ascites or in the context of bowel obstruction).

3.3 Patient outcomes

By the study end on 30th June 2009, 22 patients (71.0%) had died. 13 (60.0%) deaths were attributable to EPS. Median survival from diagnosis was 116 days (range 1-660 days, IQR 20-

297 days). The "survivors" had a median of 1076 days follow-up since diagnosis (range 63-1764 days, IQR 537-1309 days). Overall the mortality rate was 54.8% at one year after diagnosis.

3.4 Incidence of EPS

We identified 31 EPS cases in the patient cohort giving an incidence of EPS of 2.5% in this patient cohort with a minimum follow up of 1.5 years. We searched the SRR database (for International Classification of Disease codes; ICD-9/ICD-10) reported in hospital discharge statistics but no additional cases were found.

The incidence according to the duration of PD exposure is shown in Table 4. The incidence rates of EPS are higher than published previously, particularly for duration of PD exposure <5 years.

Cumulative PD Exposure	PD Cohort (n=1238)	EPS Cases (n=31)	Incidence	95% Confidence Intervals
< 1 year	470	1	0.2 %	0.1 - 1.1
1-2 years	327	3	0.9 %	0.3 - 2.6
2-3 years	198	5	2.5 %	1.1 - 5.8
3-4 years	117	6	5.1 %	2.4 - 10.7
4-5 years	63	6	9.5 %	4.5 - 19.3
5-6 years	35	6	17.1 %	8.2 - 32.8
> 6 years	28	4	14.3 %	5.8 - 31.7

Table 4. Incidence of EPS related to duration of PD exposure

3.5 Other possible "risk factors"

14 patients (45.2 %) had used high strength dextrose (3.86% or equivalent) at some point during PD treatment. 29 (93.5 %) patients had used Extraneal (Icodextrin). There was no obvious relationship to any specific brand of PD dialysate fluid. The incidence of peritonitis was similar in the patients who did and did not develop EPS. 3 of the patients who developed EPS had never had peritonitis. The spectrum of organisms causing peritonitis was comparable between the EPS cases and the PD population unaffected by EPS.

4. Discussion

4.1 Incidence of EPS

The main aim of this study was to calculate an accurate incidence of EPS and so establish the risk of EPS for patients starting PD in Scotland. This report provides a more definitive evaluation of the incidence of EPS since all of the patients in this PD cohort have a minimum of 1.5 years follow up. Our study was retrospective until June 2006 and prospective from 01 July 2006 - 30 June 2009. From previous studies it is apparent that EPS occurs very rarely if PD duration is under 18 months, and the average duration of PD exposure before the onset of EPS is 4-6 years (Kawanishi et al 2004, Rigby et al 1998, Nomoto et al 1996, Summers et al 2005, Brown MC et al 2009). Although the initial period of this study was retrospective we would expect that most cases would be reported after 2004 which is 2-3 years before we first contacted the units. In fact the first patients diagnosed from this PD cohort were in mid 2004. If any cases before 2004 were missed this would mean that the rates we report are an underestimate. We performed secondary checks of the SRR database for relevant diagnostic codes (EDTA cause of death and ICD-9 and ICD-10 codes) to identify any cases that may have been missed. However, we did not identify any other cases.

It is known from previous data that EPS often develops after stopping PD. This means that more cases from our cohort may still develop EPS and the incidence we have reported should be regarded as the minimum risk of developing EPS after PD. For this reason we are continuing to follow up the 2000-2007 PD cohort prospectively.

As our understanding of the aetiology of EPS remains poor large, prospective, multi-centred studies are required to address the clinical problems created by an apparently rising incidence of EPS. As clinicians we should be able to inform our patients of the significant risks associated with the treatments we administer. Our study allows quantification of the minimum risk of developing EPS in patients starting PD in the modern era.

4.2 Duration of PD as a risk factor for EPS

The figures reported in this study show a higher incidence of EPS after more than 3 years of PD therapy than in the earlier report after shorter follow up. This is at least in part due to the significantly more patients at risk with more than 3 years exposure to PD. The latest data suggest that after 4 years of PD therapy almost 1 in 10 patients will develop EPS. Previous studies have reported rates at 4 years PD exposure of 5% in Australia and <1% in Japan (Rigby et al 1998, Nomoto et al 1996). It is difficult to determine whether the higher rates found in this study represent an increase in the true incidence and/or increased clinical awareness of EPS or whether it reflects differences in our study design compared to previous studies. When we utilise the same method of calculating the incidence of EPS (number of cases/incident and prevalent PD patients in time period) as in previous studies, the results shown in Table 1 indicate an apparently increasing rate of EPS in the more recent studies. The rates in this report are comparable to a previous study from Manchester in the UK and to the overall incidence in the more recent studies from Japan (Kawanishi et al 2004, Summers et al 2005).

The risk of developing EPS is inversely related to the technique failure rate. A large proportion of the patients in this study with a minimum follow up period of 1.5 years were only on PD for less than 1 year so would be at low risk of developing EPS. In contrast the small portion of patients who were maintained on PD for at least 4 years has a relatively high incidence of EPS (16 of the 126 at risk patients) (Table 4).

4.3 Other risk factors for EPS

The peritonitis rates in the previous report on this incident PD cohort also showed comparable peritonitis rates between those patients who developed EPS and those patients who did not (Brown MC et al 2009). Similar peritonitis rates in patients who do and who do not develop EPS have also been shown in other studies (Hendriks et al 1997). A study of 111 patients who developed EPS showed 12 patients had no previous peritonitis episodes, 28 had one previous episode, 30 had two previous episodes and 33 had three or more previous episodes (Balasubramaniam G et al 2009). Peritonitis per se is therefore not a risk factor for the PD population although it has been reported that some patients develop an acute onset of EPS shortly after an episode of severe peritonitis (Summers et al 2005, Brown MC et al 2009).

All except two cases in our series had used Extraneal dialysate. It is very difficult to untangle whether this reflects ultrafiltration failure in the early stages of EPS or whether the use of such fluids somehow promotes the development of EPS. Only around half of the EPS patients had used high strength dextrose. Patients who develop EPS have been shown to have higher peritoneal transport rates and lower net ultrafiltration compared with matched control patients (Hendriks et al 1997) but peritoneal transport characteristics were not available in this study. It has been reported that patients with ultrafiltration failure, defined as net ultrafiltration less than 400ml after a 4 hour dwell time using 3.86% dialysis fluid, are at high risk of developing EPS if PD is continued (Sampimon et al 2011). In this recent study half of the patients with ultrafiltration failure who remained on PD for more than 3 years developed EPS (Sampimon et al 2011).

4.4 Screening for EPS

EPS may have been under-recognised in PD patients in the past and a high index of suspicion is needed in long term PD patients with symptoms due to subacute obstruction or ascites. However, it is important to avoid misdiagnosis of EPS and therefore all cases must fulfill well defined criteria in reaching a diagnosis of EPS as in this study.

At present radiological techniques are unable to establish a diagnosis of "early" EPS. CT scans which were performed coincidentally in PD patients prior to development of EPS did not show features indicating developing EPS (Tarzi et al 2008). Thus there is no evidence that regular screening of long-term PD patients by radiological techniques would be able to detect pre-symptomatic EPS or beneficially alter PD management.

Previous studies have suggested that 5 years should be the time-point for screening for EPS or discontinuing PD because of the risk of EPS (Nomoto et al 1996, Summers et al 2005, Kawaguchi et al. 2005). By 5 years 21 of the 31 cases in our case series already had developed EPS indicating that screening for EPS (if a reliable screening test was available) would already have missed two thirds of the cases and two thirds of cases would have occurred before switching dialysis modality. The data in this study lend further support to the UK EPS and ISPD guidelines on EPS which state that the optimal approach to patients on long duration PD is currently unclear but routine pre-emptive switching to haemodialysis or screening for EPS after a specified time on PD are not recommended (Woodrow et al 2009, Brown E et al 2010). Indeed many of the cases of EPS in this study and other studies (Fieren et al 2007, Korte et al 2007, de Freitas DG et al 2007, Brown M et al 2009) occurred after stopping PD. Thus pre-emptive switching to haemodialysis could potentially be associated with development of EPS rather than being preventive of EPS and at present there is no data showing any benefit from such a policy. Furthermore modality switch from PD could have significant detrimental implications for some PD patients who have social or medical reasons for not commencing haemodialysis.

5. Conclusions

Abdominal pain, vomiting, abdominal distension and weight loss are the most common symptoms at the time of diagnosis and the majority of patients in this series were diagnosed after stopping PD. Total time on PD was the main risk factor associated with EPS. Follow up of the PD patient cohort from 2000-2007 with a minimum patient follow up of 1.5 years has shown that symptomatic EPS developed in more than 1 in 10 of patients who received PD for at least 4 years.

The incidence rates reported in this study are higher than previously reported and have implications for patient education during renal replacement planning. This data may be used to inform patients of the minimum risk of developing EPS after starting PD.

6. Acknowledgements

6.1 Assistance from colleagues

The authors wish to express their thanks to the nurses, doctors and administrative staff of all the individual renal units for their assistance in identifying the cases of EPS and providing their clinical records. The authors also wish to thank the Scottish Renal Registry staff.

6.2 Disclosure of conflicts of interest

Dr. Robert Mactier wishes to declare the following potential conflicts of interest:
Study investigator for multicentre research studies conducted by Roche, Amgen and Baxter,
Member of the clinical advisory board for Baxter in 2005 and 2010
Sponsorship to attend scientific meetings from Leo, Roche and Baxter
To his knowledge, he has had no other direct support from the renal technology industry.
Dr Michaela Brown does not have any conflicts of interest to declare.

7. References

Balasubramaniam G, Brown EA, Davenport A, et al., (2009). The Pan-Thames EPS study: treatment and outcomes of encapsulating peritoneal sclerosis. *Nephrol Dial Transplant*; 24(10):3209-15. Epub 2009 Feb 11.

Brown E, Van Biesen W, Finkelstein F, et al., (2009). Length of time on peritoneal dialysis and encapsulating peritoneal sclerosis: position paper for ISPD. *Peritoneal Dialysis Int*; 29:595-600

Brown MC, Simpson K, Kerssens JJ, Mactier RA. (2009). Encapsulating peritoneal sclerosis in the new millennium: a national cohort study. *Clin J Am Soc Nephrol*; 4(7):1222-9

de Freitas DG, Augustine T, Brown EA, et al., (UK EPS Group). (2007). Encapsulating peritoneal sclerosis following renal transplantation - the UK experience. *Am J Transplant*; 7 (Suppl 2): 163

Fieren MWJA, Betjes MGH, Korte MR, et al., (2007). Posttransplant encapsulating peritoneal sclerosis: a worrying new trend? *Perit Dial Int*; 27(6):619-24

Ghandi VC, Ing TS, Daugirdas JT, et al., (1980). Failure of peritoneal dialysis due to peritoneal sclerosis. *Arch Int Med*; 140:1201-1203

Hendriks PM, Ho-Dac-Pannekeet MM, van Gulik TM, et al., (1997). Peritoneal sclerosis in chronic peritoneal dialysis patients: analysis of clinical presentation, risk factors, and peritoneal transport characteristics. *Perit Dial Int*; 17(2):136-43

Kawaguchi Y, Kawanishi H, Mujais S, et al., (2000). Encapsulating Peritoneal Sclerosis: Definition, Etiology, Diagnosis and Treatment. *Perit Dial Int;* 20(S4):S43-55

Kawanishi H, Long-Term Peritoneal Dialysis Study Group. (2001). Encapsulating peritoneal sclerosis in Japan: prospective multicentre controlled study. *Perit Dial Int;* 21 (S3):S67-71

Kawanishi H, Kawaguchi Y, Fukui H, et al.,(2004). Encapsulating Peritoneal Sclerosis in Japan: A Prospective, Controlled, Multicentre Study. *Am J Kidney Dis;* 44(4):729-737

Kawaguchi Y, Saito A, Kawanishi H, et al., (2005). Recommendations on the management of encapsulating peritoneal sclerosis in Japan 2005: Diagnosis, predictive markers, treatment, and preventative measures. *Perit Dial Int;* 25 (Suppl 4): S83-S95

Korte MR, Yo M, Betjes MG, et al., (2007) Increasing incidence of severe encapsulating peritoneal sclerosis after kidney transplantation. *Nephrol Dial Transplant;* 22(8):2412-2414

Nomoto Y, Kawaguchi Y, Kubo H, et al., (1996). Sclerosing encapsulating peritonitis in patients undergoing continuous ambulatory peritoneal dialysis: a report of the Japanese Sclerosing Encapsulating Peritonitis Study Group. *Am J Kidney Dis;* 20(3):420-7

Oules R, Challah S, Brunner FP. (1988). Case-Control study to determine the cause of sclerosing peritoneal disease. *Nephrol Dial Transplant;* 3:66-9

Perks FJ, Murchison JT, Gibson P, et al., (2004). Imaging findings in sclerosing encapsulating peritonitis. *J R Coll Physicians Edinb;* 34:116-119

Rigby RJ, Hawley CM. (1998). Sclerosing peritonitis: the experience in Australia. *Nephrol Dial Transplant;* 13:154-159

Sampimon DE, Coester AM, Struijk DG, Krediet RT. (2011). The time course of peritoneal transport parameters in peritoneal dialysis patients who develop encapsulating peritoneal dialysis. *Nephrol Dial Transplant;* 26(1):291-8. Epub 2010 Jun 21.

Scottish Renal Registry Report 2009. http://www.srr.scot.nhs.uk/Publications/scottish-renal-registry-report-2009-web-version.pdf

Slingeneyer A, (1987). Preliminary report on a cooperative international study on sclerosing encapsulating peritonitis. *Contrib Nephrol;* 57:239-47

Summers AM, Clancy MJ, Syed F, et al., (2005). Single-centre experience of encapsulating peritoneal sclerosis in patients on peritoneal dialysis for end stage renal failure. *Kidney Int;* 68:2381-2388

Tarzi RM, Lim A, Moser S, et al., (2008). Assessing the validity of an abdominal CT scoring system in the diagnosis of encapsulating peritoneal sclerosis. *Clin J Am Soc Nephrol;* 3: 1702-1710

Woodrow G, Augustine T, Brown EA, et al,, UK Encapsulating Peritoneal Sclerosis guidelines. http://www.renal.org/Libraries/Other_Guidlines/Encapsulating_Peritoneal_Sclerosis_guidelines_UK_EPS_Group_Final_July_2009.sflb.ashx

12

Biocompatible Solutions for Peritoneal Dialysis

Alberto Ortiz[1], Beatriz Santamaria[2] and Jesús Montenegro[3]
[1]IIS-Fundacion Jimenez Diaz and Universidad Autonoma de Madrid, Madrid
[2]Instituto de Investigaciones Biomédicas Alberto Sols, Consejo Superior de Investigaciones Científicas - Universidad Autónoma de Madrid (CSIC-UAM), Madrid
[3]Servicio de Nefrologia, Bilbao
Spain

1. Introduction

In 1978, a simplified technique for peritoneal dialysis (PD) using plastic bags and glucose as osmotic agent allowed PD to become accepted as a home-based renal replacement therapy. However, PD was marred by complications including peritonitis and loss of function of the peritoneal membrane. Both complications may be favored by the bioincompatibility of PD solutions. The composition of PD solutions has evolved over the years, building on a better understanding of the biocompatibility and of technical advances that enable the commercial viability of certain solutions. The main osmotic agent used to obtain ultrafiltration is glucose. Conventional glucose-containing PD solutions are lactate-buffered, acidic pH solutions presented in single chambered bags. The use of new manufacturing techniques, buffer presentation, and new osmotic alternatives to glucose have resulted in more biocompatible glucose containing PD solutions that have a lower concentration of glucose degradation products (GDP) and a neutral, more physiological pH, as well as in glucose-free solutions.

2. Composition of PD solutions

PD solutions are sterile and contain water, electrolytes, a buffer and an osmotic agent (Table 1). Electrolyte concentrations (Na^+, Cl^-, Ca^{++}, Mg^{++}) display little variation between different PD solutions.

- Water
- Electrolytes: Na^+, Cl^-, Ca^{++}, Mg^{++}
- Buffer: lactate, lactate / bicarbonate or bicarbonate
- Osmotic agent glucose, icodextrin or amino acids
- Glucose degradation products (GDPs) are not added on purpose, but are generated during heat sterilization, especially in conventional glucose-containing solutions.

Table 1. Composition of PD Solutions

PD solutions contain an osmotic agent that allows a negative balance of fluids (ultrafiltration). Glucose is the most widely used osmotic agent. The only alternative osmotic agents available are 7.5% icodextrin and a 1.1% amino acid mixture (Frampton, J. E. et al.

2003) (Tjiong, H. L. et al. 2005). Neither avoids the use of glucose as only one daily exchange of each glucose-free PD solution can be used. There are solutions with three different concentrations of glucose in order to individualize ultrafiltration. The highest concentrations of glucose obtains more ultrafiltration, but also enhances the adverse effects of glucose and in conventional solutions, of the GDPs. The glucose concentration of each of the three types of solutions varies with the manufacturer and ranges between 1360 and 4250 mg / dl, resulting in an osmolarity of 345 to 511 mOsm / L. There is some confusion in the literature regarding the concentration of glucose in the various solutions because in America it is expressed as the concentration of dextrose (glucose monohydrate with a molecular weight of 198 Da), and in Europe as the concentration of glucose (anhydrous glucose molecular weight 180 Da). Thus a dextrose concentration of 1.5%, 2.5% and 4.25% is the same as a glucose concentration of 1.36%, 2.27% and 3.86% respectively, but a concentration of glucose 1.5% corresponds to 1.65% dextrose.
Lactate is the most common buffer in PD solutions. Recently solutions buffered with lactate / bicarbonate or bicarbonate alone have been marketed, presented in bicameral bags to keep separate the bicarbonate from calcium and magnesium until just before the infusion, thereby avoiding precipitation (Fig. 1) (Montenegro, J. et al. 2006; Feriani, M. et al. 1998; Montenegro, J. et al. 2007; Tranaeus, A.2000; Schmitt, C. P. et al. 2002; Pecoits-Filho, R. et al. 2003; Otte, K. et al. 2003). Bi- or tricameral bags also allow the separation of glucose and buffer until just before the infusion. Thus, glucose is contained in a low pH chamber and the buffer in a high pH chamber. The use of acetate as a buffer was abandoned years ago due to undesirable effects including vasodilation, decreased myocardial contractility, and sclerosing peritonitis.

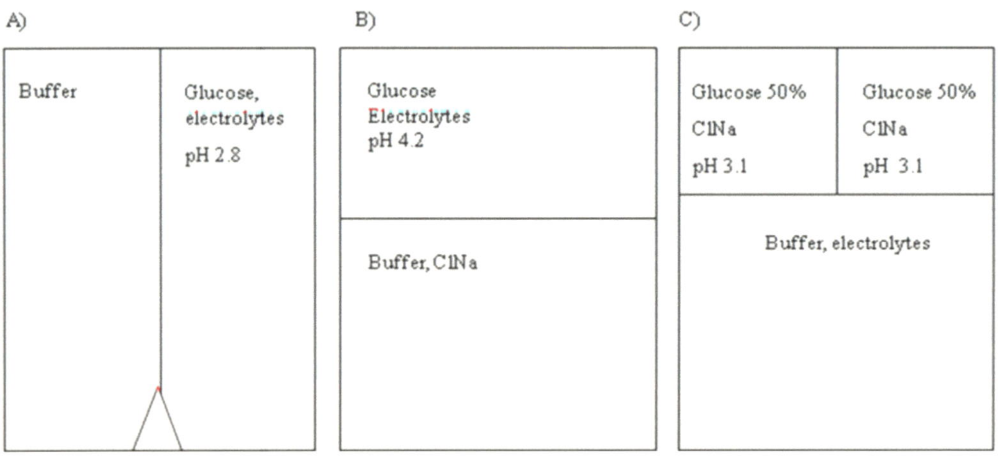

Fig. 1. **Bicameral and tricameral PD bags. A and B**) Bicameral bags. **C)** Tricameral bags. Bi- and tricameral bags are used to manufacture biocompatible PD solutions. Separating glucose form the buffer allows heat sterilization of the bags while minimizing the generation of GDPs.

3. Biocompatibility

Biocompatibility is the ability of a technique or system to fulfill its function without causing a clinically significant adverse response of the host. In PD the concept was initially applied

to the influence of PD solutions on the biological responses of peritoneal tissues and cells, and the morphology and function of the peritoneum (Holmes, C. J. et al. 2003). In addition PD solutions may also have systemic adverse effects (Pecoits-Filho, R. et al. 2003). Conventional solutions are bioincompatible mainly due to the high concentration of glucose and GDPs. The low pH, high osmolarity and the presence of high concentrations of lactate also contribute to bioincompatibility (Table 2). These factors may cause adverse effects on celular systems, including dysfunction and death of mesothelial cells and leukocytes. In this regard, GDPs are the most lethal factor (Ortiz, A. et al. 2006).
The consequences of bioincompatibility include worsening of peritoneal defense against infection and injury, loss of peritoneal mesothelial cells, epithelial-mesenchymal transformation (EMT) of mesothelial cells, fibrosis, diabetiform changes of vessels and possibly peritoneal sclerosis (Yanez-Mo, M. et al. 2003; Catalan, M. P. et al. 2001; Williams, J. D. et al. 2002). Among systemic consequences we find increased circulating advanced glycation products (AGEs), glucose metabolic effects, and poorer preservation of residual renal function (Montenegro, J. et al. 2007; Williams, J. D. et al. 2004; Kim, S. G. et al. 2008; Zeier, M. et al. 2003).

High concentration of glucose
Glucose degradation products (GDPs)
High osmolarity
Acid pH
Lactate

Table 2. Elements contributing to the poor biocompatibility of PD solutions

New solutions have been designed with a neutral pH, without lactate, lack of glucose and/or low concentrations of GDPs (Table 3)(McIntyre, C. W.2007; Montenegro, J. et al. 1993).

	Conventional	New Solutions Alternative osmotic agents	New Solutions Biocompatible dextrose
Container	Unicameral	unicameral	bi or tri-cameral
Osmotic agent	Glucose	Icodextrin, amino acids	glucose
GDPs content	High	low or no	low
pH	5.5	5.8 to 6.5	6.3 to 7.4
Buffer	lactate	lactate	lactate, bicarbonate, lactate/bicarbonate

Table 3. PD Solutions

Biocompatibility of new solutions has been amply demonstrated in studies in cultured cells and animal models and they are expected to improve peritoneal defense and survival of the peritoneal membrane function and residual renal function. Clinical experience so far in clinical trials, though still incomplete, tends to support these expectations (Table 4).
PD solutions plastic bags may also contribute to bioincompatibility, although the precise contribution has not been established. The conventional material the bags are made of is PVC (polyvinyl chloride). PVC is difficult to recycle and contains plasticizers such as phthalic acid. Phthalic acid released from the bags can eventually be absorbed from the peritoneum (Mettang, T. et al. 2000), although it is unclear whether this represents a health risk. New

materials, such as Biofine ®, a polyolefin which needs no plasticizers, Steriflex ® or Clearflex ® are thought to be more biocompatible. Conventional bags are single chambered and filled with the dialysis solution composition that is infused into the peritoneum (NO CITATION DEFINITION). The new glucose solutions are packaged in bi or tricameral bags and the contents of the chambers is mixed just before infusion into the peritoneum (Fig 1). This allows to sterilize glucose at low pH, thus decreasing the production of GDPs, and to separate the calcium and magnesium from bicarbonate to avoid precipitation.

Surrogate markers	
	Increased CA125 biomarker in the peritoneal effluent (Williams, J. D. et al. 2004; Fusshoeller, A. et al. 2004; Jones, S. et al. 2001; Haas, S. et al. 2003; Rippe, B. et al. 2001)
	Lower circulating AGEs (Fusshoeller, A. et al. 2004; Williams, J. D. et al. 2004)
	Better correction of acidosis (Montenegro, J. et al. 2006; Tranaeus, A.2000; Otte, K. et al. 2003; Carrasco, A. M. et al. 2001; Haas, S. et al. 2003)
	Better preserved residual renal function (Montenegro, J. et al. 2007; Williams, J. D. et al. 2004; Kim, S. G. et al. 2008)
	No change (Fan, S. L. et al. 2008)
Clinical Results	
	Mortality decreased (Lee, H. Y. et al. 2005; Lee, H. Y. et al. 2006)
	Decreases peritonitis rate (Montenegro, J. et al. 2007; Ahmad, S. et al. 2006)
	No change (Lee, H. Y. et al. 2006; Lee, H. Y. et al. 2005; Fan, S. L. et al. 2008; Rippe, B. et al. 2001)

[1] No clinical trials have been published whose primary objective is the study of these items

Table 4. Beneficial effects of new glucose solutions in clinical practice

3.1 GDPs

GDPs are the main contributors to the bioincompatibility of PD solutions. Heat sterilization of the solutions facilitates the formation of GDPs, especially if the pH of the glucose chamber is high. GDPs are small molecules generated from glucose (Table 5 and Fig. 2). Many GDPs are toxic and more reactive than glucose with proteins to form AGEs such as pentosidine, N (epsilon) - (carboxymethyl) lysine (CML) and others. AGEs cause protein dysfunction and activate a specific receptor (RAGE, receptor for AGE) which transmits intracellular signals that modify cell behavior. Several GDPs are toxic, but only 3,4-dideoxyglucoson-3-ene (3,4-DGE) has been shown to be lethal for leukocytes and mesothelial cells at the concentrations usually found in commercial PD bags (Justo, P. et al. 2005; Santamaria, B. et al. 2008; Catalan, M. P. et al. 2005). 3-deoxyglucosone (3-DG), the precursor of the 3,4-DGE, is also cytotoxic, although high concentrations (around 500 μM) are needed to observe cytotoxicity. These high concentrations have not been found by most authors in the PD solutions tested (Table 5).

The concentration of GDPs depends mainly on the pH of sterilization of glucose, on glucose concentration (higher GDP generation in solutions containing 4.25% glucose than in 1.5% glucose solutions) and on storage temperature (Erixon, M. et al. 2006; Erixon, M. et al. 2005; Erixon, M. et al. 2004). The lower the pH of sterilization of glucose, the lower the generation of GDPs. The optimal pH of sterilization to decrease the production of GDPs is

GDP	Conventional glucose[1]	Biocompatible glucose[1,2]	Icodextrin	Aminoacids
3-deoxiglucosone	172-425	10	4-11	<0.2
3,4-DGE[3]	10-125	0.2-0.5	3	<0.2
5-HMF	6-15	10 to 19	2	-
Methylglyoxal	2-12	<1	1.5	<0.2
Glyoxal	<3-14	<1	2.5	<0.2
Acetaldehyde	120-420	<2	37	-
Formaldehyde	7-13	<3	9	-

[1] The range represents the values for glucose solutions with concentrations around 1.5 to 4% and measurements made by different authors.
[2] Excludes Physioneal that has higher values.
[3] The wide range observed depends on the concentration of glucose as the time since the sterilization and storage conditions
Ref: (Erixon, M. et al. 2006)

Table 5. GDP content in µmol / L of different solutions PD

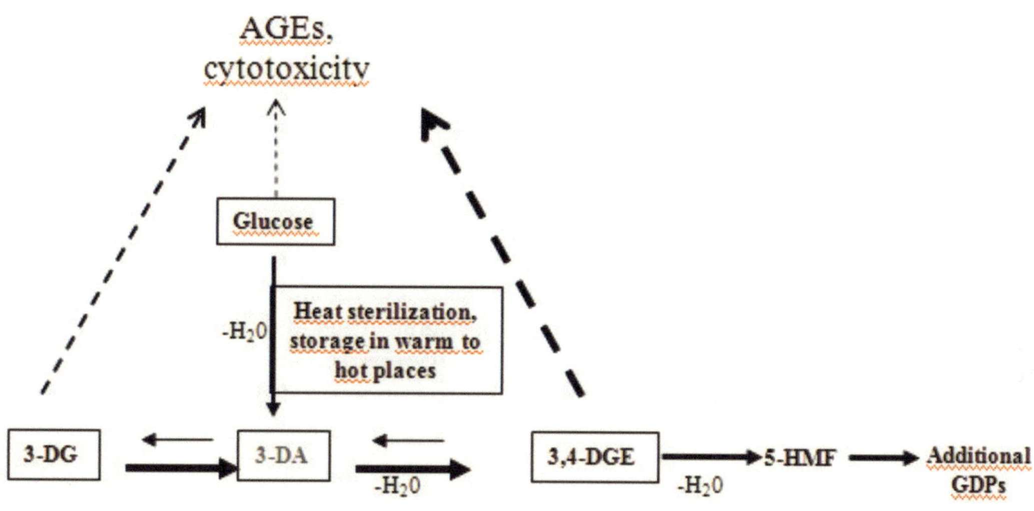

Fig. 2. **GDP generation from glucose in PD fluids during heat sterilization and storage.** Successive dehydration steps of the glucose molecule lead to initial GDPs and these are subsequently degraded into smaller molecules. There is a temperature-dependent balance between 3-DG, 3-DA and 3,4-DGE. Increasing temperature shifts the equilibrium to the right, towards the most toxic compound, 3,4-DGE. High concentrations of glucose are cytotoxic and lead to AGE formation, but 3-DG and, above all, 3,4-DGE lead to higher cytotoxicity and AGE generation. The thick dashed lines represent the ability to induce biological effects. 3-DG: 3-deoxyglucosone, 3-DA: 3-deoxyaldos-2-ene, 3,4-DGE: 3,4-dideoxyglucosone-3-ene, AGE: advanced glycation products. HMF: hydroxymethylfurfural. Adapted from reference (Ortiz, A. et al. 2006). Additional GDPs include furaldehyde, formaldehyde, acetaldehyde, methylglyoxal, glyoxal.

2.0 to 3.1 (Erixon, M. et al. 2006). It is not possible to achieve a pH so low in unicameral bags, since solutions at such low pH cannot be safely infused into the peritoneum. Therefore, conventional glucose-containing unicameral bags have a pH of approximately 5.5 and a high concentration of GDPs. The problem was solved using bi-or tricameral bags, which allow sterilization of the glucose solution in a low pH chamber, separated from the buffer which is contained in a compartment at high pH (Fig. 1). This system allows both to lower the production of GDPs and, by mixing the contents of both chambers before the infusion, to infuse a solution at more physiological pH (6.3 to 7.4).

The concentration of the most toxic GDP identified so far, 3,4-DGE, varies with storage temperature conditions: it is higher immediately post-heat sterilization, reaches a nadir at 2 months of storage at room temperature (25 ° C), but may rise again if the bag is exposed for hours at higher temperatures (Erixon, M. et al. 2005). These higher temperatures may be reached during the summer at patient's homes or during transportation. This has rekindled interest in transport and storage temperature of the solutions, especially in the summer months. This problem with sterilization and storage temperatures is not observed with the newer bicameral or tricameral having a pH <3.0 in the glucose chamber.

4. Conventional PD solutions

Conventional solutions are those contained in unicameral bags, with glucose as an osmotic agent and lactate as buffer. These solutions have a low pH and high GDP content and present the biocompatibility problems mentioned in previous sections, in addition to the continuous glucose absorption from the peritoneum and the high concentration of intraperitoneal glucose.

4.1 Glucose as osmotic agent

Glucose is the only osmotic agent which has proved safe and effective for chronic use in multiple exchanges within a 24 hour period. It is cheap and provides calories. However, it is not the ideal osmotic agent and poses several problems. Thus, the high concentrations of glucose required to induce ultrafiltration may facilitate or exacerbate:

- Hyperglycemia with hyperinsulinemia, as well as undetected peaks of hyperglycemia in diabetics
- Hyperlipidemia
- Obesity
- Conventional solutions damage the long-term peritoneal membrane, although in most studies it is not possible to tell apart the effect of glucose from the effect of GDPs (Davies, S. J. et al. 2001).

In addition, glucose-containing PD solutions are not effective in promoting ultrafiltration in patients with high peritoneal transport. This is so because the high transporters absorb glucose from the peritoneum at a faster rate, thus dissipating the osmotic gradient that favours ultrafiltration earlier. Glucose uptake varies with the type of peritoneal transport of small solutes, which is a patient-specific feature (high transporters absorb more), with the dwell time (higher amounts of glucose are absorbed in more prolonged exchanges) and the concentration of glucose in the bag. It has been estimated that the average patient on CAPD absorbs from the peritoneum between 100-200 g glucose/24 h (about 8 kcal / kg / d) (Dombros, N. et al. 2005).

4.2 pH

Conventional dextrose solutions have a pH of 5.5 (range 5-6). The low pH prevents caramelization of glucose during heat sterilization and reduces, but does not prevent the generation of GDPs. A lower pH may decrease GDP generation, but causes pain during infusion and possibly other adverse effects in the longer term. In fact, the pH of 5.5 causes pain in some patients. This pH is rapidly buffered by bicarbonate which diffuses from the circulation into the peritoneal cavity, reaching on average 7.0 in 30 minutes and above 7.30 in 90-120 minutes (Schmitt, C. P. et al. 2002). The new PD solutions with higher pH are painless during infusion and the pH is already physiological during infusion or is normalized faster.

5. New PD solutions

We distinguish two approaches to the design of new PD solutions (Table 3) (McIntyre, C. W.2007; Montenegro, J. et al. 1993). One is to use of bi- or tricameral bags to improve glucose solutions, so that GDP content decreases and final pH approaches physiological values, with or without a total or partial change of the buffer. The other is to replace glucose by other osmotic agents such as icodextrin or amino acids, keeping lactate as buffer.
The aim of this greater biocompatibility is to achieve better clinical results. The advantages of the newer, more biocompatible have been well documented in cell culture and animal studies. However, the big differences observed in basic research are more difficult to convincingly demonstrate in humans and some studies have failed to show such superiority.

5.1 Biocompatible glucose solutions presented in bi- or tricameral bags

Bi or tricameral bags allow to sterilize glucose at low pH and separate the bicarbonate (when present) from calcium and magnesium (Fig. 1). The differential characteristics of biocompatible glucose-containing solutions contained in bi or tricameral bags versus conventional, bioincompatible solutions are basically three: the low GDP concentration, a more physiological final pH, often around 7-7.4; and, in some cases, a pure bicarbonate or bicarbonate plus lactate buffer.
However, not all biocompatible glucose solutions presented in bi- or tricameral bags areequal and their impact on clinical parameters should be assessed individually. Thus, there are differences in glucose concentration, buffer (bicarbonate, bicarbonate/lactate or lactate), pH of the glucose chamber and, thus, in GDP content, and in the final pH of infusion of the solutions, once the contents of all the chambers has been mixed pre-infusion is more physiological (6.3-7.4).
Advantages and indications. The main advantage of these solutions is greater biocompatibility resulting from the low concentration of GDPs, physiological pH and, in some cases, absence of lactate. More biocompatibility suggests that these solutions should be the choice if there are resources to pay for them. Their use has resulted in improvement in surrogate parameters in clinical trials and observational studies including a higher peritoneal effluent concentration of CA125 (considered by many as a marker of mesothelial mass), lower rate of apoptosis in the effluent, lower concentration of circulating AGEs, better control of metabolic acidosis, better preservation of residual renal function, lower incidence of peritonitis, and in Registry studies, lower mortality (Table 4) (Montenegro, J. et al. 2007; Montenegro, J. et al. 2006; Williams, J. D. et al. 2004; Kim, S. G. et al. 2008; Lee, H. Y.

et al. 2005; Navarro, J. F. et al. 1999; Rippe, B. et al. 2001; Fan, S. L. et al. 2008; Ahmad, S. et al. 2006; Carrasco, A. M. et al. 2001; Fusshoeller, A. et al. 2004; Jones, S. et al. 2001; Haas, S. et al. 2003). As indicated above, the different characteristics of the various commercially available biocompatible solutions do not allow concluding that the observed effects are class effects. However, there are no direct clinical comparisons between the different solutions (from different providers) on the market and currently available information is incomplete, since not all possible effects have been studied with all the solutions. The effect on residual renal function has been the focus of three long-term randomized studies (12-18 months) with three solutions of different characteristics (Kim, S. G. et al. 2008; Fan, S. L. et al. 2008). Solutions with lower content GDPs better preserved residual renal function (Kim, S. G. et al. 2008).

Several experimental reports support the bioincompatibility of conventional PD solutions (heat-sterilized glucose-containing solutions). Prolonged exposure to conventional PD solutions exert deleterious effects on the peritoneum, including loss of mesothelial cell monolayer, submesothelial fibrosis, angiogenesis, hyalinizing vasculopathy and impaired viability and function of human peritoneal mesothelial cells (HPMC) and leukocytes (Jorres A KI 2008 (Yanez-Mo, M. et al. 2003; Vargha, R. et al. 2006; Santamaria, B. et al. 2008; Williams, J. D. et al. 2002). The adverse effects may lead, in the long-term to ultrafiltration failure and PD technique withdrawal. GDPs have been identified as the major cytotoxic agents in conventional PD solutions. GDPs impair viability, cell function, cytokine release on HPMC, induce apoptosis and promote EMT in mesothelial cells and impair leukocyte function and viability (Amore, A. et al. 2003; Witowski, J. et al. 2000; Witowski, J. et al. 2001; Witowski, J. et al. 2001; Morgan, L. W. et al. 2003) (Oh, E. J. et al. 2010). In addition, the number of mesothelial cell dying by apoptosis is increased in the effluent of patients using high GDP PD solutions vs. patients using low GDP PD solutions (Santamaria, B. et al. 2008). 3,4 deoxyglucosone-3 ene (3,4 DGE) is the main cytotoxic product in conventional PD solutions. 3,4 DGE accelerates leukocyte and HPMC apoptosis, to the same extent as conventional PD solution, retards remesothelization and may compromise peritoneal defense (Santamaria, B. et al. 2008; Catalan, M. P. et al. 2005; Morgan, L. W. et al. 2003; Linden, T. et al. 2002; Yamamoto, T. et al. 2009). The poor biocompatibility of PD solutions may also compromise peritoneal defenses and promote peritonitis or a poor resolution of peritonitis episodes. At the molecular at cellular level peritonitis is characterized by cytokine release and leukocyte recruitment to the peritoneal cavity (Zemel, D. et al. 1996; Li, F. K. et al. 1998). However neutrophils die spontaneously by apoptosis at sites of inflammation and accelerated leukocyte apoptosis may impair the peritoneal defense. Indeed bioincompatible PD solutions accelerate neutrophil apoptosis and this has been shown retard recovery from *S aureus* peritonitis in mice exposed to PD solutions (Catalan, M. P. et al. 2003). Neutrophil apoptosis is a physiologic process that limits inflammation. However, premature neutrophil apoptosis may compromise the antibacterial potential of these leukocytes. Conventional PD solutions accelerated leukocyte apoptosis in vivo and in vitro (Catalan, M. P. et al. 2003; Catalan, M. P. et al. 2005). In vitro studies, also show that 3,4 DGE accelerated neutrophils and mononuclear cell apoptosis and increased HPMC death in the same way as conventional PD solutions, but biocompatible PD solutions (low content GDPs, double chambered PD solutions) maintains low apoptosis levels as controls (Santamaria, B. et al. 2008)`79]. Mesothelial cells also die by apoptosis during peritonitis due to the combination of high levels of lethal cytokines and bioincompatible PD solutions as demonstrated in an experimental mice model of *S. aureus* peritonitis and following the intraperitoneal administration of inflammatory cytokines (Santamaria, B. et al. 2009)

Regarding the clinical evidence on the biocompatibility of glucose-based PD solutions (table 1), there is information from non-randomized observations and from clinical trials.

A retrospective observational study compared outcomes for 1100 incident CAPD patients treated with a single chamber peritoneal dialysis fluid (PDF) to the outcomes for patients treated with a low GDP double chamber PDF. Patients treated with Balance had significantly superior survival compared to those treated with the standard PDF (74% vs 62% at 28 months, p = 0.0032). This study was not stratified by age, the high number of patients with standard PDF and the absence of parameters like RRF, dialysis adequacy, transport status that are more related with survival (Lee, H. Y. et al. 2005).

A prospective non-randomized study of incident patients compared a conventional lactate solution (lactate group) to a pure bicarbonate solution (bicarbonate group) PD solution in 100 patients followed for three years in both groups (Montenegro, J. et al. 2007). The peritonitis rate was lower in patients treated with the pure bicarbonate solution than patients treated with the standard bioincompatible solution: 1 episode for each 36 patient-months versus 1 episode every 21 patient-months. At the end of the study, the RRF was significantly better preserved in patients of the bicarbonate group. Patients treated with pure bicarbonate ate more proteins according to normalized protein catabolic rate calculations and had lower markers of inflammation such as C reactive protein. Even mortality was lower in the bicarbonate group, even though this group had a higher Charlson index.

Several randomized controlled trials have focused mainly on preservation of RRF.

A crossover study compared the impact of a 25 mmol/L bicarbonate/15 mmol/L lactate buffered, solution (Physioneal) with a standard single chamber solution (Dianeal) (Fang, W. et al. 2008) on peritoneal transport and ultrafiltration. The mass transfer area coefficients (urea and creatinine) for both solutions did not differ. However net ultrafiltration was lower for Bic/Lac solution (274 ± 223 mL vs 366 ± 217 mL, p = 0.026). Physioneal avoided intraperitoneal acidity, which is present for up to 120 minutes with conventional acidic lactate solution.

The Euro-Balance trial with a crossover design and parallel arms, compared a single chamber conventional glucose-containing fluid with a lactate-buffered, low GDP double chamber glucose-containing fluid (balance) (Williams, J. D. et al. 2004). Clinical end points were RRF, adequacy of dialysis, ultrafiltration and peritoneal membrane function. Balance resulted in significantly higher effluent levels of CA125 and procollagen peptide in both arms of the study. Conversely, levels of Hialuronic acid were lower in patients exposed to balance, while there was no change in the levels of either VEGF or TNFa. Urine volume was higher in patients exposed to balance. In contrast, peritoneal ultrafiltration was higher in patients on conventional fluids. Increased extracellular volume and lower ultrafiltration in the patients with biocompatible solutions may be conditioning the results. The follow-up was short and changes in the RRF were a secondary objective.

A trial of incident patients starting PD examined changes in RRF (assessed by 24-h urine collection) over a1-year follow-up (Fan, S. L. et al. 2008). No differences were found between groups, for RRF, peritonitis rate, PD technique survival, changes in peritoneal membrane function assessed by peritoneal equilibrium test or C-reactive protein. Issues criticized in this study include the lack of statistical power to establish non inferiority as the difference of less than 1 ml / min in the RRF, use of solutions with different GDP content, inclusion of previous hemodialysis patients with little RRF and assessment of RRF at only two time points.

In 2009 three trials were published showing the benefit of biocompatible solutions in regard to RRF, ultrafiltration and tolerability.

A study of 91 incident CAPD patients for 12 months compared neutral-pH and low GDP (Balance) and conventional solutions (Kim, S. et al. 2009). Biocompatible solution preserved RRF compared with conventional solutions ($p=0.048$). Analysis by subgroups (GFR>2 ml/min) demonstrated the preservation of RRF in per protocol analysis.
In a crossover study with 26 prevalent patients treated for 3 months with lactate-based and 3 months with bicarbonate/lactate-based solution (Pajek, J. et al. 2009), switch from conventional solutions to biocompatible solution decreased ultrafiltration ($p=0.012$) and switch from biocompatible to conventional solution increased ultrafiltration solutions ($p=0.001$).
A cross over multicenter trial (Weiss, L. et al. 2009) enrolled 53 patients and compared conventional vs Bicarbonate PD fluid. Patients with biocompatible solutions had a higher concentration of CA125 ($p<0.001$) and less concentration of hyaluronic acid ($p=0.013$), TNF-α ($p<0.001$) and TGF-β1 ($p=0.016$). These biocompatibility markers suggest improvement in peritoneal membrane integrity In addition, a positive effect on RRF was observed ($p=0.011$).
Drawbacks. Biocompatible, glucose-containing PD solutions maintain the adverse effects of glucose itself.
In addition, a surprising effect of ultrafiltration has been observed that was not anticipated by experimental studies in animals. Biocompatible, glucose-containing PD solutions buffered with lactate or bicarbonate decrease ultrafiltration compared to conventional solutions in some patients: In some cases this is related to increased peritoneal transport of small molecules (Williams, J. D. et al. 2004). This effect is acute (observable with a single exchange) and reversible by discontinuing the solution. Furthermore, the decreased ultrafiltration observed with biocompatible glucose-containing PD solutions is not indicative of peritoneal injury and in this, it differs from the progressive increase in solute permeability observed over the years in PD as a result of peritoneal injury induced by conventional solutions. The results obtained when assessing the impact of lactate/bicarbonate-buffered PD solutions have not been consistent. However, a recent study showed a decrease in ultrafiltration compared to conventional solutions when compared in the same patient in a short period of time (Fang, W. et al. 2008). The interest in learning about differences in the behavior of the various solutions lies in a better understanding of the cause of these differences, which could be related to differences in pH, buffer or GDP content. A recently reported very low GDPs solution, with physiological pH and buffered with bicarbonate / lactate increased ultrafitración against a similar solution containing GDPs, pH 6.3 and lactate (Simonsen, O. et al. 2006).
An additional caveat should be made. In some patients bicarbonate-buffered solutions can overcorrect the metabolic acidosis of uremia, causing metabolic alkalosis (Vande Walle, J. G. et al. 2004; Garcia-Lopez, E. et al. 2005; Otte, K. et al. 2003).

5.2 Alternative osmotic agents

Icodextrin and amino acids are the only alternative to glucose agents that are commercially available.

5.2.1 Icodextrin

Polyglucose or icodextrin is a carbohydrate of high molecular weight obtained by hydrolysis of corn starch (Figure 3) (Frampton, J. E. et al. 2003). Icodextrin consists of a mixture of glucose polymers of different sizes (from 2 to 300 molecules of glucose) with a total average molecular weight of 13 to 19 KDa and average molecular weight per molecule of 5 to 6.5 KDa (range 0.36-54). Icodextrin is available commercially at a concentration of 7.5%.

However, icodextrin cannot be strictly considered a biocompatible solution, due to the intrinsic problems of the glucose polymer, such as generation high levels of circulating maltose in the systemic circulation. In this regard, no more than one exchange a day can be prescribed according to heath authorities.

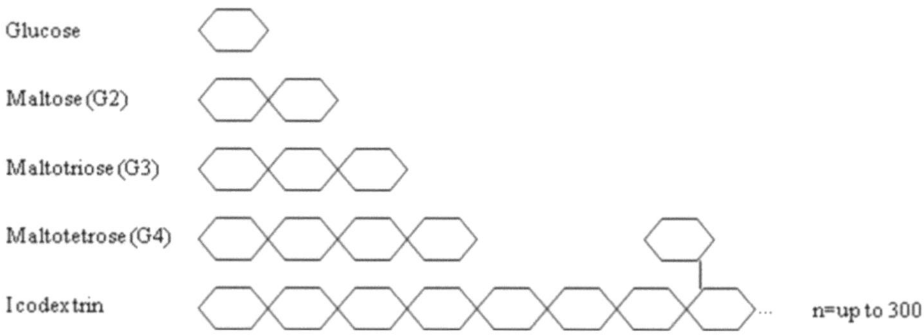

Fig. 3. Schematic representation of molecules of glucose, maltose, icodextrin polymers and intermediates.

Advantages and indications. Icodextrin-containing solutions are isosmolar and induce ultrafiltration by oncotic pressure. Icodextrin is absorbed by lymphatic vessels, more slowly than glucose. As a consequence, the oncotic pressure is durable and ultrafiltration is linear and more sustained than that induced by glucose. During an exchange of 10-16 hours 40% of icodextrin in an exchange is absorbed (Garcia-Lopez, E. et al. 2005; Moberly, J. B. et al. 2002). These features suggest the following icodextrin indications:

a. Long daytime exchange in APD (as the last cycler infusion) or the night dwell during CAPD in order to increase ultrafiltration and sodium removal (Davies, S. J. et al. 2005; Rodriguez-Carmona, A. et al. 2002; Davies, S. J. et al. 2008). In randomized controlled trials icodextrin improved the hydration status of patients ((Davies, S. J. et al. 2008; Wolfson, M. et al. 2002; Plum, J. et al. 2002). Icodextrin allows greater ultrafiltration in long exchanges than solutions with 1.5% or 2.3% glucose. Furthermore, icodextrin allows greater ultrafiltration in long exchanges than 4.25% glucose in high transporters. Since icodextrin is not a small molecule, ultrafiltration may be obtained with icodextrin in patients with failure of ultrafiltration due to high transport of small solutes. The ability to obtain ultrafiltration in these patients can prolong the life of the PD technique, delaying the transition to hemodialysis. More ultrafiltration allows a greater clearance of molecules when comparing a prolonged exchange (approx. 12 hours) of icodextrin with a glucose exchange of the same duration, especially if the concentration of glucose is 1.5% (Wolfson, M. et al. 2002). However, solute clearance is less with a long exchange of icodextrin than with two shorter glucose exchanges (approx 6 hours per glucose exchange).
b. Limit exposure to high concentrations of glucose and GDPs and absorption of glucose. This can help to preserve the functionality of the peritoneal membrane (Davies, S. J. et al. 2005). Although there are few differences in the absorption of the total amount of carbohydrates, icodextrin prevents the absorption peaks of glucose. This may contribute to less weight gain, lipid abnormalities and improved glycemic control and HbA1c levels in poorly controlled diabetic patients (Wolfson, M. et al. 2002; Babazono, T. et al. 2007).
c. Maintenance of ultrafiltration during episodes of peritonitis since the ultrafiltration capacity of icodextrin solutions is independent of peritoneal permeability to small solutes.

Peculiarities. Amylase degrades icodextrin, but in humans there is little amylase in the peritoneal cavity (unlike in some rodents). Absorbed icodextrin is degraded by circulating amylase. The consequences of icodextrin degradation by circulating amylase may be summarized as follows:

a. Increased plasma concentration of maltose (maltose 20-300 times increased over physiological levels to 120 mg/dl or 3 mM, compared to physiological glucose concentrations from 3.3 to 5.5 mM), maltotriose and other glucose polymers (Garcia-Lopez, E. et al. 2005; Burkart, J.2004; Posthuma, N. et al. 1997). These metabolites are normally excreted in the urine or degraded to glucose by tissue maltase tissue. The richest tissue in maltase is the kidney. In renal failure these two mechanisms of elimination fail, facilitating maltose accumulation. This risk of maltose accumulation limits the use of icodextrin to a single exchange within a 24 hour period. So far, no toxic effects have been identified resulting from accumulation of maltose when icodextrin is used according to the prescription data sheet.
b. Maltose and other oligosaccharides that accumulate in the blood of patients treated with icodextrin interfere with some plasma glucose monitors and test strips readings, resulting in falsely elevated glucose readings (Wang, R. et al. 2004; Wens, R. et al. 1998). In patients treated with icodextrin only glucose monitors and test strips that use glucose-specific methods should be used. These include methods based on glucose oxidase (GO), hexokinase, glucose dehydrogenase nicotine adenine dinucleotide (GDH-NAD), or glucose dehydrogenase with flavin adenine dinucleotide (GDH-FAD). Methods not to be used include glucose dehydrogenase pirrolquinolinaquinone (GDH-PQQ) or glucose-dye-oxidoreductase, which detect both glucose and maltose. After stopping the use of icodextrin it takes around 14 days for the plasma levels of icodextrin and its metabolites to return to undetectable (Plum, J. et al. 2002).
c. Mild decline in serum sodium without hypo-osmolarity to values around 135-137 mmol / L. This is associated with an increased osmolal gap due to the presence of circulating metabolites of icodextrin (which justify an increase in osmolal gap of about 8 mOsm / kg) (Plum, J. et al. 2002; Posthuma, N. et al. 1997).
d. Decrease in measured plasma amylase levels, because the circulating metabolites of icodextrin interfere with the assay (Plum, J. et al. 2002). So if pancreatitis is suspected, lipase should be assayed.

Adverse effects. The most common side effect of icodextrin in clinical trials was skin hypersensitivity (2.5-5% of exposed individuals), which usually occurs in the first 3 weeks and require discontinuation of treatment, although in some patients the rash disappears despite continued use of icodextrin (Frampton, J. E. et al. 2003; Wolfson, M. et al. 2002).

In the late 90s and early 2000s there was an epidemic of sterile peritonitis in patients treated with icodextrin. The cause was contamination of some lots with peptidoglycan, a component of the wall of gram-positive bacteria (Goffin, E. et al. 2003). New control systems of production have largely eliminated the problem and no influence has been observed of icodextrin on peritonitis incidence rates, either culture positive or negative (Vychytil, A. et al. 2008).

5.2.2 Amino acids

PD solutions containing amino acid solutions can limit the use of glucose. In addition, amino acids provide nutritional components (Tjiong, H. L. et al. 2005). The only marketed solution contains 1.1% amino acids, equivalent to an amino acid concentration of 87 mM / L (Table 6). The average molecular weight of the amino acids is 126. Approximately 65% of them (15 g/exchange) are absorbed into the systemic circulation during a 4-6h PD exchange. This is enough to replace the approximately 5-8 g/day of protein and 3 g/day of amino acids that are lost in non-aminoacid PD exchanges (Rippe, B. et al. 2007). The osmotic power of the amino acid solutions is comparable to a solution of 1.5% glucose. The osmolarity is slightly higher than the 1.5% glucose solution and a slightly higher ultrafiltration has been reported, approximately 100 ml at 4 h, despite a greater absorption of the osmotic agent. The increased uptake is probably due to the lower average molecular weight of the amino acids and to amino acid-induced vasodilation (Rippe, B. et al. 2007; Olszowska, A. et al. 2007).

Aminoacid	Concentration (mM/L)
L-Valine	11.88
L-Alanine	10.67
L-Leucine	7.79
Glycine	6.80
L-Lysine, HCl	6.51
L-Isoleucine	6.49
L-Arginine	6.15
L-Methionine	5.70
L-Threonine	5.46
L-Proline	5.13
L-Serine	4.86
L-Histidine	4.58
L-Phenylalanine	3.45
L-Tyrosine	1.66
L-Tryptophan	1.32

Table 6. Aminoacid concentration in the only commercially available aminoacid PD solution

Advantages and indications. The use of amino acids as osmotic agents decreases peritoneal glucose load and glucose uptake from the peritoneal cavity. This is especially relevant in diabetic and obese individuals. Amino acid solutions also are moderately effective as a nutritional supplement in malnourished patients. In short-term studies protein synthesis improved when amino acid solutions were associated with an adequate supply of calories, such as oral intake or by combining aminoacids with glucose in cycler (Garibotto, G. et al. 2001; Tjiong, H. L. et al. 2005; Tjiong, H. L. et al. 2007). The effect tends to be less consistent in the long-term, probably because other factors influence serum albumin such as inflammation, acidosis or inadequate calorie intake (Kopple, J. D. et al. 1995). However, in a 3-year study malnourished patients using 1.1% amino acids better maintained serum albumin (Li, F. K. et al. 2003). A decrease of serum phosphorus has also been reported and attributed to the contribution of amino acids in the absence of phosphate (Kopple, J. D. et al. 1995). In this sense, the same amount of amino acid if ingested orally, is associated with approximately 300 mg of phosphate.

Drawbacks. Amino acid solutions can only be used once daily since a higher number of bags favors acidosis (which can be compensated by oral treatment with bases or PD solutions with higher buffer content) and increases urea (Tjiong, H. L. et al. 2007; Kopple, J. D. et al. 1995; le Poole, C. Y. et al. 2005). The tendency to acidosis and uremia is more pronounced in catabolic patients, so factors that promote catabolism should be corrected and an adequate calorie intake should be maintained to prevent the catabolism of amino acids as an energy source. This can be achieved with oral caloric intake or by mixing amino acid containing PD solutions with glucose solutions simultaneously in the cycler exchanges. In addition, the methionine load from the dialysate may significantly increase plasma homocysteine levels, especially in patients with lower protein and methionine intakes (Yang, S. Y. et al. 2005). Increased plasma homocysteine levels have been associated with impaired cardiovascular outcomes. In this regard, one 6-h dwell with a commercial amino acid dialysis solution acutely impaired forearm reactive hyperemia, a marker of endothelial dysfunction, in smoking and nonsmoking PD patients (Vychytil, A. et al. 2003).

6. References

Ahmad S, Sehmi JS, hmad-Zakhi KH, Clemenger M, Levy JB, Brown EA. Impact of new dialysis solutions on peritonitis rates. Kidney Int Suppl; (103)2006 November:S63-S66.

Amore A, Cappelli G, Cirina P et al. Glucose degradation products increase apoptosis of human mesothelial cells. Nephrol Dial Transplant; 18(4)2003 April:677-88.

Babazono T, Nakamoto H, Kasai K et al. Effects of icodextrin on glycemic and lipid profiles in diabetic patients undergoing peritoneal dialysis. Am J Nephrol; 27(4)2007:409-15.

Burkart J. Metabolic consequences of peritoneal dialysis. Semin Dial; 17(6)2004 November:498-504.

Carrasco AM, Rubio MA, Sanchez Tommero JA et al. Acidosis correction with a new 25 mmol/l bicarbonate/15 mmol/l lactate peritoneal dialysis solution. Perit Dial Int; 21(6)2001 November:546-53.

Catalan MP, Esteban J, Subira D, Egido J, Ortiz A. Inhibition of caspases improves bacterial clearance in experimental peritonitis. Perit Dial Int; 23(2)2003 March:123-6.

Catalan MP, Reyero A, Egido J, Ortiz A. Acceleration of neutrophil apoptosis by glucose-containing peritoneal dialysis solutions: role of caspases. J Am Soc Nephrol; 12(11)2001 November:2442-9.

Catalan MP, Santamaria B, Reyero A, Ortiz A, Egido J, Ortiz A. 3,4-di-deoxyglucosone-3-ene promotes leukocyte apoptosis. Kidney Int; 68(3)2005 September:1303-11.

Catalan MP, Subira D, Reyero A et al. Regulation of apoptosis by lethal cytokines in human mesothelial cells. Kidney Int; 64(1)2003 July:321-30.

Davies SJ, Brown EA, Frandsen NE et al. Longitudinal membrane function in functionally anuric patients treated with APD: data from EAPOS on the effects of glucose and icodextrin prescription. Kidney Int; 67(4)2005 April:1609-15.

Davies SJ, Garcia LE, Woodrow G et al. Longitudinal relationships between fluid status, inflammation, urine volume and plasma metabolites of icodextrin in patients randomized to glucose or icodextrin for the long exchange. Nephrol Dial Transplant; 23(9)2008 September:2982-8.

Davies SJ, Phillips L, Naish PF, Russell GI. Peritoneal glucose exposure and changes in membrane solute transport with time on peritoneal dialysis. J Am Soc Nephrol; 12(5)2001 May:1046-51.

Dombros N, Dratwa M, Feriani M et al. European best practice guidelines for peritoneal dialysis. 8 Nutrition in peritoneal dialysis. Nephrol Dial Transplant; 20 Suppl 92005 December:ix28-ix33.

Erixon M, Linden T, Kjellstrand P et al. PD fluids contain high concentrations of cytotoxic GDPs directly after sterilization. Perit Dial Int; 24(4)2004 July:392-8.

Erixon M, Wieslander A, Linden T et al. How to avoid glucose degradation products in peritoneal dialysis fluids. Perit Dial Int; 26(4)2006 July:490-7.

Erixon M, Wieslander A, Linden T et al. Take care in how you store your PD fluids: actual temperature determines the balance between reactive and non-reactive GDPs. Perit Dial Int; 25(6)2005 November:583-90.

Fan SL, Pile T, Punzalan S, Raftery MJ, Yaqoob MM. Randomized controlled study of biocompatible peritoneal dialysis solutions: effect on residual renal function. Kidney Int; 73(2)2008 January:200-6.

Fang W, Mullan R, Shah H, Mujais S, Bargman JM, Oreopoulos DG. Comparison between bicarbonate/lactate and standard lactate dialysis solution in peritoneal transport and ultrafiltration: a prospective, crossover single-dwell study. Perit Dial Int; 28(1)2008 January:35-43.

Feriani M, Kirchgessner J, La GG, Passlick-Deetjen J. Randomized long-term evaluation of bicarbonate-buffered CAPD solution. Kidney Int; 54(5)1998 November:1731-8.

Frampton JE, Plosker GL. Icodextrin: a review of its use in peritoneal dialysis. Drugs; 63(19)2003:2079-105.

Fusshoeller A, Plail M, Grabensee B, Plum J. Biocompatibility pattern of a bicarbonate/lactate-buffered peritoneal dialysis fluid in APD: a prospective, randomized study. Nephrol Dial Transplant; 19(8)2004 August:2101-6.

Garcia-Lopez E, Anderstam B, Heimburger O, Amici G, Werynski A, Lindholm B. Determination of high and low molecular weight molecules of icodextrin in plasma and dialysate, using gel filtration chromatography, in peritoneal dialysis patients. Perit Dial Int; 25(2)2005 March:181-91.

Garibotto G, Sofia A, Canepa A et al. Acute effects of peritoneal dialysis with dialysates containing dextrose or dextrose and amino acids on muscle protein turnover in patients with chronic renal failure. J Am Soc Nephrol; 12(3)2001 March:557-67.

Goffin E, Cosyns JP, Pirson F, Devuyst O. Icodextrin-associated peritonitis: what conclusions thus far? Nephrol Dial Transplant; 18(12)2003 December:2482-5.

Haas S, Schmitt CP, Arbeiter K et al. Improved acidosis correction and recovery of mesothelial cell mass with neutral-pH bicarbonate dialysis solution among children undergoing automated peritoneal dialysis. J Am Soc Nephrol; 14(10)2003 October:2632-8.

Heimburger O, Blake PG. Apparatus for peritoneal dialysis. Daugirdas JT, Blake PG, Ing TS, eds.Handbook of dialysis, 4ªed, Lippincot Williams Wilkins , 339-355. 1-11-2007.

Holmes CJ, Faict D. Peritoneal dialysis solution biocompatibility: definitions and evaluation strategies. Kidney Int Suppl; (88)2003 December:S50-S56.

Jones S, Holmes CJ, Krediet RT et al. Bicarbonate/lactate-based peritoneal dialysis solution increases cancer antigen 125 and decreases hyaluronic acid levels. Kidney Int; 59(4)2001 April:1529-38.

Justo P, Sanz AB, Egido J, Ortiz A. 3,4-Dideoxyglucosone-3-ene induces apoptosis in renal tubular epithelial cells. Diabetes; 54(8)2005 August:2424-9.

Kim S, Oh J, Kim S et al. Benefits of biocompatible PD fluid for preservation of residual renal function in incident CAPD patients: a 1-year study. Nephrol Dial Transplant; 24(9)2009 September:2899-908.

Kim SG, Kim S, Hwang YH et al. Could solutions low in glucose degradation products preserve residual renal function in incident peritoneal dialysis patients? A 1-year multicenter prospective randomized controlled trial (Balnet Study). Perit Dial Int; 28 Suppl 32008 June:S117-S122.

Kopple JD, Bernard D, Messana J et al. Treatment of malnourished CAPD patients with an amino acid based dialysate. Kidney Int; 47(4)1995 April:1148-57.

le Poole CY, Welten AG, Weijmer MC, Valentijn RM, van Ittersum FJ, ter Wee PM. Initiating CAPD with a regimen low in glucose and glucose degradation products, with icodextrin and amino acids (NEPP) is safe and efficacious. Perit Dial Int; 25 Suppl 32005 February:S64-S68.

Lee HY, Choi HY, Park HC et al. Changing prescribing practice in CAPD patients in Korea: increased utilization of low GDP solutions improves patient outcome. Nephrol Dial Transplant; 21(10)2006 October:2893-9.

Lee HY, Park HC, Seo BJ et al. Superior patient survival for continuous ambulatory peritoneal dialysis patients treated with a peritoneal dialysis fluid with neutral pH and low glucose degradation product concentration (Balance). Perit Dial Int; 25(3)2005 May:248-55.

Li FK, Chan LY, Woo JC et al. A 3-year, prospective, randomized, controlled study on amino acid dialysate in patients on CAPD. Am J Kidney Dis; 42(1)2003 July:173-83.

Li FK, Davenport A, Robson RL et al. Leukocyte migration across human peritoneal mesothelial cells is dependent on directed chemokine secretion and ICAM-1 expression. Kidney Int; 54(6)1998 December:2170-83.

Linden T, Cohen A, Deppisch R, Kjellstrand P, Wieslander A. 3,4-Dideoxyglucosone-3-ene (3,4-DGE): a cytotoxic glucose degradation product in fluids for peritoneal dialysis. Kidney Int; 62(2)2002 August:697-703.

McIntyre CW. Update on peritoneal dialysis solutions. Kidney Int; 71(6)2007 March:486-90.

Mettang T, Pauli-Magnus C, Alscher DM et al. Influence of plasticizer-free CAPD bags and tubings on serum, urine, and dialysate levels of phthalic acid esters in CAPD patients. Perit Dial Int; 20(1)2000 January:80-4.

Moberly JB, Mujais S, Gehr T et al. Pharmacokinetics of icodextrin in peritoneal dialysis patients. Kidney Int Suppl; (81)2002 October:S23-S33.

Montenegro J, Saracho R, Aguirre R, Martinez I. Calcium mass transfer in CAPD: the role of convective transport. Nephrol Dial Transplant; 8(11)1993:1234-6.

Montenegro J, Saracho R, Gallardo I, Martinez I, Munoz R, Quintanilla N. Use of pure bicarbonate-buffered peritoneal dialysis fluid reduces the incidence of CAPD peritonitis. Nephrol Dial Transplant; 22(6)2007 June:1703-8.

Montenegro J, Saracho RM, Martinez IM, Munoz RI, Ocharan JJ, Valladares E. Long-term clinical experience with pure bicarbonate peritoneal dialysis solutions. Perit Dial Int; 26(1)2006 January:89-94.

Morgan LW, Wieslander A, Davies M et al. Glucose degradation products (GDP) retard remesothelialization independently of D-glucose concentration. Kidney Int; 64(5)2003 November:1854-66.

Navarro JF, Mora C, Macia M, Garcia J. Serum magnesium concentration is an independent predictor of parathyroid hormone levels in peritoneal dialysis patients. Perit Dial Int; 19(5)1999 September:455-61.

Oh EJ, Ryu HM, Choi SY et al. Impact of low glucose degradation product bicarbonate/lactate-buffered dialysis solution on the epithelial-mesenchymal transition of peritoneum. Am J Nephrol; 31(1)2010:58-67.

Olszowska A, Waniewski J, Werynski A, Anderstam B, Lindholm B, Wankowicz Z. Peritoneal transport in peritoneal dialysis patients using glucose-based and amino acid-based solutions. Perit Dial Int; 27(5)2007 September:544-53.

Ortiz A, Wieslander A, Linden T et al. 3,4-DGE is important for side effects in peritoneal dialysis what about its role in diabetes. Curr Med Chem; 13(22)2006:2695-702.

Otte K, Gonzalez MT, Bajo MA et al. Clinical experience with a new bicarbonate (25 mmol/L)/lactate (10 mmol/L) peritoneal dialysis solution. Perit Dial Int; 23(2)2003 March:138-45.

Pajek J, Kveder R, Bren A et al. Short-term effects of bicarbonate/lactate-buffered and conventional lactate-buffered dialysis solutions on peritoneal ultrafiltration: a comparative crossover study. Nephrol Dial Transplant; 24(5)2009 May:1617-25.

Pecoits-Filho R, Stenvinkel P, Heimburger O, Lindholm B. Beyond the membrane--the role of new PD solutions in enhancing global biocompatibility. Kidney Int Suppl; (88)2003 December:S124-S132.

Pecoits-Filho R, Tranaeus A, Lindholm B. Clinical trial experiences with Physioneal. Kidney Int Suppl; (88)2003 December:S100-S104.

Plum J, Gentile S, Verger C et al. Efficacy and safety of a 7.5% icodextrin peritoneal dialysis solution in patients treated with automated peritoneal dialysis. Am J Kidney Dis; 39(4)2002 April:862-71.

Posthuma N, ter Wee PM, Donker AJ et al. Serum disaccharides and osmolality in CCPD patients using icodextrin or glucose as daytime dwell. Perit Dial Int; 17(6)1997 November:602-7.

Rippe B, Simonsen O, Heimburger O et al. Long-term clinical effects of a peritoneal dialysis fluid with less glucose degradation products. Kidney Int; 59(1)2001 January:348-57.

Rippe B, Venturoli D. Peritoneal transport kinetics with amino acid-based and glucose-based peritoneal dialysis solutions. Perit Dial Int; 27(5)2007 September:518-22.

Rodriguez-Carmona A, Fontan MP. Sodium removal in patients undergoing CAPD and automated peritoneal dialysis. Perit Dial Int; 22(6)2002 November:705-13.

Santamaria B, ito-Martin A, Ucero AC et al. A nanoconjugate Apaf-1 inhibitor protects mesothelial cells from cytokine-induced injury. PLoS One; 4(8)2009:e6634.

Santamaria B, Ucero AC, Reyero A et al. 3,4-Dideoxyglucosone-3-ene as a mediator of peritoneal demesothelization. Nephrol Dial Transplant; 2008 June 3.

Schmitt CP, Haraldsson B, Doetschmann R et al. Effects of pH-neutral, bicarbonate-buffered dialysis fluid on peritoneal transport kinetics in children. Kidney Int; 61(4)2002 April:1527-36.

Simonsen O, Sterner G, Carlsson O, Wieslander A, Rippe B. Improvement of peritoneal ultrafiltration with peritoneal dialysis solution buffered with bicarbonate/lactate mixture. Perit Dial Int; 26(3)2006 May:353-9.

Tjiong HL, Rietveld T, Wattimena JL et al. Peritoneal dialysis with solutions containing amino acids plus glucose promotes protein synthesis during oral feeding. Clin J Am Soc Nephrol; 2(1)2007 January:74-80.

Tjiong HL, van den Berg JW, Wattimena JL et al. Dialysate as food: combined amino acid and glucose dialysate improves protein anabolism in renal failure patients on automated peritoneal dialysis. J Am Soc Nephrol; 16(5)2005 May:1486-93.

Tranaeus A. A long-term study of a bicarbonate/lactate-based peritoneal dialysis solution--clinical benefits. The Bicarbonate/Lactate Study Group. Perit Dial Int; 20(5)2000 September:516-23.

Vande Walle JG, Raes AM, Dehoorne J, Mauel R. Use of bicarbonate/lactate-buffered dialysate with a nighttime cycler, associated with a daytime dwell with icodextrin, may result in alkalosis in children. Adv Perit Dial; 202004:222-5.

Vargha R, Endemann M, Kratochwill K et al. Ex vivo reversal of in vivo transdifferentiation in mesothelial cells grown from peritoneal dialysate effluents. Nephrol Dial Transplant; 21(10)2006 October:2943-7.

Vychytil A, Fodinger M, Pleiner J et al. Acute effect of amino acid peritoneal dialysis solution on vascular function. Am J Clin Nutr; 78(5)2003 November:1039-45.

Vychytil A, Remon C, Michel C et al. Icodextrin does not impact infectious and culture-negative peritonitis rates in peritoneal dialysis patients: a 2-year multicentre, comparative, prospective cohort study. Nephrol Dial Transplant; 23(11)2008 November:3711-9.

Wang R, Skoufos L, Martis L. Glucose monitoring for diabetic patients using icodextrin. Perit Dial Int; 24(3)2004 May:296-7.

Weiss L, Stegmayr B, Malmsten G et al. Biocompatibility and tolerability of a purely bicarbonate-buffered peritoneal dialysis solution. Perit Dial Int; 29(6)2009 November:647-55.

Wens R, Taminne M, Devriendt J et al. A previously undescribed side effect of icodextrin: overestimation of glycemia by glucose analyzer. Perit Dial Int; 18(6)1998 November:603-9.

Williams JD, Craig KJ, Topley N et al. Morphologic changes in the peritoneal membrane of patients with renal disease. J Am Soc Nephrol; 13(2)2002 February:470-9.

Williams JD, Topley N, Craig KJ et al. The Euro-Balance Trial: the effect of a new biocompatible peritoneal dialysis fluid (balance) on the peritoneal membrane. Kidney Int; 66(1)2004 July:408-18.

Witowski J, Bender TO, Gahl GM, Frei U, Jorres A. Glucose degradation products and peritoneal membrane function. Perit Dial Int; 21(2)2001 March:201-5.

Witowski J, Korybalska K, Wisniewska J et al. Effect of glucose degradation products on human peritoneal mesothelial cell function. J Am Soc Nephrol; 11(4)2000 April:729-39.

Witowski J, Wisniewska J, Korybalska K et al. Prolonged exposure to glucose degradation products impairs viability and function of human peritoneal mesothelial cells. J Am Soc Nephrol; 12(11)2001 November:2434-41.

Wolfson M, Piraino B, Hamburger RJ, Morton AR. A randomized controlled trial to evaluate the efficacy and safety of icodextrin in peritoneal dialysis. Am J Kidney Dis; 40(5)2002 November:1055-65.

Yamamoto T, Tomo T, Okabe E, Namoto S, Suzuki K, Hirao Y. Glutathione depletion as a mechanism of 3,4-dideoxyglucosone-3-ene-induced cytotoxicity in human peritoneal mesothelial cells: role in biocompatibility of peritoneal dialysis fluids. Nephrol Dial Transplant; 24(5)2009 May:1436-42.

Yanez-Mo M, Lara-Pezzi E, Selgas R et al. Peritoneal dialysis and epithelial-to-mesenchymal transition of mesothelial cells. N Engl J Med; 348(5)2003 January 30:403-13.

Yang SY, Huang JW, Shih KY et al. Factors associated with increased plasma homocysteine in patients using an amino acid peritoneal dialysis fluid. Nephrol Dial Transplant; 20(1)2005 January:161-6.

Zeier M, Schwenger V, Deppisch R et al. Glucose degradation products in PD fluids: do they disappear from the peritoneal cavity and enter the systemic circulation? Kidney Int; 63(1)2003 January:298-305.

Zemel D, Krediet RT. Cytokine patterns in the effluent of continuous ambulatory peritoneal dialysis: relationship to peritoneal permeability. Blood Purif; 14(2)1996:198-216.